Medical Microbiology for Nurses

Medical Microbiology for Nurses
(Including Parasitology)

Prof Jacob Anthikad

MA (Psy) BEd MS (Chem) DTech (Microbiology)

Retired Wing Commander (IAF)
Visiting Professor
Hillside Group of Institutions
Kanakapura Road, Bangalore, Karnataka, India

Author of:
Psychology for Graduate Nurses
Sociology for Graduate Nurses
Psychology and Sociology for GNM
Biochemistry for Nurses
Nutrition and Biochemistry for Nurses
Practical Record Book for GNM

P Sumanaswini

MSc (Microbiology)

Hillside Group of Institutions
Kanakapura Road, Bangalore, Karnataka, India

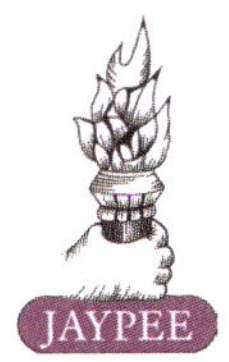

JAYPEE BROTHERS MEDICAL PUBLISHERS

The Health Sciences Publisher

New Delhi | London

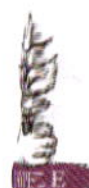

Jaypee Brothers Medical Publishers (P) Ltd

Headquarters

Jaypee Brothers Medical Publishers (P) Ltd
EMCA House, 23/23-B
Ansari Road, Daryaganj
New Delhi 110 002, India
Landline: +91-11-23272143, +91-11-23272703
+91-11-23282021, +91-11-23245672
Email: jaypee@jaypeebrothers.com

Corporate Office

Jaypee Brothers Medical Publishers (P) Ltd
4838/24, Ansari Road, Daryaganj
New Delhi 110 002, India
Phone: +91-11-43574357
Fax: +91-11-43574314
Email: jaypee@jaypeebrothers.com

Overseas Office

J.P. Medical Ltd
83 Victoria Street, London
SW1H 0HW (UK)
Phone: +44 20 3170 8910
Fax: +44 (0)20 3008 6180
Email: info@jpmedpub.com

Website: www.jaypeebrothers.com
Website: www.jaypeedigital.com

© 2013, Jaypee Brothers Medical Publishers

Inquiries for bulk sales may be solicited at: jaypee@jaypeebrothers.com

Medical Microbiology for Nurses (Including Parasitology)

First Edition: 2013

Reprint: **2024**

ISBN: 978-93-5090-279-0

Printed at Nutech Print Services - India

Dedicated to
The revered memory of
Louis Pasteur (27-12-1822 to 28-09-1895)
'Father of Medical Microbiology'

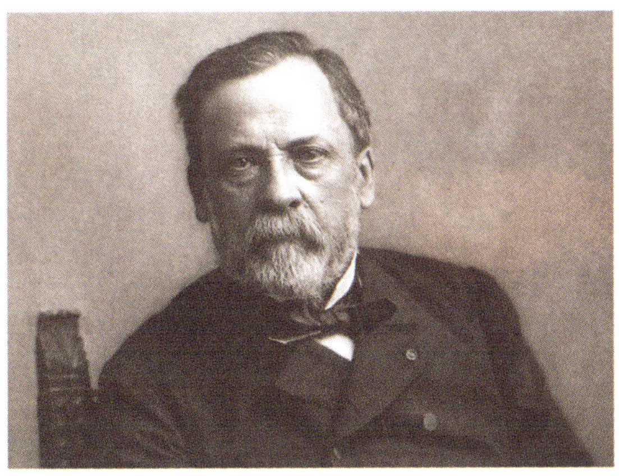

"In the field of observation, chance favours only the prepared mind."
– Louis Pasteur, French Biochemist

Foreword

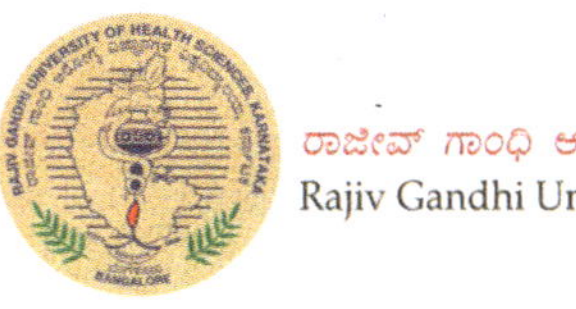

Dr. Sriprakash. K. S. M.S.(Oph.)
VICE-CHANCELLOR

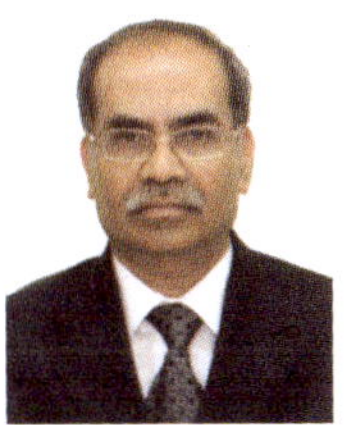

Dr Sriprakash KS
Vice-Chancellor
Rajiv Gandhi University of Health Sciences
Karnataka

It is my pleasure to write foreword to the textbook "Medical Microbiology for Nurses (Including Parasitology)" written by Prof Jacob Anthikad and Sumanaswini P. With their vast teaching experience they have written the book with authority, clarity and in a simple style.

The publication of this book is a timely and laudable venture as it strictly follows the INC and RGUHS syllabus for the nursing students at the degree level. I am glad to note that the present textbook keeps a balance between the basic essentials and advanced areas of knowledge in Medical Microbiology.

The authors are to be congratulated for the enormous pains that they have taken in compiling this very useful and concise work which will meet the learning requirements of our nursing students. I am pleased to introduce the book to the nursing students in particular and to the nursing fraternity in general.

Dr Sriprakash KS

Preface

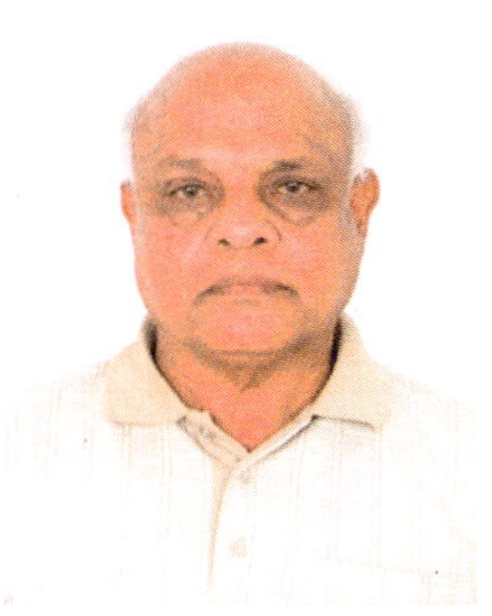

Prof Jacob Anthikad
Retired Wing Commander (IAF)
Visiting Professor
Hillside Group of Institutions
Kanakapura Road, Bangalore

This book is intended to provide an easily comprehensible, non-intimidating and concise textbook on medical microbiology including parasitology. It is written strictly as per the Indian Nursing Council syllabus for nursing courses at degree level.

A concise glossary of terms has been provided at the end of the textbook to help the student nurses to understand the meaning of keywords and their usages. A set of three model question papers is included for the three sections of the subject namely, general microbiology, clinical microbiology and parasitology. This is in addition to the large question bank of university question papers on the subject to help the students from the examination point of view. Multiple choice questions are given chapterwise to enable the students to check their own assimilation.

We hope this little book makes its modest contribution by presenting the subject of microbiology in an easy, simple and straightforward style to motivate the student nurses and stimulate academic interest.

A book such as this will always have scope for improvement. Suggestions for correction and improvement will be gratefully acknowledged, appreciated and included in future editions.

Jacob Anthikad
P Sumanaswini

Acknowledgments

We are extremely grateful to Dr Sriprakash KS, Vice-Chancellor, RGUHS, for giving an inspiring foreword for this book, fortunately. We are also thankful to the authors of publications and textbooks giving valuable details of medical microbiology and parasitology. For their constant guidance and encouragement, we are specially obliged to the following professionals:

Dr Fenny Anthikad MD, University of Pittsburgh, USA

Prof Sherly Sebastain MSC (N), New York

Ms Mini Anthikad MA M Phil, Editor: 'The Hindu'

Dr Paul Davis MD, Virginia Beach, USA

Dr Sheela Segaram FRCOG (London), Kuala Lumpur

Dr AK Augustin MD MRCP (London)

Dr Beena Augustin MD DGO MRCOG (London)

Dr Dominic Puthur MS D ORTHO, Amala Hospital, Thrissur

Dr Beemappa MS (General Surgery), Chairman, Hillside Group of Institutions, Bangalore.

We take this opportunity to specially thank Shri Jitendar P Vij Sir (Group Chairman), Mr Ankit Vij (Managing Director), Mr Tarun Duneja (Director-Publishing) of M/s Jaypee Brothers Medical Publishers (P) Ltd, New Delhi, India, Mr Venugopal V, Bangalore (Branch Manager) and Ms Sajini SV (Team Leader). Our heartful thanks are also due to Mrs Hemalata Malini BA for formatting, Ms Ramya VR, Ms Nikita G, Ms Bhavya M, Ms Sunitha P, Ms Nethra S, Mr Yogesh Kumar, Ms Lavanya H, Ms Sujatha B, for efficient proofreading, Mr Shivaprasad K Naik and Ms Shilpa K Bhat for the attractive images and Mr Venkatesha N for the excellent layout.

Contents

PART 1 - BACTERIOLOGY AND GENERAL MICROBIOLOGY

1. Introduction and History   03
Definition   3
Application of Microbiology in Health Science   3
Important Contributions   4
Classification of Microorganisms/Microbes   5

2. Microscopy   06
Size of Bacteria   6
Techniques of Microscopy   6
Hanging Drop Method   8

3. Morphology of Bacteria   09
Morphological (Shape) Classification of Bacteria   9
Bacterial Anatomy   10
Bacterial Spores   12

4. Identification of Bacteria/Staining   14
Bacterial Staining   14
Staining Techniques   14
Gram Staining   14
Acid-fast Staining: Ziehl-Neelsen Staining   15
Albert Staining   16

5. Bacterial Growth Factors   18
Factors Influencing the Growth of Bacteria   18
Bacterial Growth Curve   19
Reproduction   20

6. Culture Media   21
Classification   21
McIntosh and Fildes Jar   24
Inoculation   24
Antibiotic Sensitivity Tests   25
Antibiogram   26

7. Control of Microorganisms — Sterilization and Disinfection   27
Definitions   27
Disinfection/Sterilization   27

8. Infections—Nosocomial Infections   **35**

Classification of Infections   35
Infectious Agents   35
Sources of Infection in Man   36
Disease Transmission   37
Methods of Transfer of Infection   37
Microbial Pathogenicity   40
Nosocomial (Hospital) Infections: Hospital-Acquired Infections   41

9. Antimicrobial Therapy   **44**

History   44
Antibiotics   44
Drug Resistance   46

10. Systemic Bacteriology   **47**

Cabibi Staphylococci   47
Micrococcus   49
Streptococci   49
Pneumococci   51
Neisseria   52
Corynebacterium   53
Bacillus   55
Clostridium   56
Enterobacteriaceae   58
Vibrio Cholerae   62
Pseudomonas Aeruginosa   63
Yersinia   63
Haemophilus Influenzae   64
Bordetella Pertussis   65
Brucella   65
Mycobacterium Tuberculosis   66
Spirochetes   67
Actinomycetes   70
Chlamydia   70
Mycoplasma   71
Rickettsia   72

11. Immunology   **74**

Natural Immunity   74
Classification of Immunity   76
Antigens   78
Antibodies   79
Cells and Organs of Immune System   80
Immune Response   84
Complement System   84
Major Histocompatibility Complex   86
Harmful Effects of Immunity   86
Immune Deficiency Diseases   88
Antigen-Antibody Reactions   90

12. Immunization   95

Immunity   95
Vaccines   96
Vaccination   97

13. Serology: Antigen-Antibody Reactions   99

Antigen-Antibody Reactions   99
Precipitation Tests   99
Agglutination Reactions   102
Complement Fixation Test   104

14. Virology   107

Virus   107
Morphology   107
Viroids   110
Prion   111
DNA Viruses   111
RNA Viruses   114
Hepatitis Viruses   118
Retroviruses   121
Diseases Caused by Viruses Transmitted by Mosquito   122
Virus Infections Transmitted by Droplet Infection   123
Virus Infections Transmitted by Fecal-Oral Route   124

15. Mycology   126

Introduction   126
Superficial Mycoses   126
Deep Mycoses   127
Opportunistic Mycoses   128

PART 2 - PARASITOLOGY

16. Introduction to Medical Parasitology — Amebiasis   133

Medical Parasitology   133
Protozoa: Amoeba   134

17. Kala-azar, The Black Sickness   138

Indian Leishmaniasis   138

18. Malarial Parasites   140

Causative Agents   140
Life Cycle   140
Pernicious Malaria   143
Laboratory Diagnosis — Microscopic Examination   143

19. Filariasis   144

Wuchereria Bancrofti   144

20. Ascariasis (Roundworm Infection)   146

Ascaris Lumbricoides   146

21. Ancylostomasis (Hookworm Infection) — **148**
Ancylostoma Duodenale (Hookworm) 148

22. Stool Examination — **150**
Precautions 150
Types of Stool Examination 150
Direct Examination 150
Helminth Ova in Human Stool 151

PART 3 - CLINICAL MICROBIOLOGY

23. Normal Microbial Flora of Human Body — **155**
Types of Normal Flora 155
Location of Normal Flora 155
Advantages and Disadvantages of Normal Flora 156

24. Medical Entomology — **157**
Sources of Infection 157

25. Specimen Collection — **163**
Collection of Specimen 163

26. Hospital Waste Management — **165**
Management of Hospital Waste 165

APPENDICES

Appendix A — Terms to Know — 171
Appendix B — Model Semester Question Papers — 175
Appendix C — University Question Papers — 178
Appendix D — Multiple Choice Questions — 190

Index — 203

INC Microbiology Syllabus

COURSE DESCRIPTION

This course is designed to enable students to acquire understanding of fundamentals of microbiology and identification of various microorganisms. It also provides opportunities for practicing infection control measures in hospital and community settings.

Unit	Time (Hour)		Learning objectives	Content	Teaching/ learning activities	Assessment methods
	Theory	Practical				
I	5		Explain concepts and principles of microbiology and their importance in nursing.	Introduction: Importance and relevance to nursing Historical perspective Concepts and terminology Principles of microbiology	Lecture Discussion	Short answers Objective type
II	10	5	Describe structure, classification, morphology and growth of bacteria. Identify microorganisms.	General characteristic of microbes Structure and classification of microbes Morphological types Size and form of bacteria Motility Colonization Growth and nutrition of microbes Temperature Moisture Blood and body fluids Laboratory methods for identification of microorganisms Staining techniques, gram staining, acid-fast staining, hanging drop preparation Culture—various media	Lecture Discussion Demonstration	Short answers Objective type

Contd...

Contd...

Unit	Time (Hour)		Learning objectives	Content	Teaching/ learning activities	Assessment methods
	Theory	Practical				
III	10	2	Describe the methods of infection control program.	Infection control Infection: sources, portals of entry and exit, transmission Asepsis Disinfection types and methods Sterilization types and methods Chemotherapy and antibiotics Standard safety measures Biomedical waste management Role of nurse Hospital acquired control program Protocols, collection of samples, preparation of report and status of rate of infection in the unit/hospital, nurse's accountability, continuing education, etc.	Lecture Discussion Demonstration Visits to CSSD Clinical practice	Short answers Objective type
IV	12	4	Describe the different disease-producing organisms.	Pathogenic organisms Microorganisms Cocci gram-positive and gram-negative Spirochete Mycoplasma Rickettsia Chlamydia Viruses Superficial fungi and deep mycoses Parasites Rodents and vectors Characteristics, source, portal of entry, transmission of infection Identification of disease-producing microorganisms Collection, handling and transportation of various specimens	Lecture Discussion Demonstration Clinical practice	Short answers Objective type
V	8	4	Explain the concept of immunity, hyper-sensitivity and immunization.	Immunity Immunity types Classification Antigen and antibody reaction Hypersensitivity skin test Serological tests Immunoprophylaxis Vaccines and sera Types and classification, storage and handling, cold chain Immunization for various diseases Immunization schedule	Lecture Discussion Demonstration Clinical practice	Short answers Objective type

Bacteriology and General Microbiology

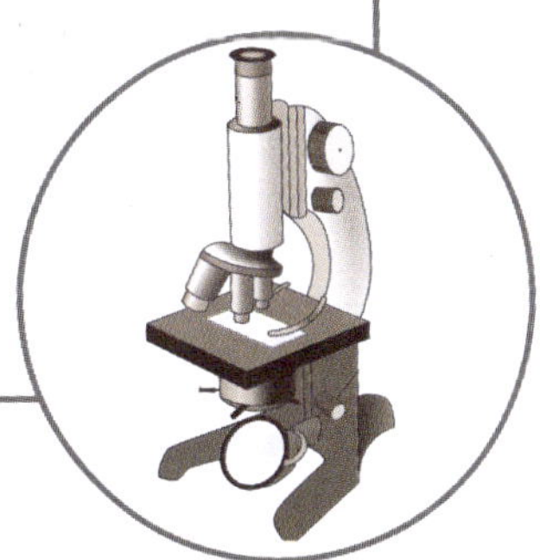

Introduction and History

DEFINITION

Microbiology (Greek; mikros = small, bios = life, logos = study of) is the science of living organisms that are visible only under the microscope.

In the second half of the nineteenth century, microbiology was differentiated into general, medical, industrial, agricultural, veterinary, food, soil and plant microbiology.

Medical microbiology has become an intensive science and it is subdivided into:

Bacteriology	=	Science of pathogenic bacteria
Virology	=	Science of infectious viruses
Serology	=	The study of reactions between antigen and antibody
Mycology	=	Study of fungi — pathogenic to man
Parasitology	=	Study of parasites — protozoa and helminths
Protozoology	=	Study of pathogenic protozoa
Helminthology	=	Study of helminths (worms)
Entomology	=	Study of insects (vectors) — transmitting diseases to man.

In addition, medical microbiology includes the study of mechanisms of infectious disease and immunity (immunology), the methods of therapy and prophylaxis of infectious diseases. Genetics is the study of heredity and variations.

Nursing microbiology is the application of the knowledge of medical microbiology at the bedside of patients during nursing care. Basic principles of various procedures are drawn from the science of microbiology.

APPLICATION OF MICROBIOLOGY IN HEALTH SCIENCE

Why should the nurse study microbiology?

Application of the basic principles of medical microbiology is essential to the practice of any medical profession. The following are some of the areas in health science where microbiological principles are applied:

1. Health: Promotion and betterment of human health. Enhancement of human life expectancy and longevity.
2. Conquest of epidemics and fatal infections: Immunization has resulted in the eradication of smallpox, control of plague, diphtheria, tuberculosis, poliomyelitis and measles.
3. Child care safe: Upbringing and prevention of infectious diseases of childhood and thus reduce infant mortality.
4. Revolutionary influences on the prevention, diagnostic methods, treatment and control of infectious diseases.
5. Improved food preservation and safe drinking water for all.
6. Effective disposal of sewage and waste.

With microbiology forming the foundation of professional nursing, the nurse has an increasing responsibility to practice and teach hygienic measures both in the care and prevention of diseases.

The study of microbiology helps the nurse in many different ways. Nurse learns how the disease-producing organisms enter into the body, how they are discharged from the body and how they spread from person to person. Nurse will understand the principles of disinfection and effect of drugs on microorganisms. Nurse recognizes the importance of proper collection of specimens for bacteriological examination in the laboratory and understands the meaning of reports received from the laboratory. In addition, nurse understands how sera and vaccines used in the treatment and prevention of diseases are prepared and their effects on the human body.

The modern study of microbiology has developed in stages. Fracastoro of Verona (1546) gave the idea that infection consists of minute particles, which are too small to be seen by the naked eye. He also described the modes of spread of infection by direct contact and by fomites.

Antonie van Leeuwenhoek, the father of microscopy (1632–1723) was the first person to see and describe microbes. He was a draper from Delft, Holland, who wanted to observe the weaving of fine cloth. He made the earliest high power microscope consisting of a single magnifying glass held in a metal frame. He was able to produce lenses with 300 to 400 magnification power. With the help of these he observed minute organisms, bacteria and protozoa, which he called 'animalcules' from rain water and tartar of teeth, some of which were mobile.

IMPORTANT CONTRIBUTIONS

Louis Pasteur (1822–1895)

French chemist considered as Father of microbiology
1. Microbial theory of fermentation.
2. Principles and practice of sterilization (steam sterilizer, hot air oven and autoclave).
3. Control of diseases of silkworms.
4. Development of vaccines against
   a. Anthrax
   b. Rabies
   c. Chicken cholera.
5. Discovery of streptococci.

Robert Koch (1843–1910)

German doctor considered as Father of bacteriology
1. Discovery and use of solid media in microbiology.
2. Discovery of the causative agents of
   a. Anthrax (1876)
   b. Tuberculosis (1882)
   c. Cholera (1883).

3. Koch's phenomenon, hypersensitivity phenomenon of *Mycobacterium tuberculosis*.
4. Koch's postulates.

Koch's Postulates

According to Koch's postulates, a microorganism can be accepted as the causative agent of an infectious disease only if the following conditions are satisfied:
a. The specific organism should always be found in·association with the given disease.
b. It should be possible to isolate the organism in pure culture from the lesions of the disease.
c. The isolated organism in pure culture, when inoculated into suitable laboratory animals, should produce a similar disease.
d. It should be possible to reisolate the organism in pure culture from the lesion produced in the experimental animal.
e. An additional criterion introduced subsequently, requires that specific antibodies to the organism should be demonstrable in the serum of the patient. However, it may not be possible to satisfy for all the postulates in every case. An important exception of not fulfilling the Koch's postulates is lepra bacillus.

Koch's Phenomenon

Koch observed that guinea pigs already infected with *Mycobacterium tuberculosis* respond with an exaggerated inflammatory response when infected with tubercle bacilli or its proteins. This hypersensitivity reaction is known as Koch's phenomenon.

Joseph Lister (1827–1912)

English surgeon considered as Father of antiseptic surgery
Lister was deeply concerned with postoperative sepsis, which took a terrible toll. Postoperative patients were dying like flies after successful surgery. By washing wounds with phenol (carbolic acid) spray and applying protective dressings, he prevented germs from entering the site of operation and thereby reduced postoperative sepsis, mortality and morbidity.

Because carbolic acid is too toxic to the tissues, it was replaced by sterilization techniques and other modern antiseptic approaches, which have revolutionized modern surgery.

Florence Nightingale (1820–1910)

Florence Nightingale organized hospitals that minimized cross-infections.

Fanny Hesse (1850–1913)

Fanny Hesse was a housewife. She suggested the use of agar as a solidifying material in microbiological media.

CLASSIFICATION OF MICROORGANISMS/MICROBES

1. Bacteria.
2. Viruses.
3. Fungi.
4. Protozoa.
5. *Mycoplasma.*
6. Rickettsiae.

Microscopy

SIZE OF BACTERIA

Most of the bacteria are so small that their size is measured in micrometer or microns.

$$1 \text{ micron } (\mu) \text{ or micrometer } (\mu m) = \frac{1 \text{ millimeter}}{1,000}$$

$$1 \text{ nanometer (nm)} = \frac{1 \text{ micron}}{1,000}$$

$$= \frac{1}{10^9} \text{ meter}$$

$$1 \text{ Angstrom unit, Å} = \frac{1}{10} \text{ nm}$$

Bacteria of medical importance measures 2 to 5 µm (length) and 0.2 to 1.5 µm (width). The resolution power of the unaided eye (naked eye) is about 200 microns. Bacteria being much smaller than the resolution limit, can be visualized only under the microscope.

TECHNIQUES OF MICROSCOPY

Microscopy and staining techniques are used to visualize and study bacteria. Various techniques of microscopy are:

1. Light microscopy.
2. Phase-contrast microscopy.
3. Fluorescent microscopy.
4. Darkfield microscopy.
5. Electron microscopy.

Light Microscopy

The ordinary microscope (monocular and binocular) give only a resolution power of 200 nm. Their resolving power can be vastly increased by the use of short wavelength.

Care of Microscope

a. Place and store the microscope in a dry, dust-free and vibration-free environment.
b. Keep the microscope and lenses clean.
c. Do not leave the immersion oil on the surface of the immersion lens.
d. Clean the microscope with lens tissue before and after use.
e. Never use spirit or alcohol to clean the lenses as these can damage them.
f. Never let the immersion lens touch the smear.
g. Use the fine focusing only, while using the oil immersion lens.
h. All the lenses should be cleaned with dry lens paper. Lens paper can be moistened with xylene, if necessary. Do not clean lens with ordinary cloth.

Adjustment System

The adjustment system in a compound microscope (Fig. 2.1) consists of the following:

Coarse adjustment screw: This is the largest screw. It is used first to achieve an approximate focus.

Fine adjustment screw: This moves the objective more slowly, it is used to bring the object into perfect focus.

Condenser adjustment screw: This is used to raise the condenser for greater illumination or to lower it to reduce the illumination.

Condenser centering screws: There may be three screws placed around the condenser: one in front, one on the left and one on the right. They are used to center the condenser exactly in relation to the objective.

Iris diaphragm lever: This is a small lever fixed on the condenser. It can be moved to close or open the diaphragm, thus reducing or increasing both the angle and the intensity of the light (Fig. 2.2).

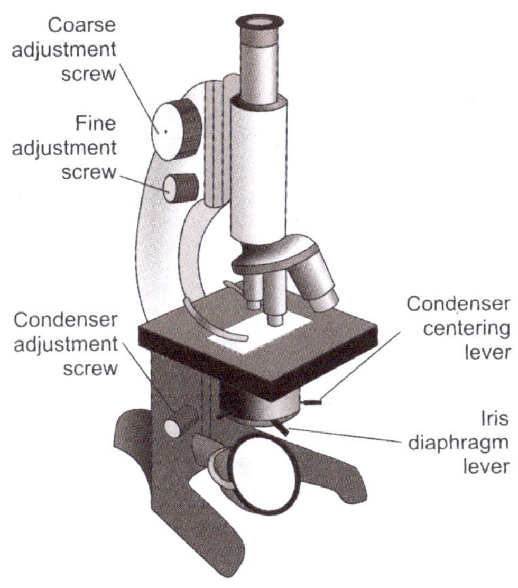

Fig. 2:1: Adjustment system in a compound microscope

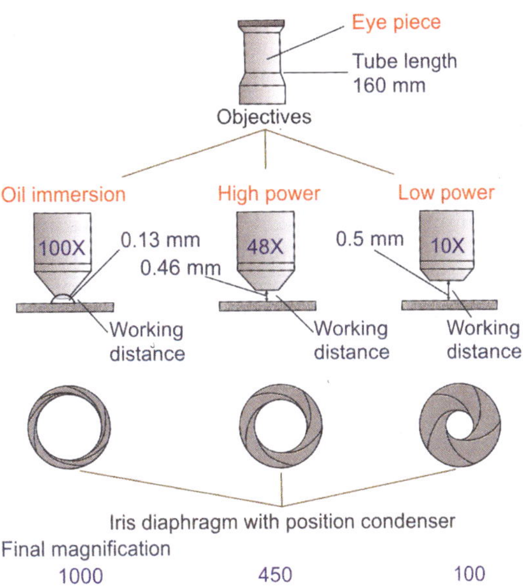

Fig. 2.2: Diagram showing working distance, iris and condenser position

How to Use the Microscope?

a. Switch on the light.

b. Place the slide on the stage.

c. Raise the condenser as high as possible.

d. Adjust the distance between the eye pieces until both the right and left images become one.

e. Focus with 45X and then with 100X lens. Using 45X lens find a suitable area of the slide to examine. The selected area should not be too thick or too thin and should have more pus cells than epithelial cells.

Place one drop of immersion oil on the stained smear. Never let the immersion oil application touch the slide.

Slowly change to the 100X lens. The oil will make a thin film between the 100X lens and slide.

Phase-contrast Microscopy

Phase-contrast microscopy enhances the refractive index differences of the cell components. This is used to study microorganisms in their living state to reveal details of internal structures as well as capsules, endospores and mobility.

Fluorescent Microscopy

Fluorescent microscopy utilizes short-wave length ultraviolet (UV) rays to examine cells after treatment with fluorescent dyes.

Uses:

a. Detection of acid-fast bacilli (*Mycobacterium*) after staining with auramine.

b. Extensively used in immunology for the detection of an antigen and antibody.

Darkfield Microscopy (Dark Ground Microscopy)

When a beam of light enters a darkened room, it renders minute particles of dust floating in the air, visible to the naked eye, which cannot be seen ordinarily in a better lighted room (Tyndall effect). Similar principle is used in darkfield illumination where the condenser is so designed (paraboloid) so that light rays do not pass directly through the object being examined, but strike it from the sides illuminating it very obliquely. This light will not pass up into the objective and the tube. It is reflected or scattered by the object. Only objects, which have a different refractive index from the medium will do this. The microscopic field becomes a dark background against which bacteria and other particles appear as bright as a silver object. Used to observe poorly refractile microbes especially treponemes in their living state.

Electron Microscopy

The principle of electron microscope resembles the light microscope. A beam of electrons replaces the conventional light sources and focusing is done by magnetic fields instead of glass lenses. ·

The material under investigation is examined in a high vaccum. The electron behave as rays of very short wavelength and will resolve objects as small as 0.001 µm. The final image in the electron microscope is projected on to phosphor-coated screen (so that it can be seen) or on to a photographic negative plate to get a negative film. From this film enlarged photographs can be developed thus increasing the magnification still further.

By this, minute structural details of bacteria and viruses can be studied.

HANGING DROP METHOD

Living bacteria can be examined, without staining them, in their natural living state. A drop of fluid containing the bacteria is placed on a very thin glass coverslip, which is then inverted over a cavity in a special glass slide. Actively mobile organisms are seen under high power objective of the microscope, darting, rolling and bumping

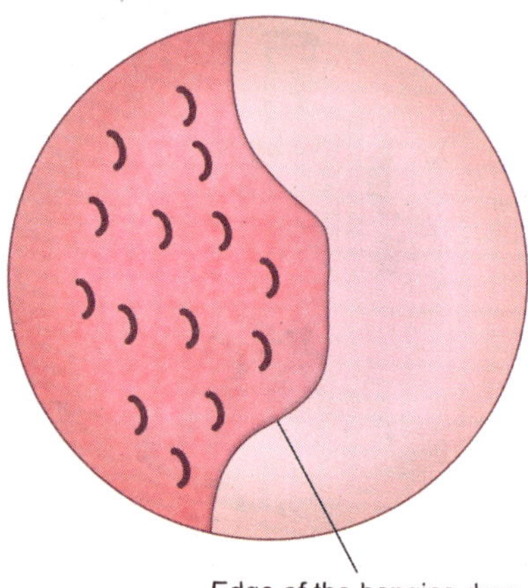

Edge of the hanging drop

Fig. 2.3: Hanging drop method

into each other. Power of movement is due to the presence of flagella. Examples of motile organisms are *Vibrio cholerae* and *Salmonella typhi*.

While observing the motility, the objective of the microscope is focused on the edge of the hanging drop (Fig. 2.3) because:

1. Due to higher oxygen tension, more organisms are at the edge.
2. In the shallow edge, the shape of the organism can better be appreciated than in the deep center of the drop.

The method of microscopy can be broadly divided into wet coverslip method and dry staining methods for which the details are given in Figure 2.4.

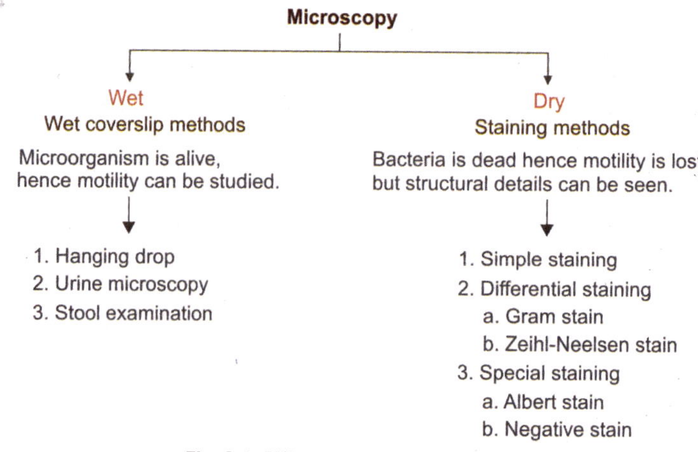

Fig. 2.4: Different microscopic methods

Morphology of Bacteria

Bacteria are unicellular free living organisms without chlorophyll having both deoxyribonucleic acid (DNA) and ribonucleic acid (RNA). They are capable of performing all essential processes of life—growth, metabolism and reproduction. They have rigid cell walls containing muramic acid.

They were originally classified under plant and animal kingdoms. This being unsatisfactory a third kingdom protista was proposed by Heckal in 1866. Protista is again subdivided into two groups (Table 3.1):

1. Prokaryotes (with primitive nucleus).
2. Eukaryotes (with true nucleus).

Bacteria and blue green algae, which can exhibit sliding movements like photosynthetic bacteria are prokaryotes. Fungi, algae, slime molds and protozoa are eukaryotes.

MORPHOLOGICAL (SHAPE) CLASSIFICATION OF BACTERIA

Depending on their shape, bacteria are classified as coccus, bacillus, vibrios, etc. (Fig. 3.1).

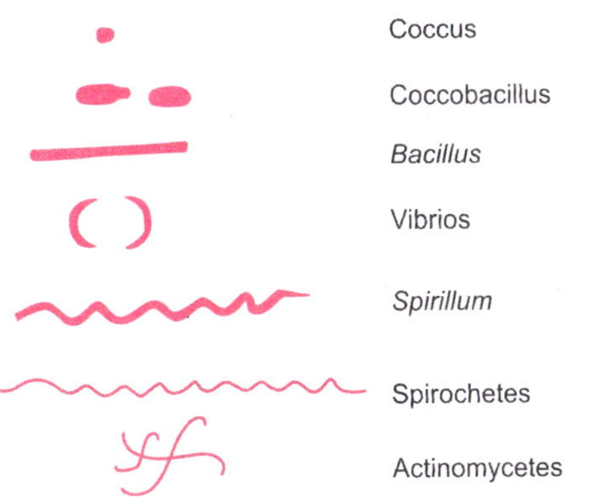

Fig. 3.1: Classification of bacteria according to shape

Coccus

Coccus (from 'kokos' meaning beri) are oval or spherical shaped cells. Cocci may be arranged in pairs (diplococci), clusters (staphylococci) and chains (streptcocci).

Bacillus

Bacillus means rod-shaped cell. Some of these bacilli may have less variable arrangement because they divide perpendicular to the long axis.

Coccobacilli: Length of the bacilli is approximately the same as its width.

Streptobacilli: Bacilli arranged in chains.

Chinese letters or curie form patterns at right angles to each other, e.g. *Corynebacterium diphtheriae*.

Table 3.1: Differences between prokaryotes and eukaryotes

Structures	Prokaryotes	Eukaryotes
Nucleus	Absent	Present
Nuclear membrane	Absent	Present
Nucleolus	Absent	Present
Chromosome	One	More than one
Deoxyribonucleoprotein	Absent	Present
Division	By primary fission	By mitosis
Cytoplasm		
Mitochondria, golgi apparatus, lysosomes, pinocytosis, endoplasmic reticulum	All are absent	All are present
Chemical composition		
Sterols	Absent	Present
Muramic acid	Present	Absent

Curved or Comma Shaped

Curved rods, e.g. *Vibrio cholerae*, derives their name from vibrating motility.

Spirilla

Rigid spiral forms, e.g. *Spirillum minus*.

Spirochetes

The word derived from 'speira' meaning coil, and chaite meaning hair. Spirochetes are slender flexuous spiral forms.

Actinomycetes

The word actinomycetes derived from two Greek words 'aktis' meaning ray and 'muketes' meaning fungus. Actinomycetes are slender, flexuous spiral, branching filamentous bacteria, resembling fungus when seen in tissue lesions, e.g. actinomycosis, nocardiasis and maduromycosis.

Mycoplasma

Mycoplasmas are cell-wall deficient bacteria and hence do not posses, a stable shape. They are round or oval bodies with interlacing filaments. Mycoplasmas are tiny bacteria smaller than large viruses, which lack cell wall, but can live independently and grow on artificial media. Diseases caused in human include atypical pneumonia and puerperal fever.

Chlamydia

Chlamydiae are microorganisms resembling viruses in size and reproducing only inside the cells, but they are in fact very small intracellular bacteria visible with light microscope. They are intracellular parasites, which are filterable and fail to grow in cell-free media. But they possess both DNA and RNA and are susceptible to usual antibiotics. Human diseases caused by chlamydiae are trachoma and lymphogranuloma venereum.

BACTERIAL ANATOMY

Cell Wall

The cell wall of bacteria is a multilayered structure and constitutes 20 percent of the dry weight of the bacterium (Fig. 3.2). The external surface of the cell wall is smooth in gram-positive bacteria whereas gram-negative bacteria have convoluted cell surfaces.

The average thickness of cell wall is 0.15 to 0.50 µm. Chemically the cell wall is composed of mucopeptide scaffolding formed by N-acetylglucosamine (NAGA) and N-acetylmuramic acid (NAMA), which are cross-linked with peptide chains (Fig. 3.3). In gram-positive bacteria, various proteins and polysaccharides are attached to peptidoglycan present in the cell wall.

The cell wall is a three-layered structure in gram-negative bacteria — outer membrane, middle layer and plasma membrane. The outer membrane consists of lipoproteins and lipopolysaccharides (LPS) components.

Functions of Cell Wall

1. Provides shape to bacterium.
2. Gives rigidity to the organism.

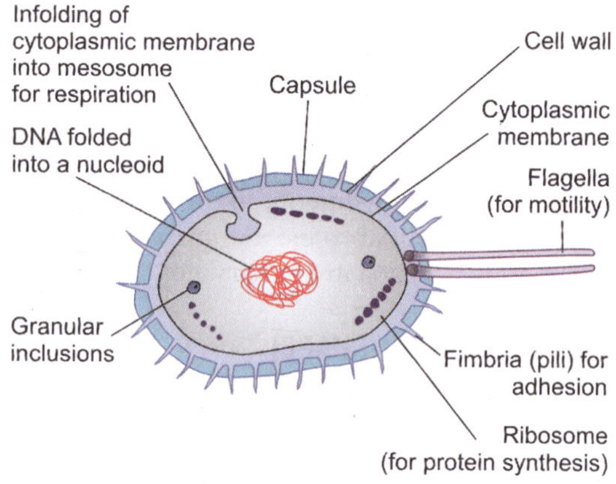

Fig. 3.2: Anatomy of the bacterial cell (DNA = deoxyribonucleic acid)

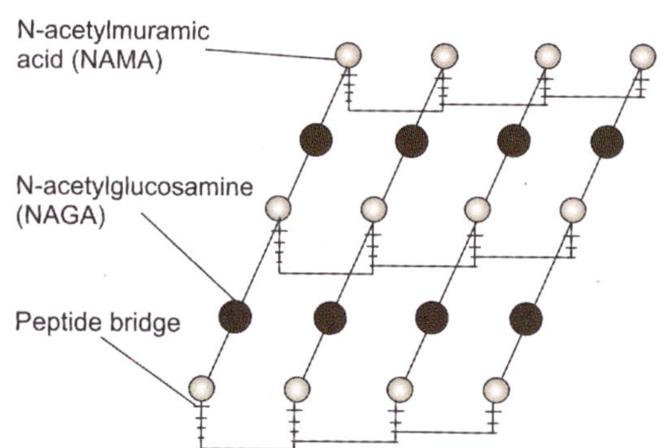

Fig. 3.3: Bacterial wall

3. Protects from environmental factors.
4. Contains receptor sites for phages.
5. Site of action of antibody.
6. Provides attachment to complement.
7. Site of action of colicine, a protein lethal to other strains of the bacterium.

Cytoplasmic Membrane

Cytoplasmic membrane is 5 to 10 µm thick elastic semipermeable layer, which lies below the cell wall separating it from the cell cytoplasm.

Cytoplasmic membrane acts as an osmotic barrier. It acts as a semipermeable membrane controlling the inflow of metabolites to and from the protoplasm. The cell wall and the cytoplasmic membrane are comparable to pneumatic tire and tube, each one having different functions.

Cytoplasm

Cytoplasm contains ribosomes, mesosomes, vacuoles and inclusions.

Ribosomes

Ribosomes are the centers of protein synthesis. They are composed of RNA and proteins.

Intraplasmic Inclusions

Intraplasmic inclusions are sources of stored energy and present in some species of bacteria.

Mesosomes (Chondroids)

Mesosomes are vesicular multilayered or convoluted structures formed as invaginations of plasma membrane into the cytoplasm. They are the principle centers of respiratory enzymes and are analogous to mitochondria of eukaryotes.

Nuclear Apparatus

Bacteria do not possess a well-defined nucleus and the nuclear region is referred to as nuclear body, nuclear apparatus or a nucleoid. Bacterial DNA represents 2% to 3% of the cell weight and 10 percent of the volume of the bacterium. The genomic DNA is double-stranded in the form of a circle, which may open under certain conditions to form a long chain of about 1,000 µm. The bacterial chromosome is haploid and replicates by binary fission. Apart from the nucleoid, bacteria may have extrachromosomal genetic material in the form of DNA, which is known as plasmid.

Adherents and Appendages/ Capsule and Slime

The basic differences between capsule and slime is in their property of firm attachment to the cell. The gel formed by the capsule adheres to the cell whereas the slime can be easily washed off. Capsule can be detected by India ink staining, which is a negative staining in which the capsule stands out as a halo (Fig. 3.4). When a suspension of capsulated bacterium is mixed with its specific anticapsular serum and examined under the microscope, the capsule appears 'swollen' due to the increase in its refractivity. This phenomenon is called capsule swelling reaction or Quellung phenomenon. Capsule are not necessary for viability.

Pneumococci are stained with India ink to show capsule (negative staining). *Klebsiella pneumoniae* and *Haemophilus influenzae* also have capsules.

Important Functions of Capsule

1. Usually capsules are weakly antigenic.
2. Protects from phagocytosis.
3. Capsulated strains are non-motile.

Flagella

Flagella are organs of locomotion and provide motility to the bacterium. With the help of flagella,

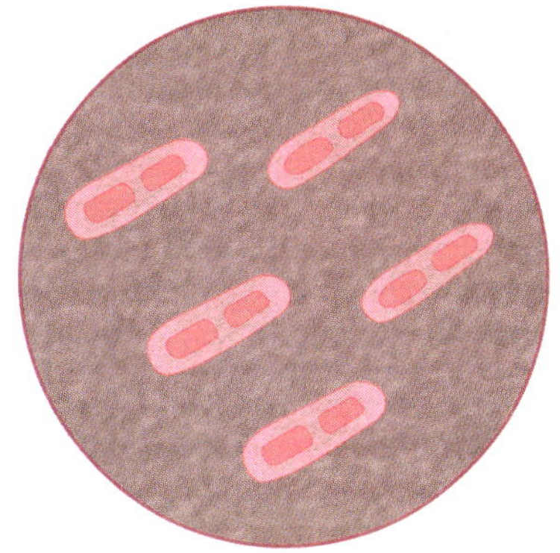

Fig. 3.4: Structure of capsule shown by negative staining

bacteria can move away from any toxic substance that may cause damage or death of the cell.

These are thread-like structures composed of a protein (flagellin), 5 to 20 µm in length and 0.01 to 0.02 µm in diameter.

Parts and Composition

Each flagellum consists of three parts:
1. Filament.
2. Hook.
3. Basal body.

The basal body contains outer and inner rings by which it is attached to the cytoplasmic membrane.

Arrangement/Types

Different arrangements of bacterial flagella are shown in Figure 3.5.

Monotrichous — single polar flagellum (at one end) e.g. *Vibrio cholerae.*

Amphitrichous — single flagellum at both ends, e.g. *Alcaligenes faecalis.*

Lophotrichous — tuft of flagella at one or both ends, e.g. *Spirillum.*

Peritrichous — flagella arranged all around the cell, e.g. *Salmonella typhi.*

Demonstration

Flagella are almost 0.02 µm in thickness and hence beyond the resolution limit of the light microscope. The following methods are used for its demonstration:
1. Dark-field illumination.
2. Special staining techniques in which the thickness of the flagella is increased by mordanting.
3. Electron microscopy.

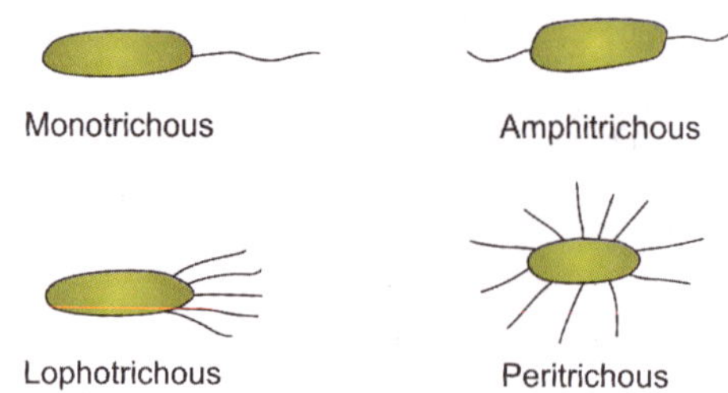

Fig. 3.5: Arrangement of flagella

4. Indirect method by which motility of the bacteria can be seen or demonstrated.
   a. Spreading type of growth on a medium, e.g. swarming growth of *Proteus* species.
   b. Motility under the microscope, e.g. hanging drop method.
   c. Spreading of bacteria in a semisolid agar, e.g. Craigie tube method.

Fimbriae

Fimbriae are hair-like appendages projecting from the cell surface as straight filaments. They are also called pili. They are 0.1 to 1.0 µm in length and less than 0.01 µm thick (shorter than and thinner than flagella). Fimbriae are composed of a protein called pilin.

Functions

1. Organs of adhesion — This property enhances the virulence of bacteria. Fimbriae help the bacteria to attach to the cells and help in invasion or penetration of bacteria into the human cells.
2. Transfer of genetic material.

Detection of functions
   a. Electron microscopy.
   b. Hemagglutination.

BACTERIAL SPORES

Bacteria belonging to the genus *Bacillus* and *Clostridium* (that cause anthrax and gas gangrene) are able to form highly resistant and resting stage within their cells known as spores. These enable the bacteria to survive adverse conditions such as heat, drying, freezing, radiation and action of chemicals. They are not reproductive structures. As bacterial spores are formed within the parent cell, they are called endospores.

Shape and Position of Spores/Morphology of Spores

The cell membrane grows inwards and forms spore wall around the core (forespore). The inner most layer of spores wall forms the spore membrane from which the cell wall of the future vegetative bacterium develops. Outside of this membrane is a thick layer, the cortex and a multilayer tough spore coat. Some spores have an additional loose coating called exosporium.

Spores are usually smooth walled or ovoid. In some species they are spherical. In bacilli, spores usually fit into the normal cell diameter except in *Clostridium* where they may cause bulging (Fig. 3.6). This bulge can be terminal (drumstick) or central. Spores do not take up ordinary stains.

Resistance

Bacterial spores (Fig. 3.7) are extremely resistant to ordinary boiling, heating and disinfectants. However, spores of all medically important bacteria are destroyed by autoclaving at 121°C and 15 pounds per square inch pressure applied for 15 minutes.

Germination

The process of conversion of spore into vegetative cell is known as germination.

Demonstration

1. Gram staining—spores appear as an unstained refractile body within the cell.
2. Modified Ziehl-Neelsen (ZN) staining with 0.25% to 0.5% sulfuric acid (H_2SO_4).

Uses of Spores

Spores of certain species of bacteria are employed as indicator for the proper sterilization, e.g. *Bacillus stearothermophilus* is destroyed in

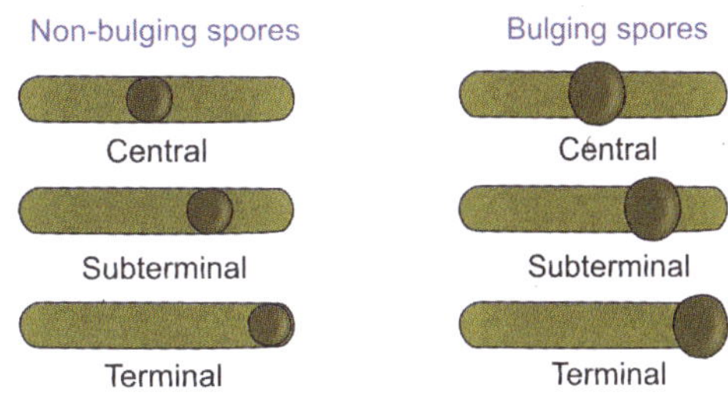

Fig. 3.6: Shape and position of spores

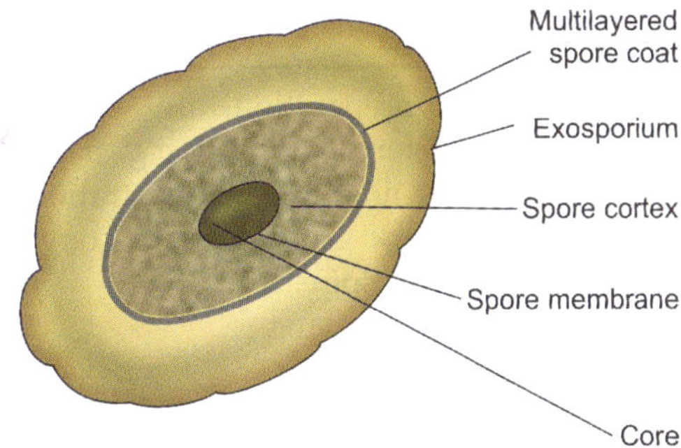

Fig. 3.7: Bacterial spore

the autoclave at a temperature of 121°C within 15 minutes when the pressure is 15 pounds per square inch. Absence of spores after autoclaving indicates proper sterilization.

Spore forming bacteria:
1. Obligate aerobes—genus *Bacillus*, e.g. *B. anthracis, B. subtilis.*
2. Obligate anaerobes—genus *Clostridium*, e.g. *Cl. tetani, Cl. welchini, Cl. botulinum.*

Identification of Bacteria/Staining

BACTERIAL STAINING

Unstained (wet) preparation are examined mainly for the bacterial motility, e.g. hanging drop preparations and for demonstration of spirochetes, e.g. dark ground microscopy for treponemes and leptospires.

Stained Preparation

Smear made from bacterial cultures or specimens is first air dried and then heat fixed by flaming the slide from underneath. Heat kills and fixes the bacteria on the slide due to coagulation of bacterial proteins. The fixed smear is stained by an appropriate staining technique.

STAINING TECHNIQUES

In their natural states, bacterial cells appear under the microscope as tiny, colorless, spheres or rods, which are difficult to see especially, if they are not mobile. To see them distinctly, they are stained with different type of dyes.

The commonly used stains are salts. Basic stains consist of a colored cation with a colorless anion, e.g. methylene blue$^+$ chloride$^-$. Acidic stains are the reverse (sodium$^+$ eosinate$^-$) of basic stains. Bacterial cells are rich in nucleic acids with negative charges as phosphate groups. These combine with the positively charged basic dyes. Acidic dyes do not stain bacterial cells and hence used to stain background materials with a contrasting color.

Special stains are used to differentiate flagella, capsules, cell walls, cell membranes, granules, nuclear region and spores.

Simple Staining

Dyes such as methylene blue or carbol fuchsin are used in simple staining. They provide color contrast, but impart the same color to all bacteria and have limited applications.

Negative Staining

Bacteria are mixed with dyes, such as India ink or nigrosin. The background gets stained and unstained bacteria stand out in contrast. This is useful to demonstrate bacterial capsule, which do not take simple stains, e.g. spirochetes.

Differential Staining

Differential staining impart different colors to different bacteria or bacterial structures. Staining procedures that make visible the differences between bacterial cells and components of a bacterial cell are termed differential staining techniques, e.g. gram staining.

GRAM STAINING

Gram stain was originally developed by the Danish histologist, Christian Gram in 1884. The method divides bacteria into two groups, gram positive and gram negative based on the nature of the cell wall.

Procedure

The method consists of four steps:

Step 1—Primary stain: The air-dried and heat-fixed smear is stained with crystal violet/gentian violet/methyl violet for 60 seconds. All bacteria, gram positive and gram negative will take up the purple color of the primary stain.

Step 2—Mordant: Wash the slide with tap water and add gram iodine (10%) as mordant. Keep for 60 seconds. The mordant fastens the stain to the cells forming a crystal violet-iodine complex.

Step 3—Decolorizer: Wash the slide with water and decolorize with 70 percent ethyl alcohol or acetone for 15 seconds. Alcohol removes the crystal violet iodine stain from gram-negative cells, which have thin cell wall. The gram-positive cells retain their purple color even after the decolorization process.

Step 4—Counterstain: Wash the slide with water and counterstain with safranin or neutral red for 60 seconds. The gram-negative cells are stained with red color of the counterstain. Wash with water.

Examine the slides under the oil immersion (cedar wood oil) objective of the microscope.

Result

The gram-positive cells (Fig. 4.1) appear purple in color. The gram-negative organisms (Fig. 4.2) appear pink red in color.

Gram staining is an essential procedure in the identification of bacteria and frequently the only one method required for studying morphology.

Mechanism of Gram Staining

1. The gram-positive cells have a more acidic protoplasm, which retain the basic dye more strongly than gram-negative bacteria. Iodine makes the protoplasm more acidic and serves as mordant, i.e. iodine combines with the dye to form an iodine complex and fixes the dye in the bacterial cell.
2. The gram-positive cytoplasmic membrane being less permeable, the dye-iodine complex gets trapped within the cell. The gram-negative cell has increased permeability to

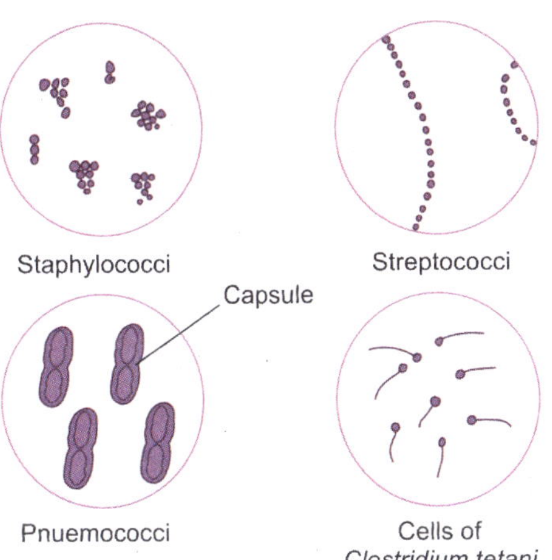

Fig. 4.1: Gram-positive bacteria

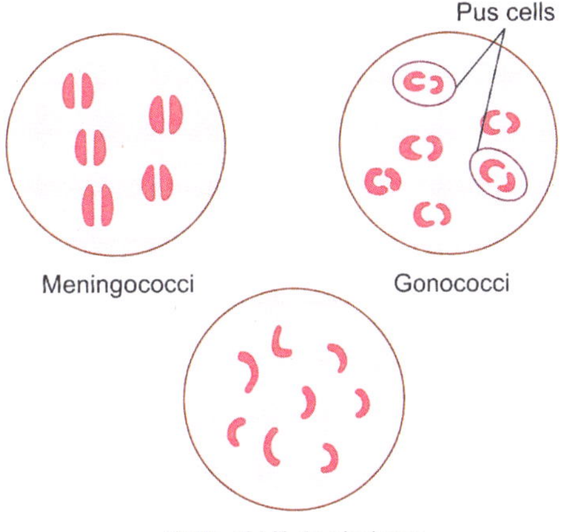

Fig. 4.2: Gram-negative bacteria

alcohol and acetone permitting the outflow of the complex during decolorization.

3. Integrity of the cell wall is essential for a positive stain. The gram-positive bacteria become gram negative when the cell wall is damaged.

Gram reactivity is of considerable importance as the gram-positive and gram-negative bacteria differ not only in staining techniques and structure, but also in several other properties such as growth requirements, sensitivity to antibiotics and pathogenicity.

Gram-positive bacteria are normally susceptible to penicillin, gram negative to streptomycin.

Gram-positive cells secrete exotoxins to the medium, which are highly antigenic in nature and extremely fatal. Gram-negative cell wall contains endotoxin in lipopolysaccharides that are highly antigenic. Different gram-positive and gram-negative organisms are listed in Table 4.1.

ACID-FAST STAINING: ZIEHL-NEELSEN STAINING

Mycobacterium tuberculosis and *Mycobacterium leprae* take up the red color when stained with a strong solution of carbol fuchsin with the application of heat and withstand decolorization with acid or alcohol. Tubercle bacilli with 20 percent sulfuric acid (H_2SO_4) *M. leprae* with 5 percent H_2SO_4. Then counterstained by a contrasting dye, methylene blue or malachite green. The acid-fast bacteria retain the fuchsin (red) color, while others take blue/green color of the counterstains.

Table 4.1: Examples for gram-positive and gram-negative organisms

Gram-positive organisms	Gram-negative organisms
Staphylococcus	Neisseria gonococcus
Streptococcus	Neisseria meningococcus
Pneumococcus	Salmonella
Clostridium`	Shigella
Corynebacterium diphtheriae	Brucella
Mycobacterium	Hemophilus
Bacillus	Enterobacteriaceae
Actinomycetes	Bordetella
	Vibrio
	Pseudomonas

Acid fastness is due to the high content and variety of lipids, fatty acids and higher alcohol (mycolic acid). Acid fastness is also due to the integrity of their cell wall.

Pulmonary tuberculosis is diagnosed by Ziehl-Neelsen (ZN) staining of the early morning sputum sample. In the procedure adopted by the Revised National Tuberculosis Control Program (RNTCP), 25 percent H_2SO_4 is used as the decolorizer.

Procedure

1. Break a broomstick into two. Pick up the large yellow purulent portion of the sputum and spread evenly onto two-third portion of the numbered slide.
2. Air dry the slide for 15 to 30 minutes.
3. Fix the dry slide by heating briefly 3 to 5 times for 3 to 4 seconds.
4. Place the slides in serial order on the staining rack. Stain the slides with 1 percent carbol fuchsin.
5. Heat the slides from below until vapors rise.
6. Let the slides stand for 5 minutes.
7. Rinse the slides with tap water. Drain off excess water.
8. Decolorize with 20 percent H_2SO_4 and let it stand for 2 to 4 minutes (allow it to stand for 3 more minutes if necessary).
9. Rinse away excess stain with tap water. Drain off the water.

10. Counterstain with 0.10 percent methylene blue and let stand for 30 seconds. Gently rinse the slides with tap water, drain the water off and allow the slides to dry.

Examine slides under the oil immersion objective of the microscope.

Result

Mycobacterium tuberculosis bacilli appear as thin bright red rods slightly beaded (Fig. 4.3A). All other organisms/cells are stained blue (if counterstained by methylene blue) or green (if counterstained by malachite green). For *M. leprae* 5 percent H_2SO_4 is used. *M. leprae* bacilli, appear as red rods in the shape of cigar bundles (Fig. 4.3B). Note: Nitric acid (HNO_3) or hydrochloric acid (HCl) can be used in place of H_2SO_4.

ALBERT STAINING

Diagnosis of Diphtheria in the Laboratory

Albert staining is performed to demonstrate the metachromatic (volutin) granules in *Corynebacterium diphtheriae* a gram-positive bacterium (the 'coryne' means club).

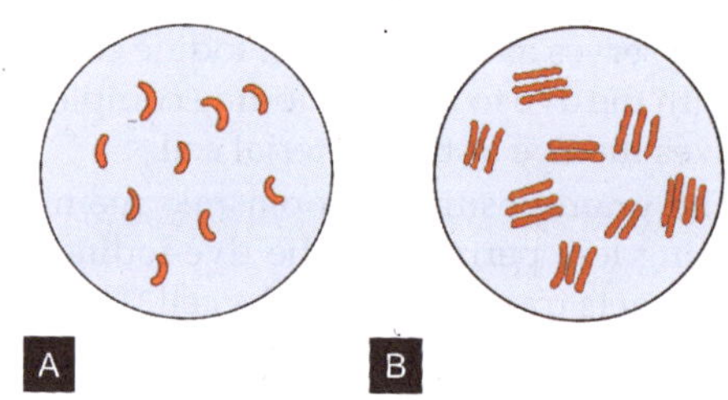

Figs 4.3A and B: Acid-fast staining. **A.** *M. tuberculosis* when stained with Ziehl-Neelsen (ZN) stain (20% H_2SO_4); **B.** *M. leprae* when stained with ZN stain (5% H_2SO_4).

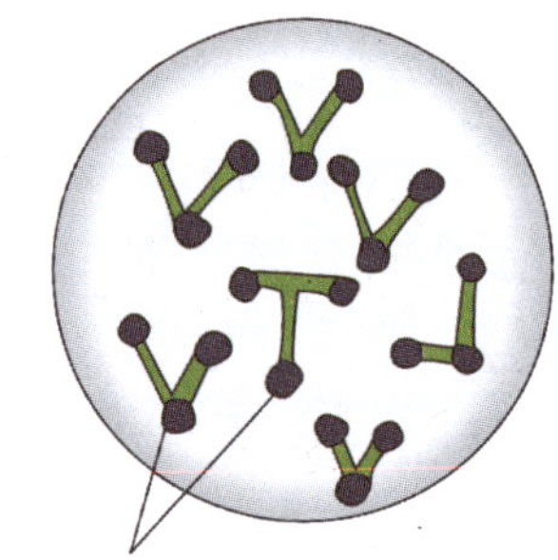

Fig. 4.4: Albert staining of *C. diphtheriae*

Principle

The volutin granules of *C. diphtheriae* take up a different color than body of the bacteria and hence they are called metachromatic granules.

Procedure

The protocol is as follows:

1. The smear is made from suspected culture or throat swab.
2. It is air dried and heat-fixed.
3. It is covered with Albert stain I for 4 to 6 minutes.
4. The smear is washed with water and blotted dry.
5. It is covered with Albert stain II and allowed to act for 1 to 2 minutes.
6. The slide is finally washed, blotted dry and examined under the oil immersion objective of the microscope.

Result

Corynebacterium diphtheriae appear as dark green bacilli with bluish black granules (Fig. 4.4). Other bacteria stain light green. *C. diphtheriae* bacilli are arranged in typical chinese letters pattern, perpendicular to each other.

Ingredients

Albert stain I: Toluidine blue 0.15 g, malachite green 0.20 g, glacial acetic acid 1.0 mL, ethyl alcohol (95%) 2.0 mL and 100 mL distilled water.
Albert stain II: Iodine 6.0 g, potassium iodide 9.0 g and 900 mL distilled water.

Bacterial Growth Factors

FACTORS INFLUENCING THE GROWTH OF BACTERIA

Moisture

Like all living things, bacteria are sensitive to their environment. Water is necessary for the growth of bacteria, because they cannot absorb food materials unless they are in solution. They cannot survive in the absence of water, this is demonstrated in the preservation of food by drying, e.g. fish, meat and fruits.

Nutrition

Bacteria obtain their nutrition from organic and inorganic matter for growth and multiplication. Most bacteria of medical importance will grow only if an organic material is available as a source of food. Such bacteria are called chemoheterotrophs. Bacteria also require a source of nitrogen and a number of salts to have a supply of potassium, magnesium, iron, phosphate and sulfate. Minor concentrations of calcium, manganese and trace quantities of copper, zinc, cobalt, nickel and chlorine are also required.

Many bacteria oxidize glucose like higher animals and some are able to build up protoplasm through complex processes. Some require vitamins such as niacin, thiamine and riboflavin and use these like human beings.

Temperature

Each species of bacteria requires a certain temperature range for its growth, called optimum temperature. Bacteria, which attack human body live best at body temperature, i.e. for most pathogenic bacteria the optimum temperature is 37°C. Most bacteria are killed at 56°C in 30 minutes. Low temperature kills them. Refrigeration for preservation of foods and sterilization by heat are based on this principle.

On the basis of temperature requirements bacteria are divided into three groups:

1. *Psychrophilic:* Bacteria grow at an optimum temperature of 10°C to 20°C with a range of 5°C to 30°C, e.g. *Flavobacterium psychrophilum.*
2. *Mesophilic:* Bacteria grow best at 20°C to 40°C with a range 10°C to 45°C. All medically important bacteria belongs to this group, e.g. *Streptococcus lactis.*
3. *Thermophilic:* Bacteria live best at 50°C to 60°C with a range of 25°C to 80°C, e.g. *Bacillus stearothermophilus.*

pH (Hydrogen Ion Concentration) or Acidity and Alkalinity

Most of the pathogenic bacteria grow best in a neutral or slightly alkaline (pH 7.2 to 7.6) medium. Acid medium prevents the growth of many bacteria. Preservation of fish, meat and vegetables by pickling in vinegar is based on the sensitivity of bacteria to the extreme acidity of vinegar (acetic acid).

Gases

Oxygen

The capacity of bacteria to grow in presence of oxygen and to utilize it depends on possession of a cytochrome oxidase system. On the basis of requirement of oxygen, bacteria are divided into aerobes and anaerobes.

Aerobes: They grow only in presence of oxygen, e.g. *Pseudomonas, Bacillus, Nitrobacter, Sarcina.* They require oxygen as hydrogen acceptor.

Facultative aerobes: They are organisms that live with or without oxygen, e.g. *Vibrio, Escherichia coli* (*E. coli*), *Salmonella*, *Shigella* and *Staphylococcus*. The microaerophilic organisms grow well with relatively small quantities of oxygen, e.g. *Haemophilus*.

Obligate anaerobes: Multiply only in the absence of oxygen, e.g. *Clostridium*. They require a substance other than oxygen as hydrogen acceptor. The toxicity of oxygen results from its reduction by enzymes in the cell (e.g. flavoproteins) to H_2O_2 and more toxic free radical superoxide.

Carbon Dioxide

The metabolic activities of some organisms like *Neisseria gonorrhoeae*, *Brucella abortus* are enhanced by the presence of extra amount of carbon dioxide (CO_2) in the atmospheric air.

Osmotic Pressure

Many bacteria are sensitive to concentrated solutions of salt and sugar because of their osmotic pressure. Preservation of food in concentrated salt solution (salted mango) or thick sugar syrup (rasugulla, gulab jamun) is based on this principle.

Light and Radiation

Light is bacteria's worst enemy. When exposed to direct sunlight they become sluggish and die rapidly. Darkness favors development of bacteria. They become very active and multiply rapidly. Mattresses, pillows and blankets of hospital wards are often disinfected by sunlight. Ultraviolet (UV) light and radiation also destroy bacteria. Special lamps, which produce UV rays also destroy bacteria and are used for the treatment of skin infections.

BACTERIAL GROWTH CURVE

When a bacterium is seeded into a suitable liquid medium and incubated, its growth follows a definite course. If bacterial counts are made at intervals after inoculation and plotted against time, a growth curve is obtained (Fig. 5.1). This curve has the following four phases.

Lag Phase

Immediately, following the seeding of a culture medium, there is no appreciable increase

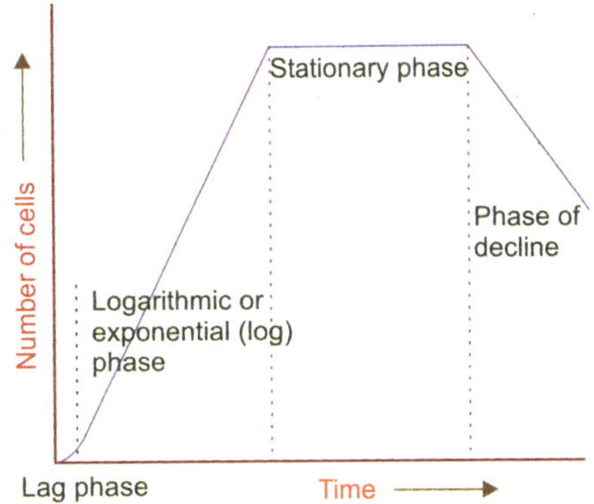

Fig. 5.1: Growth curve of a bacterial culture in a liquid medium

in the number of the cells though there may be an increase in the size of the cells. The initial period is the time taken for adaptation to the environment during which the necessary enzymes and metabolic intermediates are built up in adequate quantities for the multiplication to proceed. The duration of the lag phase varies with the species, size of the inoculum, nature of the culture medium and environmental factors such as temperature.

Log Phase (Logarithmic or Exponential Phase)

Following the lag phase, the cells start dividing and their number increase exponentially or by geometric proportions with time.

Stationary Phase

After varying periods of exponential growth cell division comes to a halt due to the depletion of nutrients and accumulation of toxic products. The number of new cells born is equal to the number of dying cells.

Phase of Decline

Population decreases due to death of cells, because of depletion of nutrients and accumulation of toxic end products. The number of bacteria dying is much more than dividing and hence there is a decline in the total number of bacteria.

REPRODUCTION

Most bacteria multiply by simple fission into two halves, a process known as binary fission. Reproduction takes place at an extraordinary rate in favorable environment. If one cell divides at the rate of once in an hour, the descendants of the cell should number nearly 20 million at the end of the day. Some bacteria may divide as frequently as in 20 minutes. The generation time for *Mycobacterium tuberculosis* is 20 hours and *M. leprae* is 20 days.

If a single bacteria divides after 30 minutes, then the total number of bacteria after 24 hours will be $N = 2^n$ (where 'n' is the number of generations).

Culture Media

A culture medium is any substance on which or in which microorganism can grow and multiply. It is essential to grow the microorganism from infected materials to identify the cause of infection. Like all other living forms, microorganism also require suitable nutrients as well as favorable environment for growth.

A culture medium:

1. Must contain nutrients essential for the growth of the given microbes.
2. Provide suitable environment for growth, e.g. proper pH, osmotic pressure, temperature and oxygen.

CLASSIFICATION

According to Their Consistency

Culture media is classified as follows according to their consistency:

- Liquid media
- Solid media.

Liquid Media

1. Peptone water.
2. Nutrient broth.
3. MacConkey liquid medium.
4. Robertson cooked meat (RCM) medium.

Peptone water: Contains peptone (hydrolysis products of proteins and contains mixtures of proteases, polypeptides and amino acids), sodium chloride (NaCl) and distilled water. It is a colorless watery solution used for:

a. Preparation of sugar media.
b. Indole production.
c. Cultivation of *Vibrio cholerae* (at an alkaline pH of 8.5).

Nutrient Broth: Fatless meat of ox heart (500 g) is minced and extracted with 1 liter of water, 10 g of peptone and 10 g of NaCl are added, pH adjusted to 7.3. Clear straw-colored transparent fluid, more nutritious than peptone water and is used for the growth of fastidious organisms like *Streptococcus, Pneumococcus, Gonococcus* and *Meningococcus.*

MacConkey liquid medium: Consists of sodium taurocholate (bile salt), peptone, NaCl, lactose and water; pink red in color. It is used to detect coliform bacilli in water sample, etc. The medium is dispensed in Durham tubes to detect gas.

Robertson cooked meat medium: RCM medium for anaerobes contain meat cooked in sodium hydroxide (NaOH), filtered and squeezed, making a layer overlayered with 10 mL nutrient broth. Finally, the medium is dispensed in McCartney bottles with cap. It is used for the growth of anaerobes and also for preservation of stock culture of aerobes. Different types of liquid media are shown in Figure 6.1.

Advantages of liquid media

1. Rapid growth of the organism.
2. Used for chemical tests.
3. To study mobility.

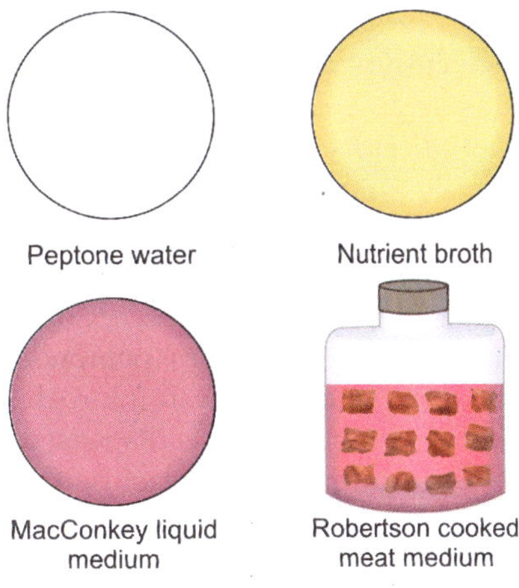

Fig. 6.1: Liquid media

Disadvantages of liquid media
1. From a mixture containing different organism individual types cannot be identified.
2. The growth of the organism does not exhibit special characteristic appearance.

Solid Media

Nutrient agar: It contains peptone, meat extract (Lab-Lemco), NaCl, agar and distilled water. Shake, autoclave it and adjust pH to 7.4. Medium should be light brown in color.

Used for:
1. The growth of common pathogenic organisms.
2. Sensitivity test.
3. Preparation of selective media, e.g. salt agar, potassium tellurite.
4. Preparation of enriched media, e.g. blood agar, deoxycholate agar.

Blood agar: It contains 7% to 10% sheep blood in nutrient agar. It is a red colored opaque medium contained in petri dishes used for the growth of most pathogens. Delicate bacteria like *Haemophilus* and *Gonococcus* also grow on this medium. Can be used as a differential medium, as it will help to differentiate hemolytic and non-hemolytic colonies. On addition of certain chemicals, e.g. potassium tellurite or neomycin, blood agar may become selective medium.

Chocolate agar: It contains 7% to 10% sheep blood in nutrient agar. The medium is kept at 30°C for about 10 minutes or till chocolate color develops. This medium is dispensed in petri dishes just like blood agar. Can be easily identified by its typical chocolate color. Chocolate agar is more enriched than blood agar and is used for culture of organisms requiring more nutrition, e.g. *Neisseria pneumoniae* and *Haemophilus influenzae.*

MacConkey agar: Certain bacteria utilize sugars like lactose and produce acid, which is detected by a suitable indicator, which changes its colors in acid conditions, e.g. MacConkey agar. MacConkey agar consists of peptone, lactose, agar, neutral red and bile salt (taurocholate). It is pinkish red in color and is dispensed in petri dishes. Used to distinguish lactose fermenters (LF) as pink colonies and non-lactose fermenters (NLF) as colorless or pale colonies. It is also called an indicator medium. The medium allows the growth of only intestinal organism; it is a selective and differential medium.

Lowenstein-Jensen (L-J) medium: Consists of beaten eggs, malachite green and mineral salts, which include asparagine, glycerol, magnesium citrate and potassium dihydrogen phosphate (KH_2PO_4) solution. It is green opaque slope dispensed in McCartney bottles; used for the growth of *Mycobacterium tuberculosis.*

Sabouraud dextrose agar medium: It consists of glucose (dextrose), peptone, agar and distilled water. It is whitish semi-transparent slope dispersed in large tubes or screw capped bottles. It is used for the isolation of fungi from clinical material. Sensitivity to antimycotic compounds also can be determined.

Different types of solid media are shown in Figure 6.2.

According to Their Functions and Uses

Culture media is classified as follows according to their functions and uses:
1. Simple media, e.g. nutrient broth, nutrient agar.
2. Enriched media, e.g. blood agar, chocolate agar.
3. Enrichment media, e.g. alkaline peptone water, selenite 'F' broth.
4. Selective media, e.g. thiosulfate-citrate-bile salts-sucrose (TCBS).

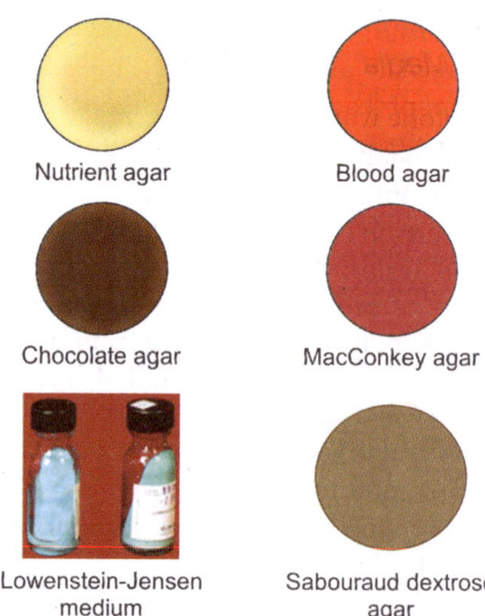

Fig. 6.2: Solid media

5. Selective and differential media, e.g. MacConkey agar.
6. Anaerobic media, e.g. RCM medium, thioglycolate broth.
7. Transport media, e.g. Stuart transport medium, Venkatraman Ramakrishnan (VR) fluid.

Simple Media

Medium contains only the basic nutrients for the growth of ordinary bacteria, which are not fastidious. It may be liquid (peptone water, nutrient broth) or solid (nutrient agar).

Peptone water: It consists of proteins, water, carbohydrates and a few mineral salts. Peptone is a water soluble yellowish granular powder, hygroscopic in nature, prepared by acid hydrolysis of cheap proteins or meat. It contains proteases, amino acids, minerals and other essential nutrients.

Nutrient broth: It is another example of simple liquid medium. It consists of peptone water and meat extract. When 2% to 3% agar is added to nutrient broth, it becomes solid nutrient agar. This is the simplest and routinely used medium in laboratory diagnosis.

Enriched Media

Media that are enriched by the addition of highly nutritious substances such as animal proteins, blood, serum or egg. May be liquid (serum broth) or solid (serum agar, blood agar and chocolate agar). Solid medium is used for isolation of bacteria and liquid medium for study of biochemical properties of pure culture. Some pathogens will not grow in simple media and will grow only in enriched media. Blood agar and chocolate (heated blood) agar are common examples of enriched media used for the growth and identification of *Streptococcus pyogenes* and *Gonococcus*.

Enrichment Media

Enrichment media are liquid media mostly used to isolate bacteria from diarrheal stools or food materials, which are suspected for contamination as in food poisoning. Some substances are added to the liquid media, which have a stimulating effect on the bacteria to be grown or inhibit its competitors. This results in an absolute increase in the number of wanted bacteria compared to others. Such media are called enrichment media, e.g. selenite 'F' broth and tetrathionate broth.

Selenite F broth: These are very useful for culture of feces when the non-pathogenic or commensal bacteria tend to overgrow the pathogenic ones, e.g. *Salmonella* type being overgrown by *Escherichia coli*.

Tetrathionate broth: It is added, which inhibits coliform bacteria and allows typhoid and paratyphoid bacilli to grow.

Selective Media

Selective media contain substances that inhibit all, but a few types of bacteria and facilitate the isolation of a particular species. These media are used to isolate a particular bacteria from specimens where mixed bacterial flora are expected. Selective medium is solid in contrast to the enrichment medium, which is liquid. Examples are:

Deoxycholate citrate agar (DCA): Addition of deoxycholate acts as a selective agent to enteric bacilli (*Salmonella* and *Shigella*).

Potasium tellurite medium for *Corynebacterium diphtheriae*. Potassium tellurite inhibits the growth of all organisms except diphtheriae.

Alkaline peptone water and TCBS (pH = 8.5) for cholera vibrio because of alkaline pH.

Lowenstein-Jensen (L-J) medium for *Mycobacterium tuberculosis*.

Selective and Differential Media

When a medium contains substances, which help to distinguish different characteristics of bacteria, it is called differential media, e.g. Mac Conkey agar. The LF form pink colonies whereas NLF form colorless colonies or pale colonies.

MacConkey agar is an enteric medium, because bile salt in the medium inhibits all others. It also differentiates LF and NLF. The acid from lactose acts on the neutralized indicator, e.g. *Salmonella typhi, S. paratyphi* and *Shigella* (bacteria producing bacillary dysentery) are NLF and colorless.

Transport Media

Transport media contain essential salts and low concentrations of nutrients, so that bacteria do not multiply before examined in the laboratory. Transport media are mainly used to collect specimens with sterile swabs and bacteria present in such swabs are maintained by putting the swabs in transport media before they are depatched.

In case of delicate organisms like gonococci, which may not survive the time taken for transport to the laboratory or may be overgrown by non-pathogens, (e.g. dysentery or cholera organisms) special transport media are used to protect the pathogens and keep them viable and prevent the over growth of non-pathogens.

Transport media most commonly used for storage and transporting of stool specimens are:

Cary-Blair medium for feces: It is useful for transport of most diarrhea producing bacteria. It is a stable semisolid medium and can be stored in sealed containers.

Stuart transport medium: For *Neisseria gonorrhoea* in which case, bedside inoculation of the medium is not necessary. This is a non-nutrient soft agar gel containing a reducing agent to prevent oxidation and charcoal to neutralize certain bacterial inhibitors.

Venkatraman Ramakrishnan fluid: It is useful for transportation of feces specimens from suspected cases of cholera. Specimens for isolation of *Vibrio cholerae* are to be collected in one ounce screw capped McCartney bottles. VR fluid preserves vibrios for more than 6 weeks and has also proved to be a very convenient medium for transportation, as it can be kept at room temperature after collection of specimen.

Buffered Glycerol Saline—for enteric bacteria for transporting fecal samples of gastroenteritis cases suspected to be due to *Shigella.*

Anaerobic Media

Robertson cooked meat (RCM) medium: Consists of fat-free minced meat (Lab-Lemco) in broth. The meat particles act as reducing substances and allow growth of anaerobes such as clostridia.

When growth of *Clostridium* causes changes in the medium, turbidity and change in color of meat pieces occur, inferences as to the organism is possible.

1. Sacrolytic clostridia: For example, *Clostridium perfringens* causing gas gangrene. Reddening of the meat pieces. The medium becomes turbid within 24 hours with production of gas.
2. Proteolytic clostridia: *Clostridium botulinum* causing food poisoning. There is blackening of the meat pieces due to break down of proteins and production of gas.
3. *Clostridium tetani*: Grows well on this medium with turbidity and gas. There is no change in the color of the meat pieces because it has no sacrolytic or proteolytic action. The meat is not digested, but turns black after prolonged incubation.

McINTOSH AND FILDES JAR

McIntosh and Fildes jar consists of glass or metal jar, with metal lid, which can be clamped air tight with screw. The lid has two tubes, one acting as a gas inlet and the other as outlet. Additionally the lid has two terminals, which can be connected to electrical supply.

Inoculated culture plates are placed inside the jar. The outer tube is connected to vacuum pump and air inside is evacuated. The outlet tube is closed and inlet tube is connected with hydrogen gas cylinder. After filling the jar with hydrogen, electric terminals are connected so that palladinised asbestos is heated. This acts as catalyst for combination of hydrogen and residual oxygen. It ensures complete anaerobiosis. At the same time, it also carries risk of explosion.

An indicator should also be kept for verifying aerobic conditions in jar. Reduced methylene blue is used for this purpose. It is colorless anaerobically and regains its color on exposure to oxygen.

INOCULATION

Once the media are prepared they must be inoculated with materials obtained from patients suspected to be suffering from disease. The method of culture used in the laboratory are the streak, lawn, stroke, stab, pour plate and liquid culture.

1. Surface plating or streak inoculation: Routinely employed for isolation of bacteria in pure culture. A platinum loop with 2 to 4 cm long wire and loop of 2 to 4 mm diameter at the other end is charged with the specimen to be cultured on the surface dry plate of solid media towards peripheral area. The inoculum is spread thinly over the plate in series of parallel lines in different segments of the plate. On inoculation we may find confluent growth at the site of the primary inoculation. Well separated colonies are obtained over the final series of streaks.

2. Lawn cultures are prepared: By flooding the surface of the plate with suspensions of bacteria. It provides uniform surface growth of bacteria useful for antibiotic sensitivity test.

In a liquid medium, if the specimen contains bacteria the whole liquid becomes turbid.

On solid media colonies appear. Study the morphology of the colony, size, shape, surface, edge, pigment, hemolysis of red blood cells (RBCs), gram stain, motility, etc.

ANTIBIOTIC SENSITIVITY TESTS

Finding out the antibiotic sensitivities of pathogens to different antibiotics helps in selecting the right antibiotic for treating the patient. There are two different methods.

Kirby-Bauer Method (Diffusion Method)

The method involves inoculating the whole surface of a dry nutrient agar plate with the organism under test. At appropriate intervals on the surface of the plate, a number of filter paper discs containing antibiotics are applied. The antibiotics diffuse out of the discs into the open medium and if susceptible, bacterial growth is inhibited in a circular zone around the discs. The zone sizes are compared, results are recorded and reported.

Interpretation

The results are interpreted as sensitive or resistant, depending on the size of inhibition for that particular antibiotic.

Sensitive: Strains affected by/amenable to treatment with conventional doses of the antimicrobial agent.

Resistant: Strains unaffected by high concentration of antibiotic and hence unlikely to be affected by any dosage of the antibiotic.

Stokes Method

In stokes method (Fig. 6.3), the test and control organization are compared against the same antibiotic disc on the same medium and under the same physical conditions. The middle third of a culture plate is seeded with the test strain, which has been grown in peptone water. On either side of the test strain, standard strain is inoculated leaving a little gap between the inoculated area. Antibiotic discs are placed in the gap and inoculated overnight at 37°C.

Result

A zone radius that is the same size or is larger than the control or is not smaller than 3 mm is reported to be sensitive to that particular antibiotic.

The advantage with this method is that the factors affecting the potency of discs and media, etc. are taken into account, while reporting the sensitivity pattern.

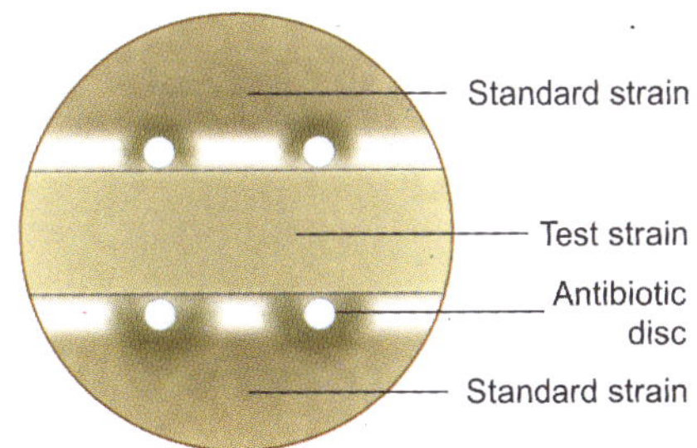

Fig. 6.3: Stokes method

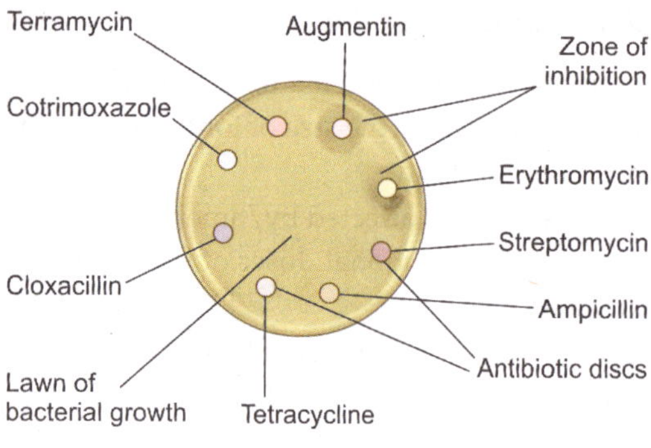

Fig. 6.4: Antibiogram

1. For testing gram-positive cocci standard strain is *Staphylococcus aureus*.

2. For testing gram-negative bacilli other than *Pseudomonas*, the standard strain is *E.coli*.

3. For testing of *Pseudomonas*, standard strain is *Pseudomonas aeruginosa*.

ANTIBIOGRAM

Antibiogram (Fig. 6.4) is the antimicrobial agent sensitivity profile for any particular organism. In order to treat or cure any microbial infection there are many antimicrobial compounds, which are used in the form of antibiotics, antifungal and antiviral drugs. Before administration of these compounds, it is necessary to verify the sensitivity of the microorganisms for that particular drug.

Control of Microorganisms— Sterilization and Disinfection

DEFINITIONS

Disinfection

Disinfection is a process of destruction of pathogenic organisms capable of giving rise to infection, but not bacterial spores. It also means slowing down of growth and activity of microorganisms that cannot be destroyed. Chemical agents are usually used in disinfection.

Sterilization

Sterilization is a process by which articles are freed of all microorganisms both in the vegetative and spore forms.

Bactericidal Agents

Bactericidal agents are those which only prevent multiplication of bacteria. Some of the bacteria may remain alive.

Sepsis or Infection

Implies the presence of pathogenic microorganisms in the living tissue.

Asepsis

Asepsis is the absence of pathogenic microorganism.

Antisepsis

Antisepsis is the destruction or inhibition of microorganisms in living tissues thereby limiting or preventing the harmful effects of infection.

Antiseptic

Antiseptic is a chemical substance applied to skin surface to kill or inhibit pathogenic organisms.

Disinfectant

Disinfectant is a chemical substance that destroys the vegetative forms of pathogenic organisms, but not spores.

DISINFECTION/STERILIZATION

Sterilization and disinfection can be accomplished by mechanical, physical and chemical means.

Mechanical Means of Control

Scrubbing

Scrubbing is usually done by soap and water. The process itself removes many microorganisms mechanically. Soap in addition acts chemically. Nurse scrubs the hands every time when she comes in contact with a contaminated article or infectious material.

Sedimentation

Sedimentation is the process by which articles suspended in a liquid settle down to the bottom of a liquid, carrying with them bacteria, which stick to them. The method can be used in purification of large amounts of water along with other methods like chlorination.

Filtration

See physical methods.

Physical Agents of Sterilization

1. Sunlight.
2. Drying.
3. Heat.
   a. Dry heat
      • Red heat

- Flaming
- Incineration
- Hot air oven.
  b. Moist heat
  - Temperature below 100°C
    - Pasteurization
    - Inspissation
  - Temperature at 100°C
    - Tyndallization
    - Hot water boiler
  - Temperature above 100°C
    - Autoclave.
4. Filtration
   a. Earthenware candles.
   b. Asbestos disc filters—Seitz.
   c. Sintered glass filters.
   d. Collodion membrane filters.
   e. Fiberglass filters—high efficiency particulate air (HEPA) filters.
5. Radiation
   a. Ionizing—gamma (γ) rays, cold sterilization, electron accelerators.
   b. Non-ionizing—ultraviolet (UV), infrared (IR).
6. Ultrasonic and sonic vibrations.

Sunlight

Light is bacteria's worst enemy. When exposed to direct sunlight, they become sluggish and die rapidly. Darkness favors the development of bacteria. They become very active and multiply rapidly. Sunlight has bactericidal activity and sterilizes under natural conditions. The action is primarily due to UV rays (most of which will be screened by glass) and the presence of ozone in the outer regions of the atmosphere. Direct sunlight as in tropics when not filtered by atmospheric impurities has an active germicidal effect due to UV rays and heat rays. Bacteria suspended in water are readily destroyed by sunlight. This is the natural method of sterilization of water in lakes, rivers, tanks and wells. Also blankets, beddings and pillows of hospital wards are disinfected by sunlight.

Drying

Water is necessary for the growth of bacteria, because they cannot absorb food material unless they are in solution. The fact that bacteria cannot grow in the absence of water is demonstrated in the preservation of food by drying, e.g. dry fruits, dry fish, dry meat.

Dry Heat

Dry heat is a less efficient process as compared to moist heat and bacterial spores are most resistant to it. Spores may require a temperature of 140°C for 3 hour to get killed.

Killing by dry heat is due to:
- Protein denaturation.
- Oxidative damage.
- Toxic effects of elevated levels of electrolytes.

Red heat: It is used to sterilize metallic objects by holding them in flame till they are red hot, e.g. inoculating wires, needles and forceps.

Flaming: The article is passed over the flame without allowing them to become red hot, e.g. mouth of culture tubes, cotton wool plugs and heat fixing of specimen on glass slides for staining process.

Incineration: Articles, which are badly contaminated and materials like sputum cups, infected dressing, bedding, pathological materials and animal carcasses can be destroyed by burning in an incinerator (or furnace). It is an economic and effective way of destroying materials by complete burning. Negative aspect is atmospheric pollution by half burnt polyvinyl chloride (PVC) plastic material.

Hot air oven: It is used for sterilization by dry heat (Fig. 7.1). Its principle is the destructive oxidation

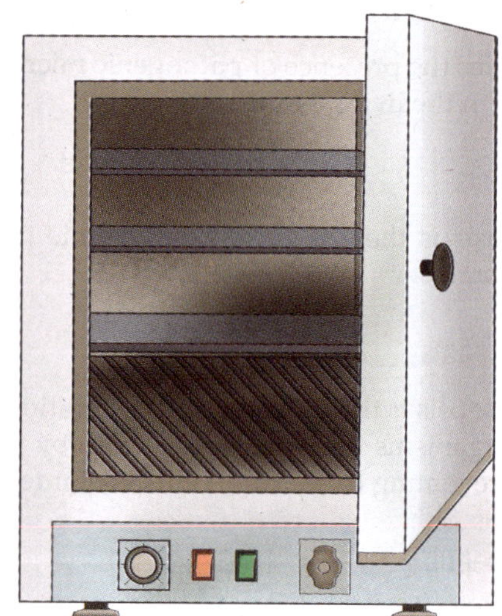

Fig. 7.1: Hot air oven

of essential cell metabolites and destruction of proteins. A number of time temperature combinations as below can be used:

- 140°C for 1½ hours
- 160°C for 1 hour
- 180°C for ½ hour.

Can sterilize glassware—all glass syringes, petri dishes, test tubes, flasks, pipettes, blunt instruments scalpel, scissors, cotton swabs and some pharmaceutical products such as liquid paraffin, sulfonamides, fats, grease, dusting powder, petroleum jelly, oils and oily injections.

Spores are also killed. It is essential that hot air should circulate between the objects to be sterilized there should be only one door to the instrument. Humidity is absent.

Hot air oven is recommended where it is undesirable/unlikely that steam under pressure (autoclave) will make direct and complete contact with the materials to be sterilized.

Moist Heat

Temperature below 100°C

- Pasteurization
- Inspissation.

Pasteurization

Pasteurization is a process of making milk and milk products and other foods safe for consumption by destroying all harmful organisms like tuberculosis bacilli, diphtheria, *Brucella*, *Salmonella* and staphylococci. Spores are not destroyed. Therefore it is a method of disinfection and not sterilization.

Temperature employed are either 63°C for 30 minutes (Holder method) or 72°C for 10 to 15 seconds (flash method) and instant cooling to 13°C or below. Pasteurized milk is not sterilized milk.

Inspissation

Principle

Inspissation is a fractional sterilization procedure for 3 consecutive days. First day heating destroys the vegetative forms of bacteria. Spores are allowed to germinate and killed in second heating. 3 days consecutive heating ensures complete sterilization without destroying the constituents of the medium.

Procedure

1. Fill water up to the appropriate level in the inspissator.

2. Usually the media to be sterilized are kept in a standing position.
3. Switch on the instrument and adjust the temperature to 80°C. Repeat the procedure for 3 consecutive days.

Used for sterilizing egg and serum containing media.

Temperature at 100°C

Tyndallization

Similar to inspissation. The medium to be sterilized is placed at 100°C in flowing steam for 20 minutes for 3 consecutive days. The vegetative cells get damaged at 100°C and the spores that germinate during the next 2 days are destroyed on the succeeding days. Used to sterilize media containing sugar and gelatin.

Boiling

Most of the vegetation forms of bacteria, fungi and viruses are killed at 50°C to 70°C in short time. For needles and instruments, boiling in water for 10 to 30 minutes is sufficient for sterilization.

Addition of a little acid, alkali or washing soda increases the sterilization power of boiling water. Spores and hepatitis B viruses are not destroyed by boiling.

Temperature above 100°C

Autoclave (steam under pressure)

Principle

Principle of autoclave or steam sterilizer is that:

1. Water boils when its vapor pressure equals to that of the surrounding atmosphere. Hence, when pressure inside a closed vessel is increased, the temperature at which water boils also increases.
2. Saturated steam has greater penetrating power.
3. When steam comes in contact with the cooler surface of the tray, it condenses to water and gives up its latent heat to that surface (1,600 mL of steam at 100°C and at atmospheric pressure condenses into 1 mL of water and liberates 518 cal of heat). The large reduction in volume, sucks more steam to the area and the process continues till the temperature of that surface is raised to that of the steam.
4. The condensed water ensures moist conditions for killing of the microbes present.

Parts of an autoclave

The autoclave consists of a vertical or horizontal cylinder of gun metal or stainless steel in a supporting sheet iron case (Fig. 7.2). The lid or door is fastened by screw clamps and made air tight by asbestos washer. The autoclave has on its lid or upper side, a discharge tap for air and steam, a pressure gauge and a safety valve that can be set to blow off at any desired pressure. Heating is done by gas or electricity.

Steam autoclave — working

Sufficient water is put in the cylinder. The material to be sterilized is placed on the tray and heating is started. The lid is screwed tight with the discharge tap open. The safety valve is adjusted to the required pressure. The steam air mixture is allowed to escape freely till all air is removed. The steam pressure rises inside and when it reaches the desired level, the safety valve opens and excess steam escapes. From this period, the holding period of 15 minutes is calculated. When this period is over, the heater is switched off and the autoclave is allowed to cool till the pressure gauge indicates that the inside pressure is atmospheric pressure. Then the discharge tube is opened slowly and air is allowed to enter the autoclave. If the tap is opened when the pressure inside is high, the liquid media will tend to boil violently and spill from the containers and some times an explosion may take place. If not opened till pressure inside has fallen below atmospheric pressure, an excessive amount of water will be evaporated and lost from the media. The domestic pressure cooker is a miniature autoclave and may be used to sterilize small articles in clinics and nursing homes.

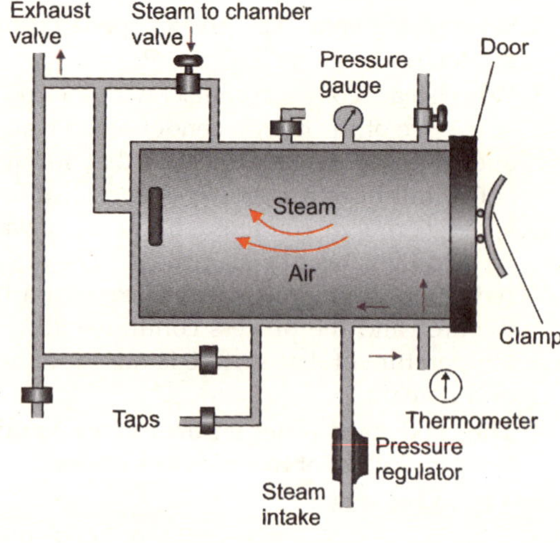

Fig. 7.2: Parts of an autoclave

Defects of autoclave:

1. The amount of air discharge is inefficient and it is difficult to decide when the discharge is complete. If air is not completely removed at the start, the required temperature of 121°C may not be achieved.
2. There is no facility for drying the load after sterilization and before taking it out.

Uses of autoclave

To sterilize surgical dressings, surgical instruments, liquids, which can withstand high temperature, culture media, discarded media with growth, rubber articles like tubing, washers, caps, gloves, aprons and all articles with spores.

Tests for the Efficiency of Autoclave and Hot Air Oven

Biological control: For determining the efficacy of moist heat sterilization, spores of *Bacillus stearothermophilus* are used as test organism. The vegetative form grows at optimum temperature of 60°C and spores are destroyed at 121°C. Paper strips impregnated with 10^6 spores are dried at room temperature and placed in paper envelopes. These envelops are inserted in different parts of the load. After sterilization, these strips are inoculated into a suitable recovering medium like nutrient broth and incubated for sterility for 5 days. If the spores are viable the broth will show turbidity due to germination and growth of vegetative forms of the bacteria. If there is no turbidity the autoclave has sterilized all the articles and is effective.

Bowie-Dick tape or autoclave tape: Adhesive autoclave tapes containing chemical strips, which is invisible before use, but turns black when the particular temperature of 121°C is reached.

Browne tubes are sealed glass tubes with a chemical substance, which turns from red to green when exposed to a temperature of 121°C for 15 minutes in an autoclave.

Thermocouple: Thermocouple can directly measure inside temperature of an autoclave by a potentiometer.

Bacterial filters: Filters are used for heat labile (destroyed by heat) liquids of microorganisms; is useful for antibiotics solutions, sera and carbohydrate solutions used in the preparation of culture media. By this technique, we can obtain bacteria-free filtrates of toxins and antibiotics. The method is also useful when we want to separate microorganisms, which are scanty in fluids and study them. The filter would retain the organism and the filter disc could be cultured. The domestic water filter with filter candles can retain bacteria, but not viruses and *Mycoplasma* as they are too small in size. Thus, the sera filtered in Seitz filters are not safe for chemical use. Filtration is done under carefully controlled positive or negative pressure.

Filtration

Various types of filters used in microbiology are:

1. Earthernware candles—do not retain viruses, e.g. Berkefeld, Mandler and Chamberland (made of unglazed porcelain); others are made of diatomaceous earth.
2. Asbestos filters—do not retain viruses, e.g. Seitz filter.
3. Sintered glass filters—also do not filter viruses.
4. Collodion or membrane filters—for heat labile liquids and solutions, e.g. toxins, antibiotic solutions, sugars, blood products and purification of water.
5. Fiberglass—HEPA filters.

Membrane filters are nowadays used widely. They are made of cellulose acetate and are most suitable for separating sterile solutions.

Other types of filters are made of porcelain, glass or fibrous materials like cotton, asbestos and paper. They do not have uniform pore size, but when thick, particles are absorbed, intercepted and settled on filter materials. Some common examples of fibrous filters are:

a. Cotton or guaze masks: Masks must be changed when they become damp from exhalation.
b. Cotton plugs in flasks, test tubes, pipettes or airlines.
c. Filters are used to prepare mixture of gases for respiratory therapy.
d. Filters in ventilation systems that provide sterile air to operation theaters.

Filters in ventilation systems

1. To provide sterile and dust-free air in operation rooms.
2. To deliver clear air to an enclosure. Development of HEPA filter had made this possible. This, together with a system of laminar airflow is now extensively used to provide dust and bacteria free air.

Laminar airflow

Flow of air in parallel stream. These parallel streams do not mingle but move along parallel flow lines.

Laminar flow hood is of two types:

1. For sterile work for preventing contamination of sterile materials, e.g. intravenous (IV) fluid manufacturing and bottling.
2. Biohazard laminar flow hood for reducing the danger of infection, while manipulating infective materials, e.g. samples containing human immunodeficiency virus (HIV), hepatitis B virus (HBV).

Radiation

Two types of radiation—ionizing and non-ionizing are used for sterilization purposes. Gamma radiation (γ) from radioactive ^{60}Co and electron accelerators are ionizing radiation. IR and UV rays are non-ionizing low energy radiation.

These rays may be absorbed by the cells often causing cell damage or death. Ionizing radiation and non-ionizing radiation are used in microbial control. This is an alternative to autoclave for sterilization of plastic petri dishes and other heat sensitive materials like disposal syringes, catheters, culture plates, rubber and fabric. Since, there is no appreciable increase in temperature the method is called 'cold sterilization'.

Ionizing radiation: γ radiations are useful in sterilization of large loads or bulky items (safety precautions to shield workers from radiation is to be provided).

Electron accelerators are less hazardous and used to sterilize small individually wrapped items.

Non-ionizing radiation: Infrared radiation (IR) is absorbed as heat. Hence, IR can be considered as a form of hot air sterilization. IR is used in rapid mass sterilization of syringes. UV radiation is used for disinfecting operation rooms, virus laboratories and small virus inoculating rooms. Germicidal effect of UV rays are dose dependent. Longer exposure and larger dose increase the vegetative cells killed.

Some bacterial spores are not killed. Therefore UV is not a sterilizing agent, but disinfecting agent. Major limitations are poor penetration power, UV light can cause severe damage to the retina of persons directly looking at the UV bulb. Also prolonged skin exposure is harmful.

Sonic and Ultrasonic Vibrations

Microorganism vary in their sensitivity for vibrations and survivors are found after such treatment. Hence, this method is unreliable and has no practical value in sterilization and disinfection.

Chemical Methods

Chemical methods make use of chemicals for disinfection. These methods are not used on live cells or human skin. But certain chemicals, which bring down the load of microorganisms are called antiseptic and are used for topical application to cure skin infections.

Question

Define disinfectant. Mention the general rules for use of disinfectants. Describe the disinfection of surfaces?

Disinfectants are chemical substances used for the destruction of all pathogens capable of giving rise to infection.

An ideal disinfectant should:

1. Have a wide spectrum of activity.
2. Be active in presence of organic matter.
3. Be effective in acid as well as alkaline media.
4. Have a speedy action.
5. Have a high penetrating power.
6. Be stable and compatible with other antibodies and disinfectants.
7. Not corrode metals or cause irritation or sensitization.
8. Not interfere with healing.
9. Not be toxic, if absorbed into the circulation.
10. Be cheap, easily available, safe and easy to use.

Types of Chemicals

The different groups of chemicals used in sterilization and disinfection are (Table 7.1):

Alcohols: 70 percent ethyl alcohol (ethanol) is used for disinfection of skin before surgery. 70 percent alcohol is more efficient than absolute alcohol.

Table 7.1: Chemical disinfectants

Functions	Chemicals
1. Interferes with membrane functions	
a. Surface active agents	Quarternary ammonium compounds, soaps, fatty acids and detergents.
b. Phenols	Cresol, Dettol, hexyl resorcinol.
c. Organic solvents	Chloroform, alcohol.
2. Denature proteins	
a. Acids and alkalies	Organic acids, inorganic acids hydrogen chloride (HCl), sulfuric acid (H_2SO_4)
b. Agents which destroy functional groups of proteins	
Heavy metals	Copper (Cu), silver (Ag), chlorine (Cl_2), iodine (I_2) mercury (Hg)
Oxidizing agents	Potassium permanganate ($KMnO_4$), hydrogen peroxide (H_2O_2),
Dyes	Acridine orange, Acriflavin
Alkylating agents	Formaldehyde gas, glutaraldehyde, ethylene oxide

Aldehydes: Common aldehydes used are as follows:

1. *Formaldehyde* is used for preservation of organs and materials. Formaldehyde gas is used in fumigation of work areas like hospital wards and sick rooms. Defects are poor penetration and high corrosion. Formalin (40%) solution is used in the disinfection of instruments, furniture, fiber, leather, wool, hide and for preparation of toxoids, for killing bacteria cultures and suspensions for fungi and tubercule bacilli.
2. *Glutaraldehyde* is used:
   i. For sterilizing delicate instruments having lenses on them, e.g. bronchoscopes and cystoscopes.
   ii. To sterilize plastic endotracheal tubes, face masks, corrugated rubber anesthetic tubes and metal tubes.

Phenols: These are common disinfectants for floors and toilets. 1 percent phenol has bactericidal action.

Phenol derivatives: Certain phenol derivatives like cresol, chlorhexidine (chlorinated phenol), chloroxylenol and hexachlorophene are commonly used antiseptics.

1. Cresol—Lysol is a solution of cresol in soap used for sterilization of infected glasswares, cleaning floor, disinfection of excreta, bed pans.
2. Chloroxylenol is an active ingredient of Dettol.
3. Chlorohexidine (Savlon) and cetrimide used as wound and for preoperative preparation of skin. Phenol coefficient of chemical disinfectant is obtained by comparing their effect with that of phenol. It is the ratio of the dilution of the disinfectant in question, which sterilizes the suspension in a given time to the dilution of phenol, which sterilizes the suspension in the same time.

Halogens: Chlorine and iodine are commonly used.

1. Chlorine is used for the disinfection of drinking water, swimming pools, etc. Chlorinated lime ($CaOCl_2$) called bleaching powder is used for wound irrigation (washing out a body cavity) and for HIV-infected materials and for the infective wastes of wards. Disinfection of chlorine compounds is due to release of chlorine.
2. Tincture of iodine (2%) is a skin disinfectant used for application on skin before surgery and on cuts. Iodophors, soluble iodine complex, do not stain and is non-irritating. It is used on burns, boils, ulcers, for surgical scrub and in preoperative skin preparation. Betadine is another commonly used iodine complex.

Dyes: Aniline and acridine dyes are used:

1. Aniline dyes: 1 percent gentian violet solution and crystal violet are used for oral thrush. Dyes like gentian violet and malachite green are active against gram-negative bacteria. They have poor penetrating power and hence bacteriostatic; used on bed sores and boils.
2. Acridine dyes: Acriflavine and acridine orange. Acriflavine is bacteriostatic and used against staphylococci and chronic ulcers and as dressing for burns.

Oxidizing agents: Potassium permanganate ($KMnO_4$) is used for disinfecting drinking water and for washing fruits, vegetables and salad vegetables.

Hydrogen peroxide (H_2O_2) is used as mouthwash and gargle, cleaning and disinfecting wounds and as ear drops.

Surface active agents: Quaternary ammonium compounds, fatty acids, soaps and detergents. They are bactericidal as well as bacteriostatic agents (Table 7.2) for gram-positive and acid-fast organisms. Detergents act by concentrating at cell membranes and thus disrupting their normal functions or it may denature proteins and enzymes.

Salts of heavy metals: Mercuric chloride ($HgCl_2$), zinc sulfate ($ZnSO_4$), silver nitrate ($AgNO_3$) and copper sulfate ($CuSO_4$) prevent the growth of many bacteria in concentrations less than one part in a million. Their action is due to affinity of certain proteins for metal ions.

Table 7.2: Different bacteriostatic and bactericidal agents

Bacteriostatic agents	Bactericidal agents
Hexachlorophene, chloroxylenol, mercurochrome, weak organic acids, common soaps.	Strong acids and alkalies, lysol, cresol, povidone iodine, formaldehyde, glutaraldehyde, sodium hypochlorite, chlorhexidine and cetrimide.

Fumigation

Fumigation is a process of sterilization of wards, operation theaters and laboratories. For sterilization of a 100 cu ft room, 50 mL of 40 percent formalin is required. This provides vapor of 2 mL formaldehyde gas per liter of air. Formalin is used on solid $KMnO_4$ in the room after doors and windows are closed and secured.

Alternatively, diluted formalin (50%) can be sprayed, which also liberates formaldehyde gas. Sterilization is achieved by condensation of gas on exposed surface.

Gases used in sterilization are:

1. Formaldehyde gas.
2. Ethylene oxide.
3. β-propiolactone (βPL).

Formaldehyde gas: Uses

    i. Disinfection of woolen blankets, wool, hides, to destroy bacterial spores.
    ii. Footwear of persons with athlete foot (fungal infection).
    iii. Fumigation of wards and operation theater. Formaldehyde gas can be produced by adding $KMnO_4$ crystals to formalin.

Ethylene oxide: It is an alkylating agent widely used in gaseous sterilization. Active against all kinds of bacteria, their spores and viruses. It can sterilize any object, but useful in sterilization of heat-labile objects, fragile heat sensitive equipment, powders, clothing as well as plastic and rubber articles, dental requirement as well as components of spacecraft, for sterilizing heart-lung machine, cystoscope, endoscope, artery and bone graft.

It is unsuitable for fumigation of rooms because of its explosive nature. It is diluted to 1 : 10 with CO_2 to reduce toxicity and inflammability. *β-propiolactone* is a condensation product of ketone and formaldehyde. More efficient for fumigation than formaldehyde. 2 percent βPL is used for inactivation of vaccines, biological products and heat-sensitive equipment. It has a rapid biocidal action, but unfortunately it is carcinogenic.

It is capable of killing all organisms and is very active against viruses. It forms a sporicidal vapor useful in combination with UV radiation to remove HBV from blood products. Sterilization and disinfection of important items are given in Table 7.3.

Table 7.3: Sterilization and disinfection of important items

Item	Method
Infected material	Incineration
Glasswares, oily fluid, diuretic powder.	Hot air oven—160°C for 2 hour or 180°C for ½ hour.
Serum fluids, vaccines	56°C water bath for 1 hour
Cystoscope, endoscope, laparoscope, catheters.	2% glutaraldehyde for 30 minute, ethylene oxide, 10 percent phenol for 4–10 hour.
Common laboratory media	Autoclaving 121°C for 15 minute
Media containing egg or serum	Inspissation at 80°C to 85°C for 30 minute for 3 consecutive day.
Media containing sugar or gelatin	Tyndallization at 100°C for 20 minute for 3 consecutive day.

Contd...

Contd...

Toxins, sugar and antibiotic solutions.	Seitz or membrane filter
Plastic and polythene tubes	2% glutaraldehyde, ethylene oxide
Sharp instruments (needles, metal caps, broken glass).	5% cresol, Lysol, 10% phenol for 10 hour.
Suture material	Autoclaving
Catgut	Ionizing radiation 2–5 minute
Disposal syringe	Ethylene oxide, ionizing radiation
Heart-lung machine	Ethylene oxide
Feces, urine, vomitus	Bleaching powder, cresols
Sputum	Incineration (burning), autoclaving
Operation theaters	Fumigation by formaldehyde gas 500 mL of 40% formaldehyde gas + 1,000 mL of water per 1,000 cubic feet of air space.
Skin	Tincture of iodine, 70% alcohol, Savlon.
Thermometer and cheatle forceps	Dip in chlorhexidine 10% + cetrimide (1%) for 10 minute after each use.
Inoculating wire	Red heat
Glasswares, syringes, petri dishes, test tubes, flasks, oily fluid (paraffin).	Hot air oven
Disposable syringes and other disposable items.	Gamma (γ) radiation
Culture media containing serum, egg	Inspissation
Milk and milk products	Pasteurization
Infected materials like soiled dressing, bedding, animal carcasses.	Incineration
Aprons, gloves, catheters, surgical instruments except sharps.	Autoclaving
Rubber, plastics and polythene tubes.	Glutaraldehyde

Chapter 8

Infections—Nosocomial Infections

Infection is the lodgement and multiplication of microorganisms in the tissue of the host.

CLASSIFICATION OF INFECTIONS

1. Primary infection is the initial infection caused by microorganisms, in the host.
2. Reinfection is the subsequent infection by the same organism in the same host.
3. Secondary infection is the new infection set up by a new organism in the host when the resistance of the host is lowered due to a pre-existing infectious disease.
4. Cross-infection is when a patient is suffering from a disease and a new infection is set up from another host or external source.
5. Nosocomial infection is the cross-infection occurring in a hospital or hospital-acquired infection (nosocomio = hospital).
6. Subclinical infection is one where clinical symptoms are not apparent.

INFECTIOUS AGENTS

The classification of microorganisms is given in Figure 8.1.

Parasites

Parasites are organisms, which live upon or within other living organisms like human beings, animals or plants. Majority of them are non-pathogens, harmless to man.

Commensals

Certain anatomical sites such as skin, nose, throat and intestines contain several harmless organisms known as commensals. However, when they migrate to other areas they behave like pathogen, e.g. *Escherichia coli* is an intestinal commensal, but when gets into urinary bladder, produces urinary tract infection (UTI). Similarly *Streptococcus viridans*, a throat commensal when gains access, (e.g. during tooth extraction) to blood and settles on already damaged heart valves cause infective endocarditis.

Saprophytes

Saprophytes are free-living organisms, which are able to live in the outside world, on dead animals and on decaying plants. They do not multiply on living matter and hence are not important for infection.

Their main activities are putrefaction and fermentation. Putrefaction is the breaking down of proteins and is very useful in decomposition of dead animals and vegetable matter. By this process, the complex substances contained in refuse are converted into simple elements, which can be used by plants as food.

Fermentation refers to the changes, which microorganisms bring about in carbohydrates, e.g. production of alcohol from sugar of fruit juice.

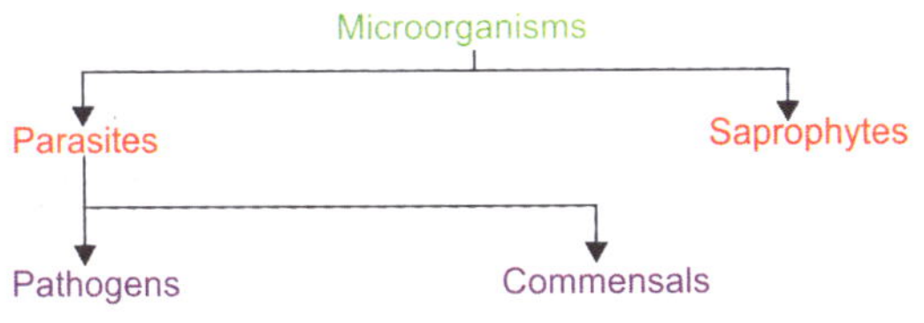

Fig. 8.1: Classification of microorganisms

$$C_{12}H_{22}O_{11} + H_2O \xrightarrow[\text{of yeast}]{\text{Invertase}} C_6H_{12}O_6 + C_6H_{12}O_6$$

Sucrose   Glucose   Fructose

$$\xrightarrow[\text{of yeast}]{\text{Zymase}} 2C_5H_5OH + 2CO_2 \uparrow$$

Alcohol

Thus, certain microorgansisms are useful in industries for the manufacture of alcohol, lactic acid, bread, butter and cheese.

SOURCES OF INFECTION IN MAN

1. Man.
2. Animals.
3. Insects.
4. Vectors acting as reservoir hosts.
5. Soil.
6. Water.
7. Food.

Man

The common source of infection for man is man himself. A parasite may originate from a patient or a carrier.

Animals

Many pathogens are able to infect both man and animals. Animals may therefore act as a source of human infections.

Zoonotic diseases in India is given in Table 8.1.

Insects

Diseases caused by insects are called arthropod-borne diseases. Insects like mosquitoes, fleas and lice that transfer infection are called vectors. Transmission may be mechanical, e.g. transmission of dysentery by housefly and they are called mechanical vector. They are called biological vector when pathogens multiply in the body of the vector, e.g. anopheles mosquito in malaria.

Mosquito-borne Diseases

- Anopheles : Malaria
- Culex : Filariasis, encephalitis
- Aedes : Dengue fever, yellow fever (in Africa)
- Mansonia : Filariasis.

Vectors

Some vectors may act as reservoir hosts, e.g. ticks in relapsing fever and spotted fever.

Table 8.1: Zoonotic disease in India

Disease	Microorganism	Animal responsible
Bacterial		
Anthrax	*Bacillus anthracis*	Cattle, sheep
Brucellosis	*Brucella abortus, B. suis*	Sheep, pig
Tuberculosis Intestine Lymph gland	*Mycobacterium bovis*	Cattle
Plague	*Yersinia pestis*	Rats
Food poisoning	*Salmonella* *Campylobacter*	Cattle, poultry
Leptospirosis	*Leptospira*	Rats, pigs, dogs, cattle
Viral		
Rabies	Rabdovirus	Dogs, fox
Parasitic		
Hydatid disease	Dog tapeworm	Dogs
Toxoplasmosis	*Toxoplasma gondii*	Cat

Soil

Soil may serve as a source of parasite infection like roundworms and hookworms. Spores of tetanus bacilli remain viable in soil for a long time. Fungi like *Histoplasma capsulatum* and higher bacteria like *Nocardia asteroides* also survive in soil and cause human infection.

Water

Water may act as the source of infection either due to contamination with pathogenic microorganisms, e.g. *Vibrio cholerae*, infective hepatitis A virus (HAV) or due to the presence of aquatic vectors (cyclops in guinea worm infection).

Water-borne Diseases

Viral: Viral hepatitis (hepatitis A), poliomyelitis.
Bacterial: Diarrhea, dysentery, typhoid and paratyphoid fevers.
Protozoal: Amebiasis.
Helminthic: Roundworm, whipworm, threadworm, tapeworm.

Food

Contaminated food may be a source of infection. Presence of pathogens in food may be due to external contamination, e.g. food poisoning by *Staphylococcus* or due to pre-existing infection in meat or other animal products (e.g. measly pork).

DISEASE TRANSMISSION

A chain of events is necessary for transmission of infectious disease. They are:

1. A causative agent: Invading organism, which may be bacterial, viral, rickettsial, protozoal, fungal or helminthic.
2. Reservoir: A place for invading agent to multiply in human, animal or non-animal.
3. Susceptible host.
4. Portal of entry: The organism into the human body.
5. A mode of transmission: Which may be direct (direct contact) or indirect through animals and vectors including inanimate fomites.
6. A portal of exit: From the reservoir such as respiratory tract or digestive tract.

The presence of an infectious disease agent does not invariably produce the disease. When the invading agent is virulent and host resistance in weak, infection results. Prevention of a communicable disease involves creating a break in the chain of events.

Portals of Entry (Gateways)

Most of the pathogenic organisms can cause disease only if they enter through their particular portal of entry, e.g. if dysentery bacilli are rubbed into a wound on the skin, they may not cause any trouble, but if the same organisms are swallowed they cause dysentery.

Skin

A large number of organism is always present on the skin, but most of them do not penetrate the unbroken skin. Staphylococci and some fungi are able to penetrate under certain conditions and cause disease in the deeper tissues.

Respiratory Tract

The air around us contains microorganisms, which have been spread widely during talking, coughing and sneezing. These enter into the repiratory tract with air inhaled, e.g. organisms causing colds, pneumonia and pulmonary tuberculosis.

Digestive Tract

Microorganism, enter the body along with food and water, e.g. organisms causing typhoid, dysentery and cholera.

Genitourinary Tract

Urinary tract infections (UTI) are caused by bacteria from urethra, perineum, etc. traveling upwards (ascending infection) and sometimes introduced through catheterization. UTI can also be through blood. Venereal diseases of genitourinary system are acquired through sexual contact.

Portals of Exit

Quite often organisms leave the body through the same system by which they entered, e.g. organism causing respiratory diseases are usually given off through nasal discharge and sputum, e.g. pulmonary tuberculosis, pneumonia and diphtheria. Organisms, which enter through the mouth usually leave the body in the feces through the rectum, e.g. typhoid, cholera, dysentery. Organisms that enter the body through skin produce pus and leave through the pus in the skin, e.g. *Staphylococcus*. Some diseases such as malaria and yellow fever enter through the skin into blood during the bite of a mosquito. These organisms leave the body by the same way when a mosquito sucks blood from a person with the disease. Malaria, syphilis and hepatitis B can leave the body through blood transfusion. Typhoid bacilli may leave through urinary tract. Syphilis and gonorrhea organisms usually leave through the genitourinary tract.

METHODS OF TRANSFER OF INFECTION

1. Direct transmission
   - i. Direct contact.
   - ii. Through inhalation.
   - iii. Ingestion.
   - iv. Inoculation.
   - v. Insects.
   - vi. Congenital (teratogenic).
   - vii. Iatrogenic and laboratory infections.

2. Indirect transmission
    i. Vehicle borne.
    ii. Vector borne.
        a. Mechanical.
        b. Biological.
    iii. Air borne.
        a. Droplet.
        b. Dust.
    iv. Fomite borne.
    v. Unclean hands and fingers.

Direct Transmission

Direct Contact

Infection may be transmitted from person-to-person either by direct contact with infected person or by contact with the secretion or excretion, e.g. organisms causing diphtheria, common cold and tonsillitis may be transferred by kissing. A nurse may contract typhoid fever or dysentery by soiling her hands with feces of the patient and not washing her hands before she prepares her food or eats with her fingers.

Through Inhalation

Respiratory infection such as influenza and tuberculosis are transmitted by inhalation of the pathogen. Such microbes are shed into the environment by patients through secretion from the nose or throat during sneezing, coughing or talking. Large drops of such secretions fall to the ground and dry there. Pathogens resistant to drying, may remain viable in the dust and act as sources of infections.

Droplet infection: A special type of direct infection is known as droplet infection. Microorganisms are thrown out into the air by coughing or sneezing fine droplets of saliva and mucus. They may be thrown as far away as 3½ feet, while talking and up to 10 feet when sneezing. Droplet nuclei (the very small amount of the substance remaining after evaporating droplet) and dust containing a variety of organisms may be carried by the air. This is an important way of spreading organisms that cause common cold, influenza, pneumonia, diphtheria and tuberculosis.

Ingestion

Intestinal infections are generally acquired by the ingestion of food or drink contaminated with the pathogens. Infection transmitted by ingestion may be water borne (cholera), food borne (food poisoning) or hand borne (dysentery). Dysentery occurs when small amounts of infective material remain on the hands generally by fecal contamination and are transmitted, while feeding as in case of nurses who may transmit diarrhea in this manner to infants.

Inoculation

Pathogens in some cases may be inoculated directly into the tissues of the host. Tetanus spores implanted in the depth of the wounds, rabies virus deposited subcutaneously by dog bites and arboviruses infected by insect vectors are examples.

Infection: Inoculation may be iatrogenic when non-sterile syringes and surgical equipment are employed. Serum hepatitis (hepatitis B) is transmitted by transfusion of contaminated blood or inoculation of material containing the virus.

Insects

Insects may act as mechanical or biological vectors of infectious disease.

Human Carriers

A person who harbors pathogenic organisms in his body and shows no signs of illness is called carrier. Carriers are often the causes of outbreaks of infection and they may be more dangerous than patients as nobody suspects that they are discharging pathogens. Carriers are of three types:

1. *Convalescent carriers* are those who have recovered from the illness, but have not got rid of all the organisms and may continue to spread the disease for a few weeks more after recovery. They may be called temporary carriers.
2. *Chronic carriers* are those who continue to carry pathogen and spread disease for a long time after recovery (1 year or more).
3. *Healthy or contact carriers* are those who never had any visible signs or symptoms of the disease, but still may spread the organisms to others. It is possible that many persons classified as healthy carriers have suffered from a subclinical or mild unorganized attack of the infection, sometimes or other.

Examples of diseases spread through contact carriers are typhoid and paratyphoid fevers, diphtheria and pneumonia.

Congenital or Teratogenic Infections

Some pathogens are able to cross the placental barrier and infect the fetus *in vitro*. This is known as vertical transmission. This may result in abortion, miscarriage or stillbirth. Live infants may be born with the manifestation of the disease as in congenital syphilis. Intrauterine infection with rubella virus especially in the first trimester of pregnancy may interfere with organogenesis and lead to congenital malformation. Such infections are known as teratogenic infection. Teratology is the study of causes and effects of congenital malformation and developmental abnormalities.

Iatrogenic and Laboratory Infections

Infections may sometimes be transmitted during procedures such as injections, lumbar puncture and catheterization, if meticulous care in asepsis is lacking. Modern methods of treatment such as exchange transfusion, dialysis, heart and transplant surgery increase the possibilities for iatrogenic infection. Laboratory personnel handling infectious materials are at great risk and special care should be taken to prevent laboratory infections.

Indirect Transmission

Vehicle Borne

Through water, food (including raw vegetables, fruits, milk products), ice, blood, serum, plasma or any other biological products like tissues and organs.

By water and food: Infection of the alimentary tract, e.g. acute diarrhea, typhoid, cholera, polio, hepatitis A, food poisoning and intestinal parasites.

By blood: Hepatitis B, malaria, syphilis, acquired immunodeficiency syndrome (AIDS) and brucellosis.

Vector Borne

Insects that spread diseases are called vectors.

Vector is defined as an arthropod or any living carrier (e.g. snail) that transports an infectious agent to a susceptible individual. Transmission by a vector may be mechanical or biological. In the later case, the disease agent passes through a developmental cycle or multiplication in the vector as in malarial parasite.

If the organism undergoes certain changes in the body of the insect as in the case of malaria parasite or multiply in the case of yellow fever virus, it is known as biological transmission and biological vectors.

If the organisms carry the disease organisms on their feet or any part of their body and deposit or drop them on food as housefly in the case of amebic dysentery, it is known as mechanical transmission and mechanical vector.

Invertebrate type of vectors include flies, fleas, mosquitoes, cockroaches, sucking lice, bugs, ticks and mites.

Vertebrate types are mice, rodents and bats.

- Man—arthropod—man (malaria)
- Mammal—arthropod—man (plague)
- Bird—arthropod—man (encephalitis).

Air Borne/Dust Borne

Some of the largest droplets, which are expelled, settle down by their sheer weight on the floor carpets, furniture, bedding and become dust. Streptococci and other pathogenic bacteria, viruses, fungal spores and skin squamous have been found in the dust of hospital wards.

Fomite Borne

Infection may be acquired indirectly through articles, which have been recently contaminated. These articles, which are likely to carry the disease organisms are called fomites (singular fomes), e.g. soiled clothes, towels, linen, handkerchief, cups, spoons, pencils, books, toys, drinking glasses, door handles, taps, lavatory chain, syringes and surgical dressings.

Diseases transmitted include diphtheria, typhoid fever, bacillary dysentery, hepatitis A, eye and skin diseases. Organisms causing gastrointestinal and respiratory infections may be transferred through fomites. Contamination of milk by the hands of those who handle milk and contamination of water by sewage are other examples of indirect infection.

Unclean Hands and Fingers

Staphylococcal and streptococcal infections, typhoid, dysentery, hepatitis A, etc. mainly spread through unclean hands and fingers. Intestinal parasites and pathogens reach from feces to food through fingers, fomites and flies (5Fs).

MICROBIAL PATHOGENICITY

Characteristics of pathogens: The organism should be able:

1. To enter the body.
2. To multiply in the tissue.
3. To damage the tissue.
4. To resist the host defence.

Factors Predisposing to Microbial Pathogenicity

Pathogenicity

Pathogenicity is the ability of the microbial strains to produce disease.

Virulence

Virulence is the ability of the microbial strains to produce disease, e.g. Polio virus has three strains of varying degree of virulence. Virulence is the sum of the following factors:

1. Invasiveness: It is the ability of the organism to spread in a host tissue after establishing infection. Less invasive organisms cause localized infection, e.g. staphylococcal abscess. Highly invasive organisms cause generalized infection, e.g. streptococcal septicemia.
2. Toxigenicity: Bacteria produce two types of toxins—exotoxins and endotoxins (Table 8.2).
3. Communicability: This is the ability of the parasite to spread from one host to another. It determines the survival and distribution of an organisms in a community. Highly virulent organisms may not exhibit a high degree of communicability due to rapid lethal effect on host. Infection in which the pathogen is shed in secretions as in respiratory and intestinal diseases are highly communicable.

Development of endemic and pandemic diseases require that the strains of pathogen posses high degrees of virulence and communicability.

Table 8.2: Comparison of exotoxins and endotoxins

Exotoxins	Endotoxins
Protiens	Protein-lipopolysaccharide (LPS) complexes
Heat labile	Heat stable
Actively secreted by cells, diffuse into surrounding medium	Form part of the cell wall. Do not diffuse into surrounding medium.
Readily separable from cultures by physical means like filtration	Obtained only by cell lysis
Action often enzymic	No enzymic action
Specific pharmacological effect for each exotoxin	Effect non-specific, action common to all endotoxins
Specific tissue affinities	No specific tissue affinity
Action in very minimum doses, e.g. 0.3 kg of *Clostridium botulinum* can kill all the inhabitants of the world	Active only in very large doses. They are much less toxic.
Highly antigenic	Weakly antigenic
Action specifically neutralized by antibody	Neutralization by antibody is ineffective
Produced mainly by gram-positive bacteria and also some gram-negative bacteria	Produced by gram-negative bacteria
Can be toxoided	Cannot be toxoided
Under the influence of formaldehyde at a temperature of 38°C to 40°C change to antitoxins (toxoid), e.g. diphtheria toxoid, tetanus toxoid (TT)	Under the influence of formalin and temperature, endotoxins are partially rendered harmless

4. Bacterial appendages: Capsulated bacteria like *Pneumococcus*, *Klebsiella pneumoniae* and *Haemophilus influenzae* will withstand phagocytosis.

Surface antigens, e.g. Vi antigens of *Salmonella typhi* and K antigen of *E. coli* will resist phagocytosis and lytic activity of complement.

Microbial Toxins

Toxins are the most important pathogenicity factor of bacteria. The comparison of exotoxins and endotoxins is detailed in Table 8.2.

Exotoxins

Exotoxins are the most potent poison known. They are proteins, which are secreted by certain species of bacteria. They readily diffuse into the surrounding media, e.g. tetanus, diphtheria.

Endotoxins

They are integral part of the cell wall of gram-negative bacteria. They are released from the bacterial surface by natural lysis of the bacteria or disintegration of the cell wall.

NOSOCOMIAL (HOSPITAL) INFECTIONS: HOSPITAL-ACQUIRED INFECTIONS

Nosocomial infections are the infections, which develop during hospitalization (nosocomio = hospital) and which were not incubating or present at the time of admission to hospital. The modes of transmission is given in Table 8.3.

The common types of hospital infections are listed in Table 8.4.

Sources

1. Endogenous   = Patients own flora.

Table 8.3: Modes of transmission

Route	Sources	Diseases
Aerial droplets (from persons), dust, skin scales	Mouth, bed making, nose, skin exudates, infected lesions.	Measles, tuberculosis, lower respiratory tract infection, pneumonia, *Pseudomonas aeruginosa* and *Staphylococcus aureus* sepsis, staphylococcal and streptococcal sepsis.
Aerial particles or aerosols (from inanimate sources)	Respiratory equipment, air conditioning plants.	Respiratory infections due to gram-negative bacilli, legionnaires disease, fungal infections.
Contact from hospital personnel—direct spread, indirect spread via equipment and materials	Respiratory secretions feces, urine, skin and wound exudates.	Staphylococcal and streptococcal sepsis, enterobacterial diarrhea, *P. aeruginosa* sepsis.
Contact (environmental sources)	Food, fluids, medicaments, equipments.	Enterobacterial sepsis *Escherichia coli*, *Klebsiella*, *Serratia* and other enterobacter species *P. aeruginosa* sepsis.
Direct contact	Blood, blood products, injury with sharps.	Hepatitis B, acquired immunodeficiency syndrome (AIDS).

Table 8.4: Common types of hospital infections

Infection	Organism responsible
Urinary tract infections	*Escherichia coli*, *Klebsiella*, *Serratia*, *Proteus* species, *Pseudomonas aeruginosa*.
Common respiratory tract infections (mostly nosocomial pneumonia)	*Haemophilus influenzae*, *Streptococcus pneumoniae*, *Staphylococcus aureus*, member of enterobacteriaceae, respiratory viruses.
Wound and skin sepsis	*S. aureus*, *E. coli*, *Proteus* species, *Enterococcus* species, aerosols, *Staphylococcus epidermidis*.
Burns	*S. aureus*, *P. aeruginosa*, *Acinetobacter* species.
Gastrointestinal infections	*S. pyogenes*, *Salmonella* species, seasonal viruses causing diarrhea.

2. Exogenous = By contact with other patients and staff.

3. Environmental sources = Inanimate objects (fomites), air and food in the hospital, surfaces contaminated by patient's secretion, excretions, blood and body fluids, animals and insects in the hospital environment.

Prevention and Control of Hospital Infections

Sterilization and Disinfection

1. Providing sterile instrument, dressing, surgical linen like face masks, gowns, theater clothing by central sterile supply department.
2. Use of single-use items like disposable syringes, needles, catheters and drainage bags are preferred.
3. Encourage use of disinfectants on walls, floors and antiseptics on the skin of the patients and hands of staff.

Hands Spread Disease

Frequent hand washing: Nurses should wash their hands frequently before any procedure for which gloves or forceps are necessary and after contact with an infected patient and after touching infective materials. Soap and water are sufficient in most circumstances, but when dealing with infected patients, antiseptic (carbolic) soap is recommended. Drying hands after washing is also important. A more prolonged and thorough scrub is necessary before commencement of surgery.

Dressing Technique

'No touch' or 'non-touch' method of dressing is the best method.

Before commencement of dressing all the materials required must be suitably placed on the top of the trolley, hands should be washed thoroughly and that neither the dressing nor the wounds are touched by hands, forceps being used to pick up the articles. Dressings removed from the infected wound should be discarded in disposable bins, lids closed and sent for incineration.

Isolation

The infectious patient is admitted to an isolation hospital or separate isolation ward. Single bedded rooms (cubicles) are necessary to avoid infection by the airborne route. Beside taking precautions, use of gowns, masks and gloves for any one coming into contact with the patient—barrister nursing.

Ward Procedure

Bed making, change of sheets and pillow cases should be completed at least 1 hour before actual dressing starts.

Transfer of germs from one patient to another as a result of contamination of mattress, blankets, pillows especially by discharging lesions could be prevented by the use of plastic covers, which could be decontaminated with disinfectants. Precautions must be taken especially in the postoperative pediatrics ward and intensive care unit (ICU).

Control of Carriers

Patients who have recovered from diphtheria, typhoid or paratyphoid fevers and hepatitis B are kept under observation. Repeated bacteriological and serological tests are conducted for them. Nursing staff may be carriers.

Cutting the Channels of Communication

Hygienic condition should be maintained in preparation of food, distribution of diet and drinking water, adequate cooking. Fruits, salad vegetables and greens, which are eaten raw are thoroughly washed. Observing cleanliness in the kitchen is very important. Handwashing with soap and water, before preparing and serving food and after visiting the toilet must be performed.

Prevention by Health Education

Continued education of medical and nursing staff in the basic concepts of infection control like hygiene in theaters, wards and kitchens. Special attention to the safe disposal of excreta and soiled dressings.

Infection Control Committee

It is essential to establish an infection control committee in the hospital. The committee should consist of physicians, nurses, administrators and laboratory personnel. The committee must meet regularly and frequently and decide about hospital policy related to infection control. Control measures include:

1. Isolation policy.
2. Personnel health program including.
   i. Immunization of hospital staff.
   ii. Use of adequate aseptic technique.
   iii. Regular in-service training program to acquaint and update all working in the hospital, of the ways to implement infection control programs.
3. Review of antibiotic policies.
4. Provision of an appropriate clean environment. Recently infection control committee and drug control committee have been made compulsory in all hospitals by environment order. Sir William Osler's aphorism that soap, water and common sense are the best disinfectants apply even today in the context of hospital infections.

Antimicrobial Therapy

Treatment of a disease with a chemical substance is known as chemotherapy. The chemical substance is known as chemotherapeutic agent. These agents are prepared in a chemical laboratory or obtained from some plants and animals. In general, naturally occurring substances, which in small amounts are detrimental or inhibitory to some other microorganisms, are called antibiotics. Now they are also synthesized artificially. Therefore, the term antimicrobial agent is used for both natural antibiotics and synthetic chemical agents.

HISTORY

Syphilis is the first known disease in which a chemotherapeutic agent was used. Mercury was used for treatment of syphilis as early as 1495, but it was not until 1910, when an arsenical compound called Salvarsan (606) was synthesized by Paul Ehrlich. Much later in 1935, the therapeutic value of a group of compounds called sulfonamides (sulfa drugs) was demonstrated by Gerhard Domagk. They are active against a large variety of pathogenic organisms even though not specific in their action. With improved research facilities, various other modifications of sulfonamides with better advantages were synthesized later.

The structure of sulfonamides and para-aminobenzoic acid (PABA) is as shown in Figure 9.1. The sulfonamides are especially useful in the treatment of infections caused by meningococci and *Shigella*, respiratory infections caused by streptococci and staphylococci and urinary infections due to gram-negative organisms. They are useful to prevent rheumatic fever, bacterial endocarditis, wound infection and urinary tract infections following surgery and catheterization.

ANTIBIOTICS

Antibiotics were known by their activities long before they were given the name. Many years ago, the Chinese used moldy soybean curd for treatment of boils. They controlled foot infections by wearing sandals with flurry of mold. Pasteur and Joubert found that pure cultures of anthrax bacilli, grew well in urine but that when certain other bacilli were present, the anthrax bacilli disappeared.

The early clinical appreciation of bacterial antagonism was the use of lactobacilli in treatment of dysentery. This was an example of replacement therapy, i.e. a harmless microbe was able to eliminate and replace one that could cause disease. Modern antibiosis is based not on replacement, but on utilization of an inhibitory principle obtained from the antibiotic producing microbe.

In 1929, Alexander Fleming noticed that an agar plate inoculated with *Staphylococcus aureus* had become contaminated with a mold and that the mold colony was surrounded by a clear zone indicating inhibition of bacterial growth or lysis

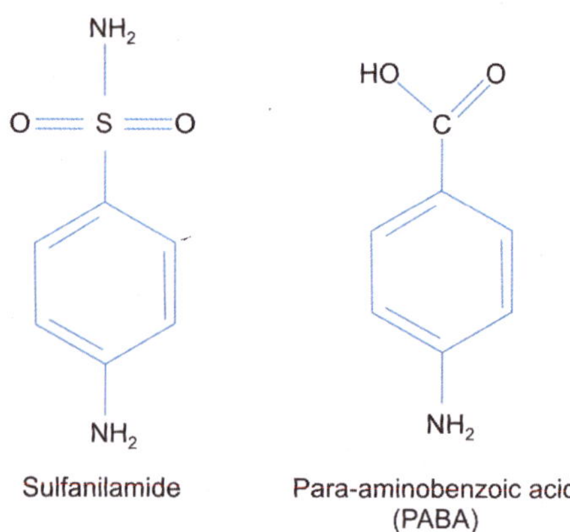

Fig. 9.1: Chemical structure of sulfa drugs

of bacteria. The contaminated drug became the 'miracle drug' penicillin, the metabolic product of *Penicillium notatum*. The second antibiotic discovered was streptomycin by Dr Selman Waksman in 1948.

Some Antibiotics in Current Use

1. Antibiotics are mainly active against gram-positive bacteria, e.g. penicillin (G and V), methicillin, cloxacillin, erythromycin, novobiocin, vancomycin, bacitracin and fucidin.
2. Antibiotics are active against gram-negative bacteria, e.g. polymyxin, aminoglycoside.
3. Antibiotics are active against both gram-positive and gram-negative bacteria, e.g. tetracycline, cephalosporin, ampicillin and chloramphenicol.
4. Antibiotics active against fungi, e.g. griseofulvin, iodides, nystatin, amphotericin B.

Spectrum of Activity of Antibiotics

Antimicrobial agents can be categorized into broad-spectrum and narrow-spectrum drugs, depending on their activity against a range of gram-positive and gram-negative bacteria. Penicillin is a narrow-spectrum agent with limited action to gram-positive bacteria. Metronidazole is also a narrow-spectrum drug because of its activity against strict anaerobes and some protozoa.

Broad-spectrum antibiotics are active against many gram-positive and gram-negative bacteria. This group includes tetracycline, erythromycin and cephalosporins.

Major Sites of Action

Four major sites of action by antimicrobial agents:

1. Inhibition of synthesis of cell wall peptidoglycan, e.g. penicillin, cephalosporins, cycloserine, vancomycin, ristocetin and bacitracin.
2. Damage to the permeability of the cytoplasmic membrane, e.g. tyrocidine, gramicidin, polymyxin and antifungal polyene antibiotics.
3. Inhibition of protein synthesis, e.g. aminoglycosides (amikacin, netilmicin, tobramycin, gentamicin, kanamycin, neomycin and streptomycin, tetracyclines and chloramphenicol). They bind to and inhibit the function of 30S ribosomal subunit.
4. Inhibition of nucleic acid synthesis, e.g. rifampicin inhibits the synthesis of messenger ribonucleic acid (mRNA) by its action on the RNA polymerase, whereas nalidixic acid inhibits deoxyribonucleic acid (DNA) replication. Other examples are novobiocin, pyrimethamine and sulfonamide.

Mechanism of Action

There are three general mechanisms of action:

1. Competition with a natural substance for the active site of the enzyme, for example,
   i. Action of sulfonamides to interfere competitively with the utilization of PABA.
   ii. Action of PABA with para-aminosalicylic acid.
2. Combination with an enzyme at a site sufficiently close to the active site as to interfere with its enzymatic function, e.g. vancomycin, ristocetin and bacitracin.
3. Combination with non-enzymatic structural components, e.g. drugs, which inhibit protein synthesis and which act by damaging cytoplasmic membrane.

Antiviral Chemotherapy

In contrast to the many of antibacterial agents available today only a few antiviral drugs have been developed. Antibacterial drugs are not effective against viruses. Viruses are intracellular. In order to attack them, the chemotherapeutic agents must enter host cells. Also the agent must not be toxic to the host cells, while exerting an inhibiting action on the viruses. This needs a high degree of selective toxicity. In case of infection by bacteria, fungi or protozoa, the infectious agent acts upon the host cells. Among the more important antiviral agents. Interferon, a small glycoprotein, which interferes with protein synthesis, acivir, idoxuridine and vidarabine are useful in the treatment of herpes simplex infections. Zidovudine is useful in acquired immunodeficiency syndrome (AIDS).

Antifungal Drugs

There are not many antifungal drugs. Nystatin and griseofulvin are the better known antifungal antibiotics. Nystatin is useful in the therapy of non-systemic fungal infections. It is produced during fermentation by a stream of *Streptomyces noursei*. Its antimicrobial activity is limited to yeasts and other fungi, e.g. *Candida, Aspergillus* and penicillin. It is fungicidal in action.

Griseofulvin is obtained from *Penicillium griseofulvum*. It is used in the treatment of many superficial fungi infections of the skin and body surfaces and is also effective in the treatment of some systemic (deep seated) mycoses. The drug is administered orally.

Antitumor Antibiotics

For example, anthramycin group. Their antitumor action is directed towards DNA structure and function.

DRUG RESISTANCE

During treatment with drugs, bacteria may acquire resistance to those drugs. Streptococci has become resistant to penicillin. Two strains of multidrug-resistant tuberculosis bacilli strains are now detected in India. *Salmonella typhi* has become resistant to commonly used drug, chloromycetin. The basis of drug resistance may be genetic or non-genetic. Drug resistance is due to:

1. Competitive inhibition between an essential metabolite and its metabolic analogue (drug).
2. Development of an alternative metabolic pathology, which bypasses some reaction that would normally be inhibited by the drug.
3. Production of an enzyme in such a way that it functions on behalf of the cell, but is not affected by the drug.
4. Alteration of ribosomal protein structure.
5. Synthesis of excess enzyme over the amount that can be inactivated by the antibiotic or drug.
6. Inability of the drug to penetrate the cell due to some alterations of the cell membrane.

Mechanisms

Following are the mechanisms of drug resistance shown by microorganisms.

Mutation

All bacteria contain drug-resistant mutants arising once in 10^7 to 10^{10} cell divisions. It is of two types:

1. *Stepwise mutation* in which a series of small step mutations results in high levels of resistance, e.g. penicillin, chloramphenicol, tetracycline and sulfonamides. This type can be prevented by giving adequate dosage of drugs.
2. *One-step mutation* in which case resistance develops suddenly even with the first exposure of drugs, e.g. tubercle bacilli developing resistance to streptomycin and isoniazid.

Transmission of Resistance

The initial appearance of resistance is supposed to be the result of a change in a single bacterial gene that conferred resistance to the bacterium. The evidence that this takes place during sulfonamide therapy is convincing. Another explanation is that in some gram-negative bacteria, the resultant organism has an additional gene whose functions is to protect the bacterium from the bactericidal effect of the drug or antibiotic, e.g. such a gene is responsible for penicillinase production by penicillin-resistant staphylococci. In some cases, the bacteria carry the resistant gene at the time of infection and their propagation is encouraged, while sensitive strains are inhibited or killed.

The resistance factor (R factor) is present in plasmids, which are single extrachromosomal self-replicating extranuclear DNA units.

Development of Resistance

Development of drug resistance can be minimized by:

1. Avoiding indiscriminate use of antibiotics when they are of real clinical use.
2. Avoiding use of antibiotics commonly employed for generalized infections for tropical applications.
3. Using correct dosage of the proper antibiotics to overcome an infection quickly.
4. Using combinations of antibiotics of proven effectiveness.
5. Using a different antibiotic when an organism gives evidence of becoming resistant to one used initially.

Systemic Bacteriology

CABIBI STAPHYLOCOCCI

Staphylococci are gram-positive cocci. The name *Staphylococcus* means 'bunch of grapes'. They are named so because they occur in grape-like clusters.

Morphology

Shape : They are spherical cocci.

Size : Their size is approximately 1 µm in diameter.

Arrangement : They are arranged in grape-like clusters. The cluster formation is because the daughter cells after division remain in close proximity. They do not show any motility and sporulation.

Cultural Characteristics

Temperature and pH: They generally grow within 10°C to 42°C, the optimum is 37°C. 7.4 to 7.6 is the pH range for staphylococci.

Oxygen (O_2) requirement: They are aerobes and facultative anaerobes.

Biochemical Reactions

On fermenting sugar, staphylococci produce only acid, gas is not produced. *Staphylococcus* usually exhibit following characteristics:

1. Coagulase positive.
2. Show β-hemolysis on blood agar.
3. Produce golden yellow pigmentation (Table 10.1).
4. Liquify gelatin.
5. Produce deoxyribonuclease enzyme.
6. Produce tellurite.
7. Reduce tellurite.

Resistance

Staphylococci are more resistant among non-sporulating bacteria. Their thermal death point is 62°C for 30 minutes, some require 80°C for 1 hour.

They also show resistance towards penicillin antibiotic producing penicillinase enzyme.

Table 10.1: Growth of staphylococci on various media

Media	Growth
Nutrient agar	Most strains produce golden yellow pigment
Nutrient agar slope	They show oil-paint appearance
Blood agar	They show β-hemolysis
Liquid medium	They show uniform turbidity
Mannitol salt agar 　Mannitol—1% 　(8%–10% NaCl) 　Phenol indicator It is known as selective medium for staphylococci	Yellow-colored colonies are seen

Pathogenesis and Virulence

Staphylococci produces disease in two types of infections or intoxications. Hence the virulence factors can be classified as antigenic structures, toxins and enzymes.

Antigenic Structure

Capsule : The capsule containing strains are virulent and inhibit phagocytosis.

Peptidoglycan : It provides rigidity to bacterial cell.

Teichoic acids : It helps cocci to attach to the host cells.

Protien A : Shows antiphagocytic and anticomplementary effects.

Toxins

They are classified as exotoxins and endotoxins

1. Hemolysin: Staphylococci produces an enzyme called 'hemolysin'. Four different hemolysins are produced—alpha, beta, gamma and delta.
2. Leukocidin.
3. Enterotoxin.
4. Toxic shock syndrome (TSS) toxin.
5. Exfoliative toxin.

Enzymes

Staphylococcus produces number of enzymes—coagulase, phosphatase and deoxyribonuclease (DNase) out of which coagulase is more important.

Coagulase: This enzyme clots human or rabbit plasma. It is also known as 'clumping factor'. It is named as clumping factor because this enzyme along with coagulase reacting factor in plasma convert fibrinogen to fibrin thus clumping plasma.

The test for coagulase can be done by two methods slide coagulase test and tube coagulase test. This test differentiates between pathogenic strain, *Staphylococcus aureus (S. aureus)* from non-pathogenic strains.

Slide coagulase test: A clean glass slide is taken and few colonies of bacteria are emulsified in normal saline and mixed with drop of undiluted human or rabbit plasma. Positive strains show clumping.

Tube coagulase test: This test is performed for detection of extracellular free coagulase. 0.1 mL of an overnight culture is mixed with 0.5 mL of one in five dilution of human or rabbit plasma. The tubes are then incubated at 37°C for 3 to 6 hours. The plasma clots does not flow when tube is inverted in case of positive test. Control can be set by taking only diluted plasma in another test tube.

Pathogenesis

Staphylococcal diseases can be classified as following infections/conditions.

Cutaneous infections: Superficial infections include pustules, boils, carbuncles, abscesses, styes, impetigo wound and burn infections.

Deep infections: These include osteomyelitis, tonsillitis, pharyngitis, sinusitis, pneumonitis, meningitis, bacteremia, septicemia.

Food poisoning: This is caused by ingesting contaminated food containing enterotoxin. Food poisoning follows after 2 to 6 hours.

Skin exfoliative diseases: It produces exfoliative toxin, which damages superficial layers of skin from underlying tissue.

Toxic shock syndrome: It is a multisystem disease with fever, hypotension, vomiting, diarrhea and erythematous rash.

Bacteriophage Typing

Bacteriophages are the viruses, which attack bacteria. This can be used as basis to type bacteria. It can be done by inoculating strain on a plate of nutrient agar to form lawn culture. After drying, phages are applied over marked squares in a fixed dose (routine test dose). After overnight incubation, culture will be lysed by some phages, but not by others. The strain is named after phages, which lysed it, e.g. if strain is lysed by 52, 79 and 80 it is called 'phage type 52/79/80'.

Laboratory Diagnosis

Specimen should always be collected in specific containers (Table 10.2) and transported to the laboratory immediately.

Table 10.2: Staphylococci smear and diagnosis

Laboratory diagnosis	Staphylococci input smear
Specimen collection	The specimens are collected according to the nature of lesion
Suppurative lesion	Pus
Respiratory lesion	Sputum
Septicemia	Blood
Urinary tract infection	Midstream urine
Meningitis	Cerebrospinal fluid
Food poisoning	Feces or food

Direct microscopy: Gram staining is the basic one where staphylococci show their cluster arrangement (Fig. 10.1). But it is preferred only to pus samples.

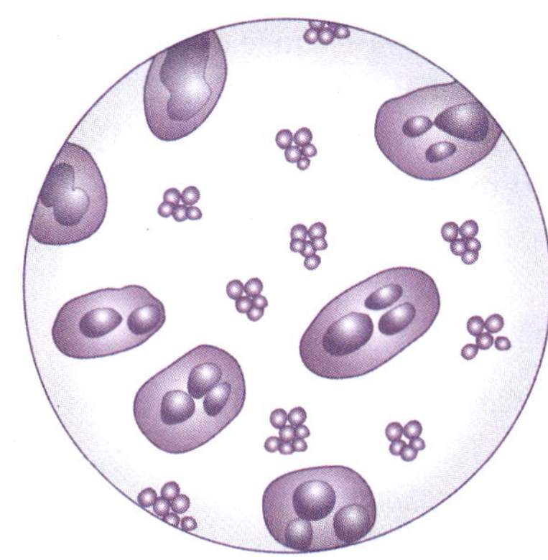

Fig. 10.1: Cluster arrangement of staphylococci

Culture: Blood agar and peptone water are generally used specimens with scanty staphylococci should be (feces) inoculated on Ludlam or Robertson cooked meat medium.

Biochemical tests: Staphylococcus show positive reaction to the tests such as coagulase, methyl red and Voges-Proskauer, catalase.

Antibiotic sensitivity by Kirby-Bauer method, bacteriophage typing can be done to diagnose staphylococcal infections.

Treatment

Benzyl penicillin is the most effective antibiotic, *Staphylococcus* shows drug resistance by producing β-lactamase enzyme. Methicillin was first compound developed to combat penicillinase, but methicillin resistant strains of *S. aureus* (MRSA) became common, vancomycin, topical applications of bacitracin or chlorhexidine may also be used.

MICROCOCCUS

They are gram-positive cocci which occur in tetrads or irregular clusters. Colonies are white in color. They are parasitic. They form small colonies. They do not ferment carbohydrates instead they oxidize them.

STREPTOCOCCI

Streptococci are gram-positive cocci arranged in chains or pairs. Some are human pathogens and some are normal flora of human and animals.

Morphology

Shape	: They are spherical or oval in shape.
Size	: Their size ranges between 0.5 to 1.0 µm in diameter.
Arrangement	: They are arranged in chains. They do not show motility and sporulation and some strains possess capsules.

Classification

Streptococci are classified into aerobic, obligate, anaerobic and facultative anaerobic (Fig. 10.2). Aerobic streptococci and facultative anaerobic streptococci are classified further based on their hemolytic properties on blood agar medium. They are:

1. Alpha (α) hemolytic streptococci: They show partial hemolysis and produce greenish coloration.
2. Beta (β) hemolytic streptococci: These streptococci produce a clear, colorless zone due to

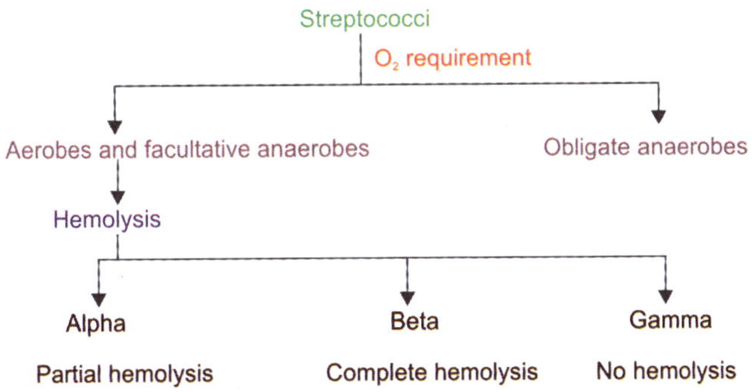

Fig. 10.2: Classification of streptococci

presence of streptolysin O and streptolysin S; most of the pathogenic streptococci fall into this group, e.g. *Streptococcus pyogenes*.

3. Gamma (γ) or non-hemolytic streptococci: They do not exhibit hemolysis, e.g. *Streptococcus faecalis*.

Cultural Characteristics

Temperature: They grow best at temperature of 37°C, crystal violet blood agar permit growth of streptococci.

Biochemical Reactions

They are catalase-negative and ferment several sugar producing acid, but no gas.

Antigenic Structure

Capsule

Hyaluronic acid capsule acts as antigen and inhibits phagocytosis.

Cell Wall

The cell wall is composed of outer layer of protein and lipoteichoic acid, middle layer of group specific carbohydrate and an inner layer of peptidoglycan or mucoprotien and is responsible for cell wall rigidity.

Several protein antigens have been identified and they are M, T and R.

Toxins and Other Virulence Factors

Streptococcus pyogenes forms several exotoxins and enzymes.

Exotoxin

Hemolysins: Streptococci produce two hemolysins streptolysin 'O' and 'S'. Streptolysin 'O' is O_2 liable streptolysin. It is oxygen stable and is responsible for hemolysis seen around colonies. Whereas streptolysin 'O' is important in virulence.

Pyrogenic exotoxin: The primary effect of the toxin is induction of fever.

Enzymes

Streptokinase: It promotes lysis of human fibrin clots by activating a plasma precursor.

Deoxyribonucleases (DNase): Streptodornase or streptococcal DNase cause depolymerization of deoxyribonucleic acid (DNA).

Nicotinamide adenine dinucleotide (NAD): This acts on coenzyme NAD and liberates nicotinamide.

Hyaluronidase: It breaks hyaluronic acid of tissues.

Pathogenesis

Streptococcus pyogenes produce following infections:

Respiratory infections: Sore throat (pharyngitis) is the most common disease and also produce scarlet fever, which causes sore throat and erythematous rash.

Skin and soft tissue infection: The two typical streptococcal infections of skin are erysipelas and impetigo. It also causes infections of wounds and burns.

Genital infection: They are normal inhabitants of female genitalia, which cause puerperal sepsis and other supportive infections. *Streptococcus pyogenes* cause abscesses of brain, lungs, liver, kidneys and also septicemia and pyemia.

Non-suppurative complication: Acute rheumatic fever and acute glomerulonephritis are two important non-suppurative complications.

Laboratory Diagnosis

Suppurative infections are diagnosed by culture where as non-suppurative complications are demonstrated by antibodies.

Acute suppurative infections: Specimens such as pus, blood, swab are collected and plated immediately on pikes medium (blood agar containing 1 in 1,000,000 crystal violet and 1 in 16,000 sodium azide. Blood agar can also be used).

Non-suppurative infections: Antistreptolysin O (ASO) titration is the routine test done where streptolysin 'O' antigens are neutralized with antibodies to streptolysin 'O'. This titre value is high in rheumatic fever where as glomerulonephritis is low.

Microscopy: Gram staining is generally performed.

Serology: Precipitation, agglutination, fluorescent antibody technique are generally employed.

Treatment

Penicillin 'G' is the drug. Erythromycin and cephalexin can also be used.

PNEUMOCOCCI

Pneumococci are lanceolate, gram-positive diplocccus, formerly classified as *Diplococcus pneumoniae*, has been reclassified as *Streptococcus pneumoniae*, but differ from streptococci in morphology, bile solubility and possess polysaccharide capsule. They are normal habitats of the upper respiratory tract of human beings.

Morphology

Shape   : They are slightly elongated cocci.
Size   : They are typically small (1 µm).
Arrangement : They are generally arranged in pairs with one end broad and other pointed, showing flame shape or lanceolate appearance (Fig. 10.3). They are non-motile, non-capsulated and non-sporing.

Cultural Characteristics

Temperature: The optimum temperature for growth is 37°C (25°C to 42°C).
pH: They grow best at 7.8 (range 6.5–8.3).
O_2 requirement: They are aerobes and facultative anaerobes and growth is improved by 5% to 10% CO_2.

The important character of colonies is they appear flat with raised edges and central umbonation and appear as carrom coin or show Draughtsman appearance on liquid media. They produce uniform turbidity (Table 10.3).

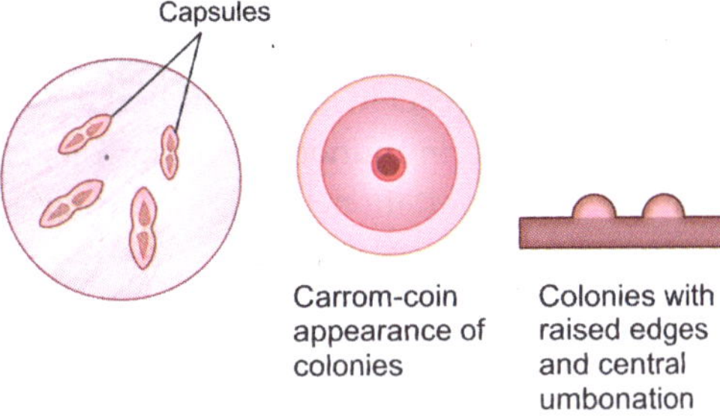

Fig. 10.3: Draughtsman appearance of pneumococci

Biochemical Reactions

It ferments sugars forming acid, it also ferments inulin, which is a differentiated character from streptococci. Pneumococci are catalase and oxidase negative. They are bile soluble.

Antigenic Structure

The *Pneumococcus* produces capsular polysaccharide. Based on capsule, pneumococci can be typed by quellung reaction or capsule swelling reaction described by Neufeld where suspension of pneumococci is mixed on slide with a drop of antiserum. In presence of homologous antiserum, an apparent swelling can be observed under microscope. M protien and C-reactive protein (CRP) are other important somatic antigens.

Pathogenesis

The most common infections are otitis media and sinusitis. They also cause pneumonia, both lobar and bronchial. It causes pyogenic meningitis, common in children.

Laboratory Diagnosis

Specimens: Sputum, cerebrospinal fluid (CSF), blood, fluid from middle ear are generally collected for diagnosis.

Table 10.3: Differentiation between *Pneumococcus* and *Streptococcus viridans*

Features	Pneumococcus	Streptococcus viridans
Morphology	Capsulated, lanceolate, diplococci	Non-capsulated oval or round cells in chains
Quellung test	Positive	Negative
Colonies	Draughtsman colonies	Dome shaped
Growth in liquid media	Uniform turbidity	Granular turbidity
Inulin fermentation	Positive	Negative

Microscopy: Gram staining is generally performed in acute lobar pneumonia. Rusty sputum contain only pneumococci in large numbers.

Serology: Counter immunoelectrophoresis, agglutination, precipitation, radioimmunoassay are generally employed.

Treatment

Penicillin, amoxicillin, vancomycin, cephalosporin are drugs of choice.

Difference between *Pneumococcus* and *Staphylococcus* is given in the Table 10.3.

NEISSERIA

The *Neisseria* genus contains two important pathogens, *Neisseria meningitidis (N. meningitidis)* and *Neisseria gonorrhoeae (N. gonorrhoeae)* many other species occur as commensals in mouth or upper respiratory tract.

Neisseria Meningitidis

Morphology

Shape	: They are oval or spherical cocci.
Size	: They are 0.6 to 0.8 μm.
Arrangement	: They are arranged in pairs with adjacent sides flattened. They are non-motile, mostly fresh isolates and possess capsules.

Cultural Characteristics

Temperature: The optimum temperature for growth is 35°C to 36°C.

pH: Optimum pH is 7.4 to 7.6. Modified Mayer-Martin (vancomycin, colistin and nystatin) is a selective medium. Blood agar, chocolate agar and Mueller-Hinton agar are commonly used media.

Biochemical Reactions

They ferment glucose and maltose and are catalase and oxidase positive. For identification, oxidase test is performed.

Antigenic Properties

Capsule outer membrane proteins and polysaccharides—act as antigens.

Pathogenesis

Neisseria meningitidis mainly causes cerebrospinal meningitis and meningococcal septicemia. Infection is acquired through droplets in some cases, site of entry may be conjunctiva. The incubation period of the disease is about 3 days. Meningococcemia, presents as acute fever with chills, malaise and prostration. A few develop fulminant meningococcemia (Waterhouse-Friderichsen syndrome) and is usually fatal.

Laboratory Diagnosis

Specimens: Nasopharyngeal swab, CSF, blood petechial lesions are the specimens generally collected. The samples collected should be immediately transported, generally Stuart medium is used.

Microscopy: Gram-staining is performed. In this case, CSF sample is made into three portions. With the first centrifuged portion, gram-staining is performed. Second and third portions are inoculated on blood chocolate and glucose broths respectively.

Serology: Latex agglutination, counter immuno-electrophoresis are generally performed.

Treatment

Sulphonamides, penicillin G, chloramphenicol are drugs of choice. Monovalent and polyvalent vaccines are also available containing the capsular polysaccharide, but induce good immunity in older children and adults, but of little value in infants.

Neisseria Gonorrhoeae

Neisseria gonorrhoeae (N. gonorrhoeae) causes veneral disease gonorrhea.

Morphology

Shape	: Gonococci are oval-shaped gram-negative cocci.
Size	: Their size ranges 0.6 to 0.8 μm.
Arrangement	: They always occur in pair with adjacent sides concave.

Cultural Characteristics

Temperature: N. gonorrhoeae grow best at 35°C to 36°C in 5% to 10% CO_2.

pH: Their pH range is 7.2 to 7.6.

They grow best on media like chocolate agar, Thayer-Martin medium, Mueller-Hinton agar medium.

Biochemical Reactions

They ferment glucose with acid and are oxidase positive.

Antigenic Structure

The surface structures of *N. gonorrhoeae* act as antigens. They are:
1. Polyphosphate capsule.
2. Pili—helps in attachment.
3. Lipopolysaccharide—acts as endotoxin and toxicity is largely due to lipopolysaccharides.
4. Outer membrane proteins.

Pathogenesis

Gonorrhea is a veneral disease. Infection is initiated by adhesion of bacteria to the urethra with the help of pile. They penetrate through intercellular spaces and reach connective tissue by third day. In men, infection extends along urethra to prostate seminal vesicles and epididymis.

In women, infection involves urethra, Bartholini glands, endometrium and fallopian tubes.

Ophthalmia neonatorum is a non-veneral gonococcal conjunctivitis in new born through infected birth canal.

Laboratory Diagnosis

Specimens: Urethral discharge in men and cervical discharge in females are collected. The specimens collected should be transported and processed immediately and if not specimens should be collected with charcoal swabs and transported in Stuart medium.

Microscopy: Gram staining is generally performed, but fluorescent antibody techniques by microscopy increases specificity, sensitivity for identification (Fig. 10.4).

Culture: Mueller-Hinton agar, Thayer-Martin medium are the media of choice and growth is identified by morphology and biochemical reactions.

Serology: Complement fixation test can be used.

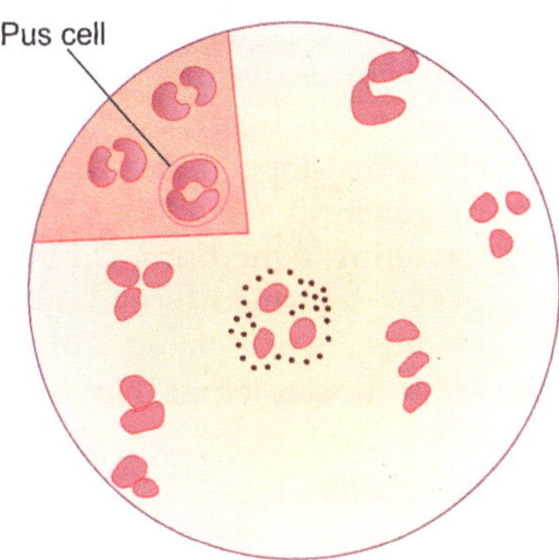

Fig. 10.4: Gonococci in mixed culture

Prophylaxis

Vaccination has no place. Health education, early detection are general measures.

Treatment

Penicillin, ceftriaxone, ciprofloxacin are the drugs of choice.

CORYNEBACTERIUM

Corynebacterium are gram positive club-shaped bacteria. The important genus *Corynebacterium diphtheriae (C. diphtheriae)* causes diphtheria.

Morphology

Shape	:	They are slender rod-shaped bacteria clubbed at one or both ends.
Size	:	They measure approximately 3 to 6 µm × 0.6 to 0.8 µm.
Arrangement	:	They usually appear in pairs, palisades resembling V or L letters known as 'chinese letter' or 'cuneiform arrangement'. They also contain granules made up of polymetaphosphate and are known as metachromatic, volutin or Babes-Ernst granules or polar bodies (as they are often situated at poles of bacilli). They are encapsulated, non-acid fast and non-motile.

Cultural Characteristics

Temperature: The optimum temperature for growth is 37°C.

pH: The optimum pH is 7.2.

O_2 *requirement:* It is an aerobe and facultative anaerobe.

Media: Loeffler serum slope and tellurite blood-agar media are generally used based on colony morphology on tellurite medium. Diphtheria is divided into gravis, intermedius and mitis. Gravis and intermedius are associated with high fatality, while mitis are less lethal (Fig. 10.5).

Biochemical Reactions

Diphtheria ferment acid glucose, galactose, maltose with acid. Hiss's serum water do not hydrolyse urea.

Antigenic Properties

Diphtheria, virulent bacilli produce an exotoxin. Avirulent strains are frequent among convalescents, carriers and contacts.

Pathogenesis

Diphtheria after entry remain confined to site of entry and produce toxin, which causes local necrotic changes. The site of infection may be:

1. Facia.
2. Laryngeal.
3. Nasal.
4. Otitic.
5. Conjunctival.
6. Genital.
7. Cutaneous.

Laboratory Diagnosis

Specimens: Generally throat, nose, larynx, ear, conjunctiva, vagina or skin lesions swabs are collected one for culture and other for smear.

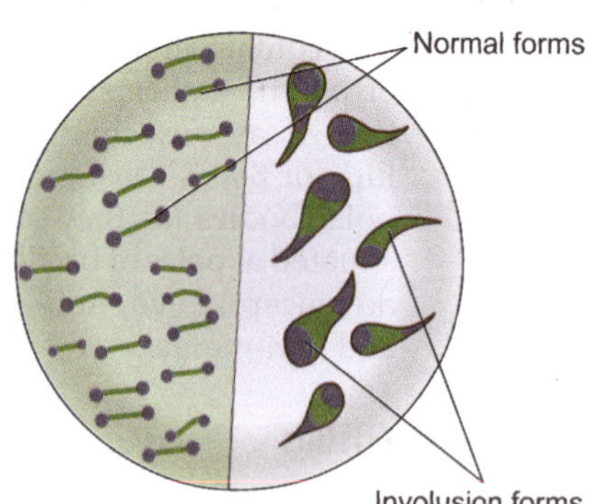

Fig. 10.5: *Corynebacterium diphtheriae*

Microscopy: Gram stain or Neisser stain and Albert stain are generally used.

Virulence tests

Virulence test may be done by *in vivo* or *in vitro* methods.

In vivo tests: Subcutaneas test — Loeffler slope culture is emulsified in 2 to 4 mL broth and 0.8 mL is injected into two guinea pigs subcutaneously, but one is protected with 500 units of antitoxin. If the strain is virulent, unprotected animal will die within 4 days.

Intracutaneous test: The 0.1 mL of culture is inoculated intracutaneously into two guinea pigs one should receive 500 units antitoxin previous day, the other 50 units 4 hour after test to avoid death. Positive reaction can be observed after 48 to 72 hours.

In vitro test: Elek gel precipitation tests — Rectangular antitoxin dipped filter paper strip is placed on surface of 20 percent normal horse serum agar, while it is fluid. Then narrow streaks of strains are made at right angles and incubated. In positive reaction, precipitation line can be observed (Fig. 10.6).

Tissue culture: The toxigenicity of diphtheria bacilli can be demonstrated by incorporating strains in agar overlay of cell culture monolayers. The toxin produced diffuses into cells below and kills them.

Prophylaxis

Three methods of immunization are available — active, passive and combined.

Active Immunization

Diphtheria vaccine is given as triple vaccine and is given in three doses; two doses 4 to 6 weeks apart, followed by third dose a year after wards. A fourth dose (booster dose) at school entry.

Passive Immunization

Subcutaneous administration of 500 to 1,000 units of antitoxin (antidiphtheritic serum [ADS]) is given as immunization.

Combined Immunization

First dose of absorbed toxin is given on one arm, while ADS on another arm to be continued by full course of active immunization.

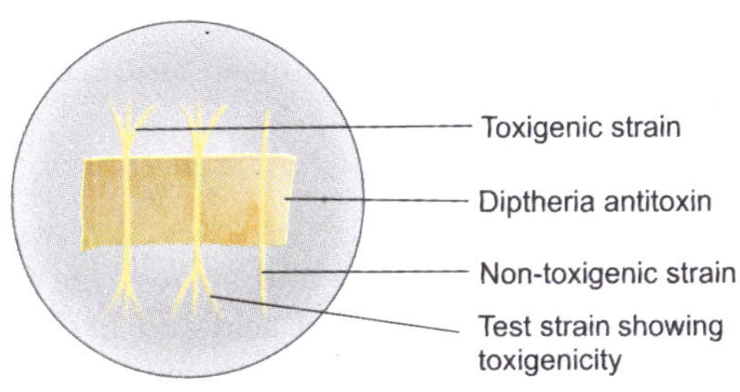

Fig. 10.6: Elek test

Ideally all cases that receive ADS prophylactically should receive combined immunization.

Treatment

Penicillin, erythromycin are generally preferred.

BACILLUS

Rod-shaped spore forming bacteria are classified into two groups, aerobic bacilli and anaerobic. Clostridia bacillus consists of aerobic, heat resistant and spore forming two major pathogenic species and are gram positive.

Bacillus Anthracis

Morphology

Shape	:	These are largest rod-shaped pathogenic bacteria.
Size	:	The size of the bacterium is about 3 to 10 µm × 1 to 1.6 µm.
Arrangement	:	Bacilli are arranged end to end in long chains and appear as 'bamboo stick'. They are non-motile, sporylating capsulated bacteria.

Cultural Characteristics

Temperature: The optimum temperature for growth is 12°C to 45°C.

O₂ requirement: Is an aerobe and facultative anaerobe.

Under microscope, bacilli resemble as locks of matted hair called 'medusa head appearance'. Polymyxin, lysozyme, ethylenediaminetetraacetic acid and thallous acetate (PLET) acts as selective media (Fig. 10.7).

Biochemical Reactions

Glucose, maltose, sucrose are fermented producing only acid; can reduce nitrates.

Antigenic Structure

Two virulence factors have been identified—capsular polypeptide and anthrax toxin.

Pathogenesis

Anthrax is zoonotic, animals like cattle, sheep, less often horses and swine are infected by ingestion of spores. Human anthrax is contracted from animals and disease may be:

1. Cutaneous—hide porter's disease.
2. Pulmonary—woolsorter's disease.
3. Intestinal—rare and caused due to improperly cooked meat.

Cutaneous causes a necrotic lesion known as 'malignant pustule'. It is seen mainly on dock workers as they carry loads of hides and skins on their backs hence known as 'hide porter's diseases'.

Laboratory Diagnosis

Specimens: Swabs, fluids, pus, sputum, blood are generally collected.

Microscopy: Gram staining is generally done. For capsule Indian-ink staining method can be done.

Serology: Complement fixation, enzyme-linked immunosorbent assay (ELISA), polymerase chain reaction (PCR) are the common serological tests to identify *Bacillus* antigen.

In the case of animals, inoculation autopsy should be done.

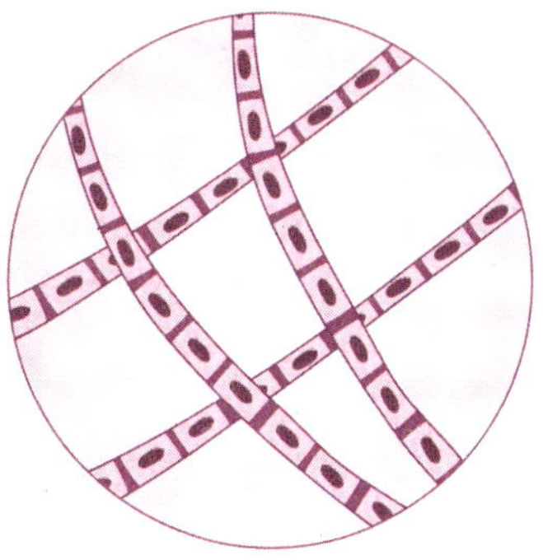

Fig. 10.7: *Bacillus anthracis*

Treatment

Penicillin, streptomycin are the drugs of choice.

Bacillus Cereus

Morphology

Bacillus cereus (*B. cereus*) resembles *Bacillus anthracis* (*B. anthracis*) in all aspects except:
- It is motile
- It is not capsulated.

Pathogenesis

It produces two patterns of foodborne disease.
1. First type is mainly associated with cooked meat and vegetables. It causes diarrhea and abdominal pain after 8 to 16 hours ingestion of contaminated foods.
2. The second type is associated with consumption of cooked rice from Chinese restaurants and it causes nausea and vomiting after 5 hours.

It can be isolated from mannitol egg-yolk phenol-red polymyxin agar (MYPA) and requires no treatment.

CLOSTRIDIUM

The genus *Clostridium* are gram-positive anaerobic spore forming bacilli. *Clostridium perfringens* (*C. Perfringens*), *Clostridium tetani* (*C. tetani*) and *Clostridium botulinum* (*C. botulinum*) are found to be pathogenic.

Clostridium Perfringens

Morphology

Shape : They exist as straight rods with parallel sides and rounded ends.

Size : Their size ranges about 4 to 6 µm × 1 µm.

Arrangement : They occur singly and in chains or bundles; are capsulated, non-motile, sporulating bacteria.

Cultural Characteristics

O_2 *requirement:* They are anaerobes, but can grow under microaerophilic conditions.

Temperature: They usually grow at a range of 37°C to 45°C.

pH: Their pH range is of 5.5 to 8.0.

Culture: Robertson cooked meat broth, blood agar are generally used.

Biochemical Reactions

Glucose, maltose, lactose and sucrose are fermented with production of acid and gas. Hydrogen sulfide (H_2S) is also produced.

Toxins

Alpha, beta, epsilon and iota are the four major toxins produced by *C. perfringens*. Besides toxins it also produce enzyme such as neuraminidase.

Pathogenesis

Clostridium perfringens produces following human infections:
1. Gas gangrene.
2. Food poisoning.
3. Necrotising enteritis.
4. Urogenital infections.

Laboratory Diagnosis

Specimen: The specimens collected are:
1. Erudites from depths of wounds.
2. Necrotic tissue and muscle fragments.
3. Films from muscles at the edge of affected area.

Microscopy: Gram staining is generally performed on rod-shaped gram-positive bacilli; without spores indicates *C. perfringens*.

C. perfringens infections can be identified by Nagler reaction. *C. perfringens* is grown on medium containing 6 percent agar, 5 percent peptic digest of sheep blood and 20 percent human serum, with antitoxin on one half and colonies without antitoxin on another half, which will be surrounded by a zone of opacity. Opacity will not be seen on another half of the plate with antitoxin due to neutralization. This is known as 'Nagler reaction'.

Prophylaxis and Therapy

Damaged tissues should be removed. Metronidazole IV surgery is preferable. Gentamicin and amoxicillin are also advisable.

Clostridium Tetani

Morphology

Shape : They are slender gram-positive bacilli with parallel sides and rounded ends.

Size : The size of the bacterium ranges from 4 to 8 μm × 0.5 μm.

Arrangement : They occur singly or in chains with spherical spores giving drumstick appearance. They are non-capsulated and non-motile.

Cultural Characteristics

Temperature: The optimum temperature is 37°C.

pH: They grow best at 7.4.

O_2 requirement: It is an obligate anaerobe.

Media: It grows well on Robertson cooked meat broth. On blood agar it exhibits hemolysis due to production of hemolysin (tetanolysin).

Biochemical Reactions

They cannot ferment any sugar and are indole positive and methyl red (MR), Voges-Proskauer (VP) negative.

Antigenic Structure

Clostridium tetani produce two toxins: hemolysin (tetanolysin) and neurotoxin (tetanospasmin).

Pathogenesis

Clostridium tetani can enter into body under favourable conditions such as reduced or potential foreign bodies or concurrent infections. The toxin is absorbed by motor nerve endings and causes neurotransmitters resulting uncontrolled spread of impulses.

Laboratory Diagnosis

Specimen: Pus samples, excised bits of tissues from wounds are generally taken as specimen.

Microscopy: Gram staining is generally done and observed for 'tennis-racquet' appearance (Fig. 10.8).

Culture: Cooked meat tubes with polymyxin B, acts as selective media for clostridia.

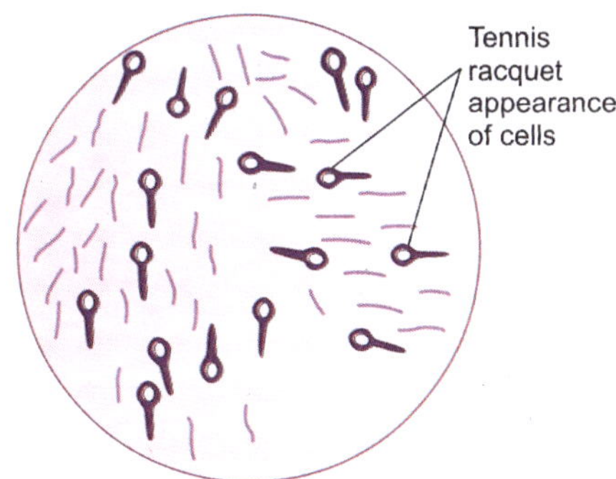

Fig. 10.8: *Clostridium tetani*

Toxigenicity testing can be done on blood agar plates with antitoxin on one half of the plate and *C. tetani* shows hemolysis of another half without antitoxin.

Prophylaxis

The three methods are:

1. Surgical attention.
2. Antibiotics.
3. Immunization—passive, active or combined.
   a. Surgical prophylaxis removes blood clots, necrotic tissue and foreign bodies.
   b. Penicillin, bacitracin or neomycin are the antibiotics generally used.
   c. Passive immunization is done by injecting antitetanus serum as antitoxin.

Active immunization is done by giving diphtheria, pertussis, tetanus (DPT) vaccine. Combined immunization is done by tetanus immune globulin (TIG) injection.

Treatment

Penicillin or metronidazole are the drugs of choice.

Clostridium Botulinum

Morphology

Size: The gram-positive bacteria measures about 5 μm × 1 μm.

These bacilli are non-capsulated and non-motile, sporulating bacteria.

Cultural Characteristics

Temperature: Optimum temperature for growth is 35°C.

pH: 7.4 is the optimum pH.

Antigenic Structure

Antigenic structure produces a powerful exotoxin and is a strong neurotoxin. It generally blocks acetylcholine and weakness muscles.

Pathogenesis

Botulism is of three types—foodborne botulism, wound botulism and infant botulism.

Foodborne botulism is due to ingestion of preformed toxin; vomiting, thirst, constipation are symptoms after 12 to 36 hours.

Wound botulism is produced at site of infection and the symptoms are same as foodborne botulism.

Infant botulism occurs in infants below 6 months, manifestations are constipation after period of normal development, poor feeding, weakness and loss of head control.

Laboratory Diagnosis

Diagnosis may be confirmed by demonstration of the bacillus or the toxin in food or feces. Gram-positive sporing bacilli may be demonstrated in smear made from food.

Control

Botulism is mainly due to canned and preserved food and control can be achieved by canning and preservation. Polyvalent antiserum may be administered.

ENTEROBACTERIACEAE

Enterobacteriaceae are important aerobic bacterial flora of large intestine of human beings and animals. They exhibit similar morphological and biochemical properties, they are gram-negative, non-sporing, non-acid, motile and non-motile, capsulated and non-capsulated, aerobic and facultatively anaerobic bacilli.

Escherichia Coli

Morphology

Shape   : They are straight rod-shaped bacteria.

Size   : They measure about 1 to 3 μm × 0.4 to 0.7 μm in size.

Arrangement : They are arranged singly or in pairs. They are non-sporing, but some strains are capsulated and mostly exhibit motility.

Cultural Characteristics

Temperature: Temperature ranges from 10°C to 40°C, but optimum growth temperature is 37°C.

Growth on ordinary media: Colonies appear circular, moist, smooth and non-mucoid on solid media where as on liquid media it shows uniform turbidity.

Growth on MacConkey media: Colonies appear pink due to lactose fermentation.

Biochemical Reactions

The four biochemical tests employed in classification of enterobacteria are indole, methyl red (MR), Voges-Proskauer (VP) and citrate utilization tests or IMViC tests. *Escherichia coli (E.coli)* is positive for indole and MR; negative for VP and citrate.

Antigenic Structure

Two types of virulence factors have been recognized—surface antigens and toxins.

Surface antigens: Lipoplysaccharide surface O-antigen being endotoxin protects from phagocytosis and in fimbriae it also acts as virulence factors.

Toxins: Hemolysins and enterotoxins are the two exotoxins produced. Enterotoxins are important in pathogenesis. Three types of enterotoxins are present—heat labile toxin (LT), heat stable toxin (ST) and verotoxin (VT).

Pathogenesis

Escherichia coli causes four types of clinical infections:

1. Urinary tract infection.
2. Diarrhea.

3. Pyogenic infections.

4. Septicemia.

Urinary tract infection: E. coli are responsible for majority of naturally acquired urinary tract infections.

Diarrhea: Five different *E. coli* are recognized — enteropathogenic, enterotoxigenic, enteroinvasive, enterohemorrhagic and enteroaggregative *E. coli*.

1. Enteropathogenic *E. coli* (EPEC): Associated with diarrhea in infants and childhood.
2. Enterotoxigenic *E. coli* (ETEC): It is common in local populations and is known as 'travelers diarrhea'.
3. Enteroinvasive *E. coli* (EIEC): Apart from diarrhea they also cause keratoconjunctivitis in guinea pigs.
4. Enterohemorrhagic *E. coli* (EHEC): They cause hemorrhagic colitis (HC).
5. Verocytotoxin producing *E. coli* (VTEC): Hemolytic uremic syndrome (HUS).

Pyogenic infections: E. coli causes neonatal meningitis.

Septicemia — is seen in hospitals.

Laboratory Diagnosis

Specimen collection:
- Urinary infections — urine
- Diarrhea — fecal and rectal swab
- Pyogenic infection — pus and wound swab
- Septicemia — blood.

Microscopy: Gram staining is generally done, but in the case of urine it is centrifuged and deposit is examined. Motility — hanging drop method can be done.

Culture: MacConkey and blood agar are the common media used to isolate *E. coli* and is identified by colony morphology.

Biochemical reactions: Sugar tests such as glucose, lactose, sucrose are done (Table 10.4).

Table 10.4: Identification on IMViC biochemical tests

E. coli	Indole (I)	Methyl red (M)	Voges Proskauer (V)	Citrate (iC)
	+	+	-	-

Serological tests: ELISA, agglutination tests are generally done for the identification of *E. coli*.

Antibiotic sensitivity test: E. coli and other common urinary pathogens develop multiple drug resistance. Antibiotic sensitivity is necessary to administer proper antibiotics.

Klebsiella

Morphology

Shape : They are short, plump, straight rods.

Size : The size of this gram-negative bacteria ranges about 1 to 2 µm × 0.5 to 0.8 µm.

They are non-motile, capsulated, non-sprouting bacteria.

Cultural Characteristics

Temperature: Klebsiella grow well at 37°C.

pH: The optimum pH range is 6.8 to 7.

Growth on MacConkey media: On MacConkey agar colonies appear mucoid (due to slime) and pink to red in color.

Biochemical Reactions

Klebsiella ferment sugar (glucose, lactose, sucrose, mannitol) with production of acid and gas. They show positive for both VP test and citrate test (*Klebsiella pneumoniae* [*K. pneumoniae*]).

Antigenic Structure

Capsule and enterotoxin produced act as antigens.

Pathogenesis

Klebsiella is the popular aerobic bacterial flora of human intestine and is important to cause nosocomial infection. *K. pneumoniae* causes:

1. Pneumonia.
2. Urinary infection.
3. Pyogenic infection.
4. Septicemia.

Laboratory Diagnosis

Diagnosis is made by biochemical reactions. Antibiotic sensitivity should be done.

Treatment

Cephalosporins, trimethoprim, nitrofurantoin and gentamicin are generally used.

Proteus

Morphology

Shape: They are rod-shaped gram-negative bacteria. They are non-capsulated, non-sporing and motile bacteria and can be differentiated from other by a test called 'phenylpyruvic acid reaction'. They produce an enzyme phenylalanine deaminase, which converts phenylalanine to phenylpyruvic acid.

Size : Their size ranges from 1 to 3 μm × 0.5 μm.

Cultural Characteristics

Temperature: These aerobic and facultative anaerobic bacteria grow best at 37°C.

pH: They grow best at pH 6.8 to 7.2.

Growth on ordinary media: Proteus show swarming growth due to vigorous motility of bacteria.

Antigenic structure: The bacilli possess 'O' somatic and 'H' flagellar antigens.

Biochemical Reactions

Biochemical reations shows phenylpropanolamine (PPA), urease, MR, H_2S and indole positive.

Pathogenesis

Proteus are widely distributed in nature as saprophytes and causes infections such as urinary, pyogenic, respiratory and nosocomial infections.

Laboratory Diagnosis

Specimens: Urine, pus samples can be collected.

Microscopy: Gram staining, motility by hanging drop are generally done.

Culture: MacConkey agar, peptone water inoculation are generally performed.

Antibiotic susceptibility test: It should be done because proteins exhibits resistance to most common antibiotics.

Treatment

Amikacin and ciprofloxocin are generally effective in treatment.

Shigella

The causative agent of bacillary dysentery, belongs to genus *Shigella.*

Morphology

Shape: They are rod-shaped gram-negative bacteria. *Shigella* are non-motile, non-sporing and non-capsulated.

Size: Their size ranges about 0.5 μm × 1.3 μm.

Cultural Characteristics

Temperature: The optimum temperature for growth is 37°C.

pH: The grow is best pH 7.4.

Culture: These aerobic or facultatively anaerobic bacteria grow on deoxycholate citrate agar (DCA) and sodium selenite broth.

Biochemical Reactions

Shigella are MR positive and reduce glucose, mannitol and nitrates to nitrites.

Antigenic Structure

Shigella possess somatic 'O' antigens and some strains produce endotoxin.

Pathogenesis

Infection occurs by ingestion, bacilli can resist gastric acidity and infect epithelial cells of villi spreading to adjacent cells and penetrate to lamina propria leading to necrotic patches of epithelium. Human beings are the only natural hosts. Clinical features include passage of loose, scanty feces containing blood mucus with abdominal cramps.

Laboratory Diagnosis

Specimens: Feces sample is generally collected.

Transport: Fresh feces sample should be transported in suitable medium such as Sachs glycerol saline.

Microscopy: Saline and iodine preparation of faces show large number of pus cells, erythrocytes and macrophages. Parasitic causes of dysentery may also be excluded by this examination.

Culture: Selective media like DCA and selenite broth are used. Colonies are further confirmed by gram staining, hanging drop and biochemical reactions.

Serology: Slide agglutination tests can be performed.

Treatment

Bacillary dysentery is a self-limiting conditions. Dehydration has to be corrected promptly, particularly in infants and young children.

Salmonella

The genus *Salmonella* are parasites in intestines of vertebrates and cause enteric fever, gastroenteritis septicemia. The most important member of this genus is *Salmonella typhi (S. typhi)*.

Morphology

Shape: *Salmonella* are gram-negative rods.
Size: Their size ranges about 1 to 3 μm × 0.5 μm.

They are motile, non-capsulated and non-sporulating organisms.

Cultural Characteristics

Temperature: These aerobic and facultatively anaerobic organisms grow at temperature 15°C to 40°C.
pH: The pH ranges between 6 to 8.
Culture media: Selenite F and tetrathionate broth are commonly employed enrichment media.

Biochemical Reactions

Salmonella ferment glucose, mannitol and maltose. They are MR and citrate positive.

Antigenic Structure

Salmonella produce flagellar 'H', somatic 'O' and surface 'Vi' antigens.

Pathogenesis

Salmonella cause following clinical symptoms in human beings. They are:

1. Enteric fever.
2. Septicemia.
3. Gastroenteritis and food poisoning.

Enteric fever: The term enteric fever includes typhoid fever caused by *S. typhi* and paratyphoid fever caused by *Salmonella paratyphi (S. paraty-* *phi)*. The sources of infection are patient and carrier.

Typhoid fever: The infection is acquired by ingestion through contaminated water and food. The characteristic features are hepatosplenomegaly, step-ladder pyrexia with leucopenia. Skin rashes known as rose spots may appear during second or third week.

Paratyphoid fever: Paratyphoid fever resembles typhoid fever, but is milder.

Septicemia: It is caused by *S. paratyphi*. It produces local suppuration in different agar.

Gastroenteritis: It is caused by ingestion of food like meat, milk, egg. It is most frequently isolated in food poisoning.

Laboratory Diagnosis

Bacteriological diagnosis consists:

1. Isolation of bacilli.
2. Demonstration of antibodies.

Isolation of Bacilli

Blood, feces, urine, duodenal fluid are collected.

Blood culture: Bacteremia occurs early in disease. About 5 to 10 mL of blood is collected and incubated in bile broth overnight at 37°C and subcultured on MacConkey agar. If *Salmonella* are not obtained from the first subculture from taurocholate broth, subculture should be done every other day up to 10 days before declaring report as negative.

An alternative to blood culture is clot culture. In clot culture, 5 mL of blood is withdrawn into test tube and allowed to clot and broken clot (streptokinase is incorporated) added to bile broth.

Feces culture: Fecal samples are plated directly on MacConkey agar, DCA, Wilson-Blair media and inoculated to selenite broth, tetrathionate borth and then incubated.

Urine culture: *Salmonella* are shed in urine irregularly. Clean voided samples are centrifuged and the deposit is inoculated into enrichment and selective media.

Other examples like bone marrow, rose spots, autopsy from gallbladder, liver, spleen and mesenteric lymph nodes can also be used.

Demonstration of antibodies

Widal reaction: This the most widely used test for measurement of H and O agglutinins. Two types of tubes are used — a narrow tube with conical bottom for H antigen and a short round bottomed tube for O antigen. To these tubes serially diluted serum are added and incubated in water bath at 37°C overnight. H agglutination leads to the formation of loose cotton wooly clumps, while O agglutination is seen as disc like pattern at bottom of tube.

Serology: Agglutination test is generally performed.

Treatment

Chloramphenicol, fluoroquinolones, cephalosporins, cefotaxime are generally recommended.

Prophylaxis

1. Carriers should not be engaged in food preparation.
2. Sanitary measures should be taken properly (heat killed *S. typhi* and *S. paratyphi* A and B)
   a. Typhoid-paratyphoid A and B (TAB) vaccines is given subcutaneously in two doses of 0.5 mL at an interval of 4 to 6 weeks followed by booster dose every 3 years.
   b. Live oral vaccine of three doses are given on alternate days (avirulent mutant strain of *S. typhi*).

VIBRIO CHOLERAE

Morphology

Shape: They are curved or comma-shaped gram-negative rods (Fig. 10.9).

Size: Their size ranges about 1.5 µm × 0.2 to 0.4 µm.

They are motile (polar flagellum), non-sporulating and non-capsulating bacteria.

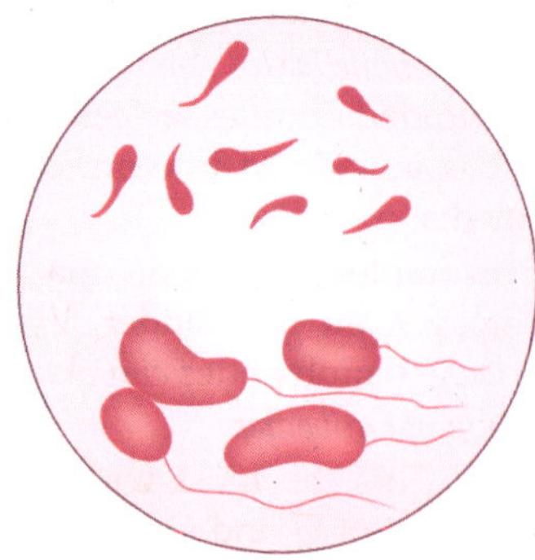

Fig. 10.9: *Vibrio cholerae*

Cultural Characteristics

Temperature: These aerobic bacteria grows at a range of 16°C to 40°C.

pH: Optimal growth is seen at pH 6.4 to 9.6.

Culture: Growth on solid media—On MacConkey agar colonies are colorless, but become reddish on prolonged incubation. Venkatraman Ramakrishnan (VR) medium and Cary-Blair medium acts as transport media.

Biochemical Reactions

Vibrio cholera (V. cholera) ferment glucose, mannitol, maltose, mannose, sucrose and produce acid. They show positive reactions towards indole and nitrate.

Pathogenesis

In human, vibrio enter orally through contaminated water or food. It produces enterotoxin. It has two fractions 'A active fragment' and 'B binding fragment'. The B subunit binds to ganglioside receptor on intestinal epithelial cell. The active A fragment enters the cell and is cleaved to its subunits A1 and A2. Stimulates adenyl cyclase and converts adenosine triphosphate (ATP) into cyclic adenosine monophosphate (cAMP), which causes hypersecretion of water and electrolytes and also inhibition of reabsorption of sodium chloride resulting in diarrhea.

Laboratory Diagnosis

Specimens: Stool and rectal swabs are generally collected as specimens. Preservation of specimens is necessary, VR fluid and Cary-Blair medium can be used.

Microscopy: As it shows characteristic darting, motility, it can be demonstrated under dark field or phase contrast microscope.

Culture: MacConkey, thiosulfate-citrate-bile salts-sucrose (TCBS) agar are generally preferred.

Serology: Slide agglutination is performed.

Prophylaxis

General Measures

1. Purification of water supplies.
2. Better provision for sewage disposal.
3. Infected patients should be isolated.

Specific Measures

Killed parental vaccine: Injections are given intra-muscularly at an interval of 4 weeks.

Killed oral vaccine: B subunit vaccine—contain cholera toxin, B subunit given orally.

Live vaccine: It is recombinant DNA vaccine where *V. cholerae* will be attenuated.

PSEUDOMONAS AERUGINOSA

Morphology

Shape : They are slender, rod-shaped bacteria.

Size : Size of this gram-negative bacillus ranges between 1.5 to 3 μm × 0.5 μm.

They are non-capsulated, non-sporing, motile bacteria. *Pseudomonas* possess polar flagellum.

Cultural Characteristics

Temperature: These strictly aerobic bacteria grow best at 37°C, but has wide range of 5°C to 42°C.

pH: The optimum pH is at 7.2.

Media: Cetrimide agar acts as selective medium and on nutrient agar they produce greenish blue pigment.

Pigment production:
- Pyocyanin—bluish green pigment
- Fluoresin—greenish yellow pigment
- Pyrubin—reddish brown pigment.

Biochemical Reactions

Biochemical reactions utilize glucose with acid production. *Pseudomonas aeruginosa are oxidase* positive and utilize citrate as source of carbon.

Pathogenesis

It mainly causes nosocomial infections. The other common infections caused by it are:
1. Urinary tract infections.
2. Acute purulent meningitis.
3. Septicemia in debilitated patients.
4. Wound and burn infections.
5. Eye infections.
6. Infantile diarrhea.

Laboratory Diagnosis

Specimens: Urine, sputum, pus, blood and CSF samples are collected.

Microscopy: Gram staining and hanging drop methods are perfomed.

Culture: Nutrient agar, blood agar, MacConkey agar cetrimide agar are generally used.

Antibiotic sensitivity method: Antibiotic sensitivity method is useful to select proper antibiotic, as multiple resistance to antibiotic is quite common.

Treatment

Ciprofloxacin, cefotaxime, ticarcillin, gentamicin are used in treatment.

YERSINIA

Morphology

Shape : They are short, plump, ovoid bacillus with rounded ends and convex sides.

Size : *Yersinia* are gram-negative bacillus about 1.5 μm × 0.7 μm.

Arrangement : *Yersinia* are arranged singly in short chains or in small groups. It is non-motile, non-sporing, non-capsulated bacteria.

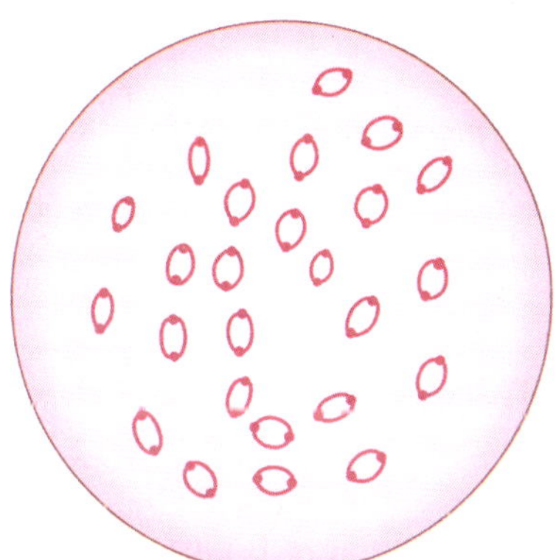

Fig. 10.10: *Yersinia*

Cultural Characteristics

Temperature: The optimum temperature for growth is 27°C.

pH: Growth occurs over a range of pH 5 to 9.6, but optimum pH is 7.2.

Biochemical Reactions

Yersinia ferments glucose, maltose, mannitol with the production of acid, but no gas. It is MR and catalase positive.

Antigens/Toxins

Heat-labile protein envelope antigens, bacteriocin, toxins such as endotoxins (protein, lipopolysaccharide in nature) are produced by *Pseudomonas*.

Pathogenesis

Yersinia pestis (Y. pestis) is the causative agent of plague and is natural pathogen of rodents. Infection is transmitted from one animal to another by bite of flea. Plague occurs in three forms—bubonic, pneumonic and septicemic.

Bubonic Plague

As the plague bacillus usually enters through the bite of infected rat fleas on the legs, the inguinal lymph nodes are involved, hence the name bubonic. The inguinal lymph nodes become enlarged and suppurated.

Pneumonic Plague

Pneumonic plague is highly infectious form of plague involving the lungs producing hemorrhagic pneumonia. It can be transmitted from man to man by droplet infection and is virtually always fatal.

Septicemic Plague

The presence of bacteria in blood denotes septicemic plague. It is terminal event of bubonic and pneumonic plague.

Laboratory Diagnosis

Specimen: Pus, sputum, blood, CSF are generally collected.

Microscopy: Detection of bacilli can be done by using methylene blue where bipolar stained bacilli can be observed (Fig. 10.10).

Serology: Fluoroscent antibody technique is of use in identifying plague bacilli.

Treatment

Streptomycin, tetracycline, chloramphenicol and gentamicin are effective.

HAEMOPHILUS INFLUENZAE

Morphology

Shape   : It usually exists as coccobacillus.

Size   : The size of bacteria ranges about 1.0 μm × 0.3 μm.

Arrangement : They usually occurs as clusters.

Cultural Characteristics

Temperature: These aerobic bacteria grow best at 37°c.

pH: The optimum pH for growth of *Haemophilus* is 7.3.

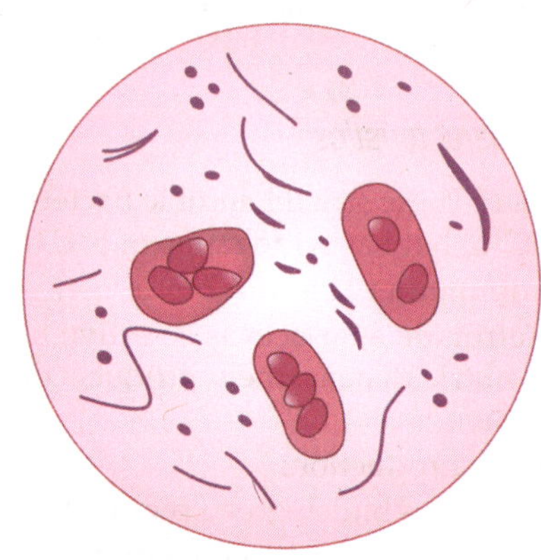

Fig. 10.11: *Haemophilus influenzae*

The bacillus requires performed growth factors in blood, X factor (hemin) and V factor (coenzyme) for its growth and the growth is directly proportional to the concentration of these factors.

Biochemical Reactions

Glucose, xylose are fermented with acid production. It shows positive reaction towards oxidase and catalase.

Antigenic Properties

Capsular polysaccharide, outer membrane protein and lipopolyssaccharides acts as antigens.

Pathogenesis

Haemophilus is an obligate human parasite and causes following infections:

1. Meningitis.
2. Epiglottitis.
3. Pneumonia.
4. Bronchitis.
5. Suppurative lesions.

Laboratory Diagnosis

Specimens: CSF, blood, throat swab, sputum, pus are generally collected. Specimens should be collected in sterile containers under aseptic conditions.

Microscopy: Gram staining is generally performed. The other method for diagnosing is by observing satellitism after overnight incubation (Fig. 10.11).

Treatment

Cefotaxime, ampicillin, co-trimoxazole are the drugs of choice.

BORDETELLA PERTUSSIS

Morphology

Shape : *Bordetella pertussis (B. pertussis)* are gram-negative ovoid coccobacilli. They are non-motile, non-sporing, capsulated bacteria.

Size : It is small bacterium of length 0.5 μm.

Cultural Characteristics

Temperature: These aerobic bacteria grow best at 35°C to 36°C.

Bordet-Gengou medium (potato-glycerol-blood agar) is the common media used for cultivation.

Biochemical Reactions

Bordetella pertussis shows positive for oxidase and catalase. It also form indole and reduce nitrates.

Antigenic Structure

Capsular K antigen, pertussis toxin are the important antigens.

Pathogenesis

Bordetella pertussis causes whooping cough—source of infection in patient. Onset is with fever and dry irritating cough.

Laboratory Diagnosis

Specimen: Swab from nasal cavity is generally preferred. Cough droplets can also be collected.
Microscopy: Fluorscent antibody technique can be employed.
Culture: Bordet-Gengou plates are generally used to cultivate.
Serology: Serological diagnosis is not helpful. ELISA has been proposed as a diagnostic method.

Prophylaxis

Three intramuscular injections of killed *B. pertussis* at intervals of 4 to 6 weeks are given before the age of 6 months followed by booster dose at the end of first year of life.

Treatment

Erythromycin, chloramphenicol, ampicillin are drugs of choice.

BRUCELLA

Morphology

Shape : These gram-negative bacteria are coccobacillary or short rod-shaped.

Size : *Brucella* size ranges between 0.5 to 0.7 μm × 0.6 to 1.5 μm.

Arrangement : They are arranged singly or in short chains. They are non-sporing, non-capsulated, non-motile bacteria.

Cultural Characteristics

Temperature: These strict aerobic bacteria grow best at temperature of 37°C (range 20°C–40°C).
pH: They grow at a pH range of 6.6 to 7.4.

Biochemical Reactions

Carbohydrates are not fermented, but produce catalase, oxidase and urease.

Pathogenesis

Brucellosis is a zoonotic disease and it may be acute or chronic.

Acute Brucellosis

Acute brucellosis causes muscular pains, asthmatic attacks, constipation and chills may occur for weeks.

Chronic Brucellosis

Chronic brucellosis causes hypersensitivity, joint pains and lasts for years.

Laboratory Diagnosis

Blood is the most commonly collected specimen.
Culture: Castaneda method—It has an advantage, Where liquid (tryptic soy broth) and solid (tryptic soy agar) media are taken in same bottle. Blood is inoculated in liquid medium and incubated in upright position. For subculture, bottle is tilted so that broth flows over surface of solid agar and is again incubated in upright position. This method reduces chances of contamination.
Serology: ELISA, immunofluorescent test, agglutination tests are commonly employed.

Treatment

Tetracyline along with streptomycin are given.

MYCOBACTERIUM TUBERCULOSIS

Morphology

Shape   : These are acid fast straight or slightly curved bacilli with rounded ends.

Size   : *Mycobacterium tuberculosis (M. tuberculosis)* measures 1 to 4 μm × 0.2 to 0.8 μm.

Arrangement : They occur singly, in pairs or in small clumps. They are non-sporing, non-capsulated, non-motile organisms. They are gram-positive, but difficult to stain with gram stain.

Cultural Characteristics

Temperature: The optimum temperature required is 37°C and fails to grow below 25°C or above 40°C.

pH: The optimum pH is 6.4 to 7.0.
Culture: These obligate aerobic bacteria are routinely cultured in Lowenstein-Jensen medium with starch.

Antigenic Structure

The virulence of *M. tuberculosis* have been correlated with formation of long cord like structures, which are glycolipid in nature.

Pathogenesis

The source of infection is due to direct inhalation of bacteria released through cough, sneeze, etc. Tuberculosis can be classified as primary and post primary.

Primary

The inhaled bacteria settle in lungs and forms aggregation of macrophages called 'tubercles'. This leads to lung tissue destruction. The infection remains localized. It is usually inapparent and appear to end. But the initial infection hypersensitized the individual to bacteria or their products.

Post Primary

Post primary is done for the reactivation of latent infection and differs in following ways:

1. It affects upper lobes of lungs.
2. Involves lymph nodes.
3. The necrotic materials break out leading to sputum, which is the main source of infection.

Laboratory Diagnosis

Specimen: Sputum, CSF are generally collected, sometimes bacteria is carried to meninges also.
Microscopy: Fluorescent microscopy and acid-fast staining are generally performed. A positive report can be given only if two or more bacilli have been seen (Table 10.5).

Table 10.5: Grading of smears of bacilli

SI No	Grade	Bacilli
1.	1 +	3–9
2.	2 +	10 or more
3.	3 +	20 or more

Culture: Bottles of Lowenstein-Jensen medium are used and bacilli grow in 2 to 8 weeks.

Tuberculin test: Tuberculin test is diagnostic test where protein fraction extracted from *M. tuberculosis* is injected intradermally into hypersensitive individual, which elicits immune response in 1 to 3 days. The reaction is characterized by hardening and swelling. A positive test indicates that individual has been exposed to organism.

Prevention and Treatment

Bacilli Calmette-Guérin (BCG) vaccination is available.

Isoniazid 5 mg/kg daily for 6 to 12 months is usual course. It reduces risk of developing active tuberculosis by 90 percent.

Rifampicin, isoniazid, streptomycin, pyrazinamide and thiacetazone are given atleast for 6 to 7 months.

SPIROCHETES

Spirochetes are gram-negative free living saprophytes. They are called hair-like structures and 5 to 500 µm in size. The characteristic feature is presence of endoflagella. The important human pathogens are found in the genera *Treponema*, *Borrelia* and *Leptospira*.

Treponema Pallidum

Treponema pallidum (T. pallidum) is the causative agent of syphilis. It is 10 µm long and 0.4 to 0.2 µm wide with tapering ends. It is motile and cannot be seen under the light microscope so generally. Phase contrast or dark ground microscopes are used. It can be stained by negative staining (Indian ink) and silver impregnation methods. The treponemas reduce silver nitrate to metallic silver that is deposited on surface enlarging the diameter of organisms.

Cultural Characteristics

They cannot be grown in artificial culture media, but strains can be maintained by serial testicular passage in rabbits.

Pathogenesis

Natural infection, syphilis, occurs in human beings, veneral syphilis is acquired by sexual contact. Through minute abrasions on skin or mucosa, it enters the body. The three clinical stages are primary, secondary and tertiary stages.

Primary lession called hard chancre occurs at genital area, mouth and nipples. It is painless, avascular indurated superficially ulcerated lesion.

Secondary syphilis sets in 3 months and the lesion are due to entry of spirochetes into blood.

Tertiary lesions contain few spirochetes and may lead to delayed hypersensitive reactions, congenital syphilis is also seen where infection is transmitted from mother to fetus. A woman with early syphilis can infect her fetus more commonly.

Laboratory Diagnosis

Diagnosis involves two important steps:

1. Demonstration of treponemas under microscope.
2. Serological tests.

Microscope: Serum is the sample generally preferred. Generally dark ground microscope is done where slender spiral structures showing slow movements can be observed (Fig. 10.12).

Serological tests

The tests may be classified as follows:

   i. Non-specific reagin antibody tests:
   a. Venereal Disease Research Laboratory (VDRL) test.
   b. Rapid plasma reagin (RPR) test.
   c. Group specific test.

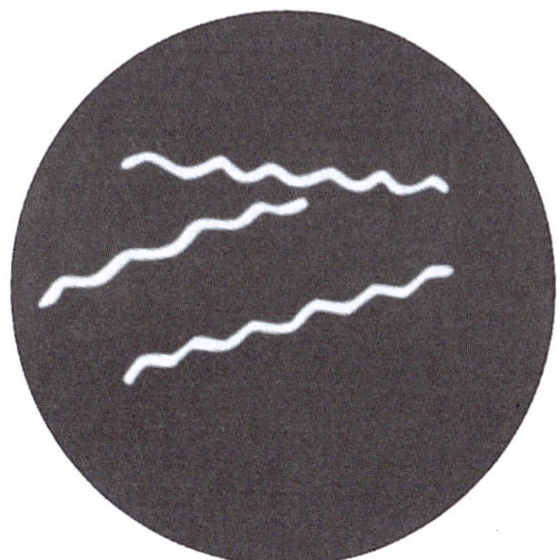

Fig. 10.12: *Treponema pallidum*

ii. Non-veneral treponematosis: They occur in communities with poor standards of hygiene. These include yaws, pinta, endemic.
   • Reiter protein complement fixation (RPCF) test.
iii. Specific tests using pathogenic treponemes (*T. pallidum*):
   a. *Treponema pallidum* immobilization (TPI) test.
   b. Fluorescent treponemal antibody absorption (FTA-ABS) test.
   c. *Treponema pallidum* hemagglutination assay (TPHA) is a major serological tests for syphilis.

Non-specific reagin antibody tests: These are standard tests for syphilis where cardiolipin and lipoidal antigen reacts with antibody reagin.

Veneral Disease Research Laboratory test: This test is developed by Veneral Disease Research Laboratory. In the VDRL test, inactivated serum (heated at 56°C for 30 minute) is mixed with cardiolipin antigen on a special slide and rotated for 4 minutes. In positive samples, it forms visible clumps with reagin antibody where as in negative samples it remains the same. Rapid plasma reagin is another test similar to that of VDRL.

Group-specific treponemal tests: In order to avoid false positive reactions these tests are developed by using cultivable treponemas. Reiter protein complement fixation test is mostly commonly employed one, which uses a lipopolysaccharide-protein complex antigen from treponeme.

Specific Treponema pallidum tests: The test serum is incubated with complement and *T. pallidum*, if the antibodies are present, the *Treponema* is immobilized in a complex anaerobic medium. It can be observed under dark ground illumination. There test are known as *Treponema pallidum* immobilization test and fluorescent treponemal antibody test. It is an indirect test where smears of killed *T. pallidum* (Nichols strain) are prepared on slides and fixed. The patients serum is allowed to react with smear. The antibodies that bind to fixed smear are detected with fluorescein-labeled antihuman immunoglobulin.

Fluorescent treponemal antibody absorption: In this modified test, serum is preabsorbed with Reiter treponemes to eliminate group specific reactions.

Treponema pallidum hemagglutination assay: Tanned erythrocytes are sensitized extract of *T. pallidum*, when these with sonicated erythrocytes are mixed with patient's serum, the erythrocytes clump together.

Treatment

Primary, secondary and latent infections can be treated by using benzathine benzylpenicillin and doxycycline.

Syphilis

Yaws: The causative agent is *T. pertenue*, which is morphologically and antigenically similar to *T. pallidum*. Papule enlarges and form ulcerating granuloma. Laboratory diagnosis and treatment are similar.

Pinta: It is caused by *T. carateum*. The disease is acquired by direct person to person. Causative agent is *T. carateum*. Non-ulcerating papule develops into lichenoid patch. Treatment is similar to that of syphilis.

Endemic syphilis: The disease is caused by *T. pallidum* by sharing common contaminated utensils. Mucous patches and skin eruption are common. Laboratory diagnosis and treatment are same.

Borrelia

Morphology

Borrelia are large motile refractile spirochetes with irregular, wide open cells. They are usually 10 to 30 μm long and 0.3 to 0.7 μm wide. They are gram-negative (Fig. 10.13).

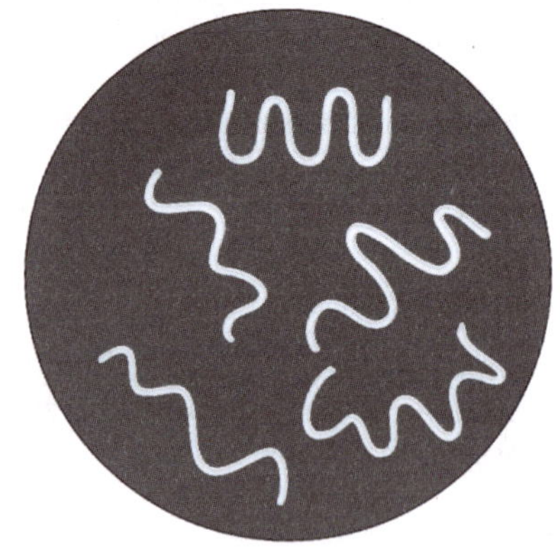

Fig. 10.13: Borrelia

Relapsing Fever

The causative agent is *Borrelia recurrentis* (*B. recurrentis*) and is transmitted through body lice (*Pediculus humanus corporis*). It is 8 to 20 μm long and 0.2 to 0.4 μm wide and is gram-negative.

Cultural Characteristics

They are microaerophilic and optimum temperature for growth is 28°C to 30°C.

Pathogenesis

Relapsing fever is transmitted through body lice and is characterized by febrile episode of sudden onset and fever subsides after 3 to 5 days. Splenomegaly is common—3 to 10 relapses are generally seen.

Laboratory Diagnosis

Blood sample is usually collected and examined under dark ground microscope. Giemsa and Leishman stains can be used. Serological tests are not that reliable.

Treatment

Tetracycline, chloramphenicol, penicillin and erythromycin are effective.

The other pathogenic *Borrelia* of medical importance include:

Borrelia vincentii—Vincents angina.
Borrelia burgdorferi—lyme disease.

Leptospira

Leptospira are actively motile, delicate and possess large number of closely wound spirals with hooked ends.

Morphology

Leptospira are about 6 to 20 μm long and 0.1 μm thick. Their ends are hooked and are actively motile. They may be stained with Giemsa stain (Fig. 10.14).

Cultural Characteristics

They can be grown in media enriched with rabbit serum. Optimum temperature is 25°C to 30°C and optimum is pH 7.2 to 7.5.

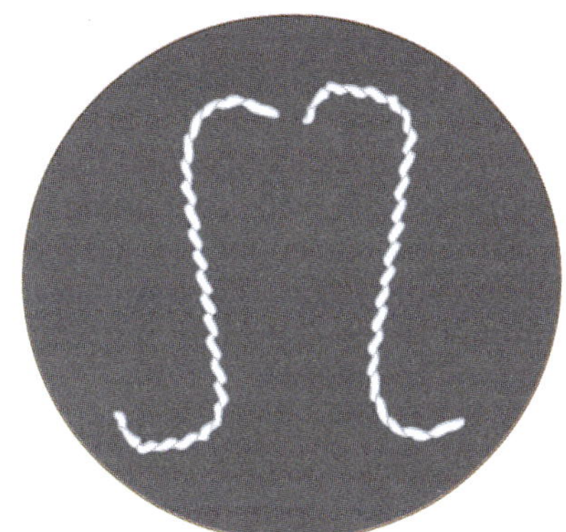

Fig. 10.14: Leptospira

Pathogenesis

Humans are infected when leptospiras in water are contaminated by urine of carrier animals, which enters the body through cuts or abrasions on skin mucosa. The clinical manifestation include pyrexia to severe fatal illness. Serotype icterohemorrhagiae causes fever, conjunctivitis, albuminurea, jaundice and hemorrhage.

Laboratory Diagnosis

The diagnosis depends on demonstration of leptospira in blood by dark ground microscopy. Urine samples can also be taken.

Culture: Blood during first week and urine in second week can be cultured. Media are generally incubated at 28°C to 32°C.

Animal inoculation: The blood and urine from patient is inoculated into guinea pigs, peritoneal fluid from third day is examined by dark ground illumination.

Serological tests: Two types are in use. They are:

1. Screening tests: Complement fixation test, hemagglutination, ELISA, indirect immunofluorescence are capable of detecting immunoglobulin M (IgM) and immunoglobulin G (IgG).

2. Serotype specific tests: Serotype specific tests identify infecting serovar by demonstrating specific antibodies. Microscopic and macroscopic agglutination tests are used for this purpose.

ACTINOMYCETES

Actinomycetes are the organisms, which exhibit both bacterial and fungal characters, i.e. like fungi they form mycelial network and like bacteria they posses cell walls containing muramic acid, prokaryotic nuclei and are susceptible to antibacterial antibiotics. They are gram-positive, non-motile, non-sporing, non-capsulated free living soil organisms.

Actinomyces is the major pathogenic genus whereas *Streptomyces* cause disease rarely, but is the major source of antibiotics, *Nocardia* genus of actinomycetes are acid-fast bacteria.

Actinomyces

Actinomyces are anaerobic or microaerophic, non-acid fast bacteria and causes actinomycosis. It causes indurated swelling in connective tissue and discharge sulfur granules. These species are present as commensals in the bodies, but poor oral hygiene, trauma may favor infection.

Actinomycosis occur in four forms in human beings:

1. Cervicofacial.
2. Thoracic.
3. Abdominal.
4. Pelvic.

It also causes inflammatory diseases of gums leading to root surface carries.

Laboratory Diagnosis

Generally pus and sputum samples are collected. Sulfur granules are usually demonstrated. They appear white and yellowish from minute specks to about 5 mm.

Under microscope these granules are observed as gram-positive filaments surrounded by peripheral zone of swollen radiating club-shaped structures giving sunray appearance.

Treatment

The treatment have to be continued for several months and supplemented by surgery. Generally penicillin or tetracycline were given.

Nocardia

Nocardia resemble *Actinomyces* but are aerobic. They are usually found in soil. It causes cutaneous, subcutaneous or systemic lesions in humans. Diagnosis is by demonstrating branching filaments microscopically and show wrinked, granular growth on ordinary media.

Cotrimoxazole, amikacin, cefotaxime, minocycline are effective.

CHLAMYDIA

Chlamydia are gram-negative obligate intracellular bacterial parasites of humans, animals and birds and grow in squamous epithelial cells and macrophages of respiratory and gastrointestinal tracts. They are also known as 'psittacosis-lymphogranuloma-trachoma' (PLT) agents. Due to their filterability they were considered as viruses. But they differ from viruses in many respects.

1. They possess both DNA and RNA.
2. They have cell walls, ribosomes.
3. They replicate by binary fission.
4. They are susceptible to bacterial antibiotics.

The major bacterial characters, which they lack are peptidoglycan in cell walls and enzymes of electron transport chain. So they depend on host cells for ATP.

The four important species of *Chlamydia* are *C. trachomatis, C. psittaci, C. pneumoniae* effects humans and *C. pecorum* effects ruminants.

Morphology and Growth Cycle

They occur in two forms elementary body (ER) and reticulate body (RB). Elementary body is infective form (200–300 µm) and reticulate is intracellular replicative form (500–1,000 µm) in size. Infection is initiated in cells, after 8 hours they transform into large reticulate bodies and start binary fission till 40 hours, but by 24 hours reticulate bodies start transforming into elementary bodies and are ultimately released from host cell (Fig. 10.15). The developing chlamydial colony is known as 'inclusion body'.

Pathogenesis

Chlamydia trachomatis cause ocular and genital infections.

Ocular infections include trachoma, inclusion conjunctivitis and ophthalmia neonataram.

Genital infections include miscellaneous urogenital syndrome and lymphogranuloma venereum.

It can also cause pneumonia in infants around 4 to 16 weeks of age.

Chlamydia psittaci causes psittacosis in parrots, can be transmitted to human beings mostly seen in poultry patients.

Chlamydia pneumoniae cause respiratory disease in older children and adults worldwide. Its clinical symptoms include pharyngitis, sinusitis, bronchitis, pneumonia.

Laboratory Diagnosis

Scrapings of mucosa, blood, sputum, respiratory secretions are collected as samples.

Microscopy: Inclusion bodies are usually detected by Giemsa stain.

Serology: Immunofluorescence and ELISA are the routine serological tests performed.

Isolation: It may be isolated from diseased animal (mice intranasal) in yolk sac of chick embryo or by tissue cultures. In cells from MacConkey agar, inclusion bodies can be easily detected.

Treatment

Tetracycline, erythromycin, sulfonamides are the drugs of choice.

MYCOPLASMA

Mycoplasma lack cell wall and are pleomorphic. These organisms were previously termed as pleuropneumonia-like organisms (PPLO) named after the first member identified of this group. Later it is replaced by *Mycoplasma* (Myco means fungus like, plasma means plastivity).

Morphology

The smallest free living organisms. They occur as granules (range from 100–1,000 μm in size) and filaments (slender). They are gram-negative non-motile, non-sporulating and reproduce by binary fission.

They show bulbous enlargement with a different tip by which they attach to host. Generally they are facultative anaerobes and aerobes. Colony shows fried egg appearance, central opaque granular area surrounded by a flat

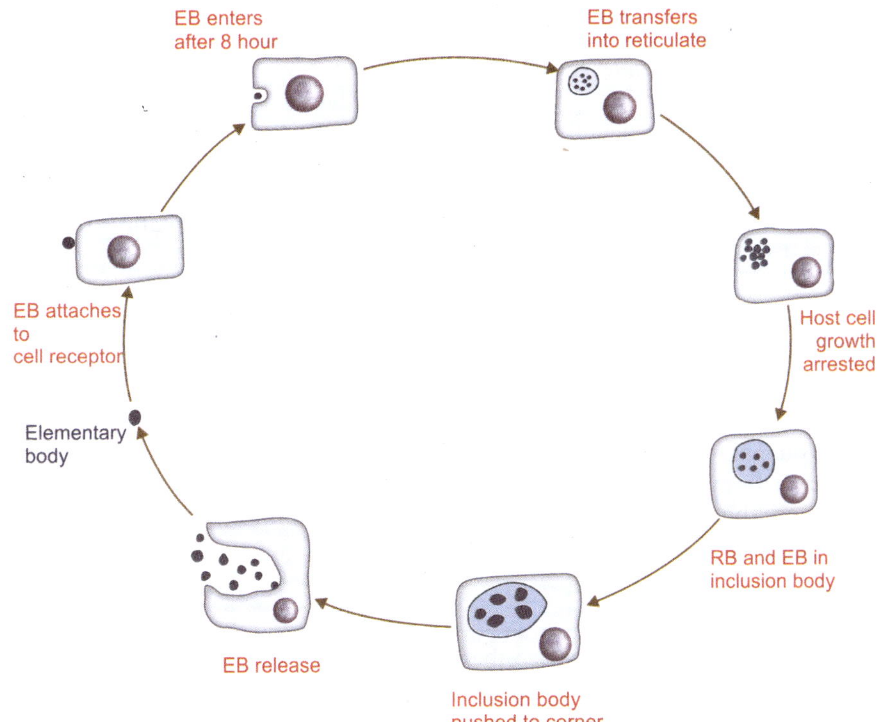

Fig. 10.15: Growth cycle of *Chlamydia* (ER = Elementary body; RB = Reticulate body).

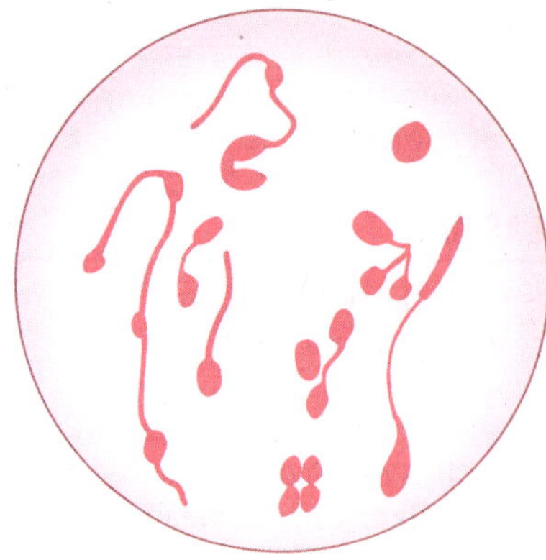

Fig. 10.16: Mycoplasma

translucent peripheral zone. The unique feature of these organisms is that they require cholesterol and sterols for their growth (Fig. 10.16).

Pathogenesis

Mycoplasma cause two types of diseases in humans. Pneumonia and genital infections. Mycoplasmal pneumonia is caused by *Mycoplasma pneumoniae* (*M. pneumoniae*). The symptoms are fever, malaise, headache and sore throat. Rashes, meningitis, encephalitis, hemolytic anemia are other complications seen.

Mycoplasma hominis (*M. hominis*) and *Ureaplasma urealyticum* (*U. urealyticum*) cause genital infections. They are transmitted by sexual contacts. *U. urealyticum* strain is usually isolated from urogenital tract and form tiny colonies of size 15 to 50 μm in size. Hence they were called 'T-strain' or 'T-form' mycoplasmas (T for tiny). Mycoplasmas cause severe infections in HIV patients.

Laboratory Diagnosis

Throat swabs and urine samples are generally taken. They can be inoculated in media containing glucose and phenol red, growth is indicated by acid production. Immunofluorescence, complement fixation are the serological tests generally used to diagnose the disease.

RICKETTSIA

Rickettsia are small gram-negative bacteria that are obligate intracellular parasite and, except 'Q' fewer, are transmitted to humans by arthropods, which serve as vector and reservoir.

They are minute organisms having properties in between bacteria and viruses. Their general properties are:

1. Contains both DNA and RNA in a ratio 1 : 3 : 5.
2. Contains muramic acid in the cell wall.
3. Contains enzymes for metabolic functions.
4. Multiplies by binary fission.
5. It is a cocobacilli, measures 300 × 600 μm in size. Visible under light microscope.
6. It is gram-negative though it stains poorly.
7. Sensitive to many antibiotics.

Morphology

Rickettsia are pleomorphic coccobacilli, non-motile, non-capsulated and gram-negative. Stains purple with Giemsa stain (Fig. 10.17).

Cultural Characteristics

Does not grow on artificial media. It is cultivated in yolk sac of developing chick embryo.

Pathogenesis

Rickettsial diseases include:

1. Typhus (spotted fever).
2. Scrub typhus.
3. Trench fever.
4. Q fever.

Rickettsial diseases develop after infection through skin or respiratory tract. Ticks and mites transmit the agents of spotted fever and scrub typhus by inoculating the *Rickettsia* directly into the dermis during feeding. The louse and flea, which transmit typhus, deposit infect-

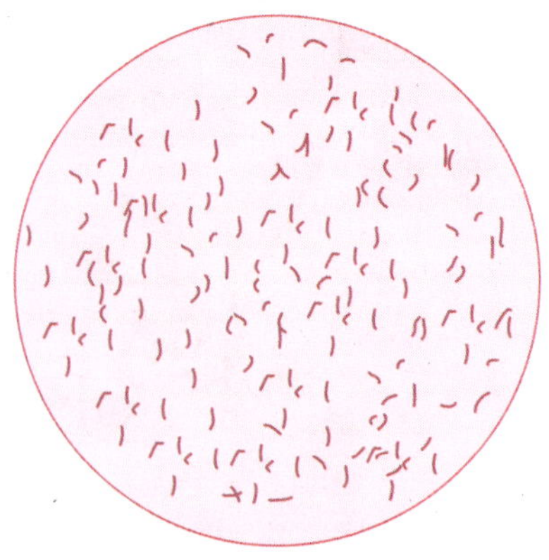

Fig. 10.17: Rickettsia

ed feces on the skin and infection occurs when organisms are rubbed into the puncture wound made by the arthropod. The *Rickettsia* of Q fever gain entry to the respiratory tract when infected dust is inhaled. After multiplication at the local sites, these enter the bloodstream.

Clinical Features

Except Q fever in which there is no skin lesions, rickettsial infections are characterized by fever, headache, malaria, prostration, skin rash and enlargement of spleen and liver. Q fever resembles influenza.

Laboratory Diagnosis

Either by isolation of the *Rickettsia* or by serology.

Serological diagnosis depends on demonstration of special antibodies in serum specimens and an increase in the antibody titers on the disease progress (Weil-Felix reaction).

Immunology

Immunology is the study of how the body protects itself against the harmful effects of pathogenic microorganisms and their toxins. It also deals with certain harmful consequences of immune mechanism such as allergy of hypersensitivity, a condition of over activity of immune system, autoimmune disorders and immune deficiency disorders. Immunity is the ability of the body to resist infection.

NATURAL IMMUNITY

Natural immunity is the resistance that is not acquired through a contact with antigen. It is non-specific and includes barriers to infectious agents, e.g. skin and mucous membranes, natural killer (NK) cells, phagocytosis, inflammation and a variety of other non-specific factors. It may vary with age and with hormonal and metabolic activity.

Defence Mechanism

Defence mechanism of body has many means of self-protection against invaders and they are considered in two categories.

Specific Defence Mechanism

Specific defence mechanism results in an immune response. The body can destroy them conferring resistance to specific microbes by hormones and/or cell-mediated immune processes.

Non-specific Defence Mechanism

The non-specific defence mechanism is against the invaders. The factors of non-specific defence mechanism are as follows:

1. Genetic factors.
2. Physical and mechanical barriers.
3. Biochemical factors.
4. Cellular factors.

1. Genetic factors

Race or strain: Blacks are more susceptible to tuberculosis than whites in the USA. But blacks have more resistance than whites to diphtheria, gonorrhea and influenza.

Sex: There are apparent differences in susceptibility between males and females due to hormonal differences.

Nutrition: Low-protein calorie diets produce a significant decrease in resistance to infection. Vitamin deficiencies cause problems. Vitamin A deficiency allows skin infection and blindness. Folic acid deficiency lowers the use of T cells. Thiamine and riboflavin deficiency lowers B-cell activity. Vitamin C deficiency causes increased bacterial infections.

Overnutrition can also be harmful. It may increase susceptibility to viruses and bacteria. When viral infection occurs, more viruses are produced in healthy cells rather than malnutritional cells. Also many bacteria need iron for growth. When the body has excess iron some of it becomes available for bacterial growth.

Hormone-related resistance: There is a relationship between hormonal imbalances and immunological response. Staphylococcal, streptococcal and fungal diseases occur more rapidly in people with diabetes. Similarly, pregnancy is associated with not only marked hormonal changes, but also an increase in the incidence of urinary tract infection (UTI) and poliomyelitis.

Age: The age of an individual has a marked influence on immunity. The very young and old are more susceptible due to gradual warning of their immune responses. The fetus *in vitro* normally is protected from maternal infection by placental barrier. But pathogens like umbella cross this barrier causing infection resulting in fetal death or malformation. This is due to immaturity of the immunal apparatus.

2. Physical and mechanical barriers

Skin: Very few organisms are capable of penetrating the intact skin, but can enter sweat or sebaceous glands, hair follicles and establish themselves there. Sweat and sebaceous secretions by virtue of their acid pH and certain chemical substances (especially fatty acids) exhibits antimicrobial properties that tend to eliminate pathogenic organisms. Lysozyme, an enzyme that dissolve some bacterial cell walls, is present on the skin and provide protection against certain microorganism. Lysozyme is also present in tears, in respiratory and cervical secretion.

Skin resistance: It may vary with age, e.g. children are highly susceptible to ring worm infection. After puberty, resistance to such fungal infections increases markedly with the increased content of fatty acids in sebaceous secretions. When skin is destroyed by burn or cuts, infection readily occurs.

Mucous membrane: In the respiratory tract a film of mucus covers the surface and is constantly being driven upwards by ciliated cells towards natural orifices. Bacteria tend to stick to this film. In addition, mucus and tears contain lysozyme and other substances with antimicrobial properties. For some microorganisms, the first epithelial cells show defence by means of bacterial surface proteins, e.g. pili of *Gonococcus* and *Escherichia coli.*

3. Biochemical factors

Lysozyme an enzyme in tears, saliva and sweat kills some bacteria. Other chemical barriers are sebaceous secretions (oil secreting glands of the skin) and sweat, which are acidic. Gastric juice contains HCl and so it is antibacterial.

Inner defense: Germs gaining access to the body barely causes infection, because of the effective clearing action of the body fluids and phagocytic cells.

Complement system: It is a complex system of proteins normally present in the serum. Once activated bys the immune mechanism, it promote phagocytosis, destruction of microbes with cytolysis (destruction of living cells by destruction of outer membrane). It also stimulates inflammatory reaction.

Interferons: Interferons are a group of proteins produced by a variety of cells infected by a virus. They confer protection on other cells and have a broad antiviral action.

4. Cellular factors in innate immunity

Phagocytosis: It is the recognition, engulfment and digestion of some particles by cells. To initiate this process, agents that can attract phagocytic cells to the particles must be present in the tissue. Substances that can act on chemical attractants include soluble bacterial products, histamine, compounds derived from complement system, F cells and their products. Molecules called opsonines are needed to promote the attachment of a phagocytic cell to the target particles. The most effective opsonin is the antibody to the foreign particles such as leukins is extracted from humoral factors.

Engulfment occurs when plasma membrane of phagocytic cells, flows completely around the particles followed by ingestion of the particles. This is facilitated by acid, a variety of hydrolytic enzymes stored within the phagocytes and oxidizing agents like H_2O_2, OH^- and superoxide anion radical, Cl_2.

There are two types of phagocytic cells derived from bone marrow. The granulocytes (neutrophils, eosinophils and basophils), which circulate only in the blood and migrate to the site of inflammation and the macrophages, which are found in blood and tissue. Macrophages are much more diverse in its function and respond more than granulocytes. The relative levels of phagocytic activity are macrophages, neutrophils, eosinophilis and basophils. In addition to taking part in phagocytosis, macrophages help to regulate the immune responses of the cells, for complement they help to bind antibodies and secrete several compounds in immune response.

   i. Macrophages includes:
      a. Histiocytes (wandering ameboid cells in tissue).
      b. Fixed reticuloendothelial cells.
      c. Monocytes.
   ii. Microphages, e.g. polymorphonuclear (PMN) leukocytes or white blood cells (WBCs).

Inflammation: Tissue injury or irritation initiated by the entry of pathogens or other irritants leads to inflammation, which is an important non-specific mechanism of defence.

The polynuclear leukocytes escape into the tissues and accumulate in large number, attracted by the chemattractive substances released at the site of the injury. Microorganism are phagocytosed and destroyed. There is an out pouring of plasma, which helps to dilute the toxic product present. A fibrin barrier is laid, serving to wall off the site of infection.

Fever: A rise of temperature following infection is a natural defence mechanism and helps not only to accelerate physiological processes, but in many cases it actually destroy the infecting pathogens. Therapeutic induction of fever was employed for the destruction of *Treponema pallidum* in syphilis patients before penicillin. Fever stimulates the production of interferon and helps in the recovery from virus infections.

Adaptive specific factors are humoral due to antibodies and cell-mediated immunity.

CLASSIFICATION OF IMMUNITY

The resistance exhibited by the host against any foreign body (antigen) such as microorganisms is called immunity. This resistance can be either natural or acquired. Immunity is broadly classified into two, natural or innate and acquired (Fig. 11.1).

Innate Immunity

If the host exhibits resistance as a natural phenomenon it is called innate immunity, an individual possess it from birth. This is the first response exhibited by the body towards any antigen.

The mechanisms involved are as follows:

Skin: The dense normal flora on skin is always regulated by low pH due to sebum, desiccation, etc. If these properties are altered infection through skin may occur.

Mucous membranes: Mucous membranes of various body systems such as respiratory, gastrointestinal, genitourinary and eye prevent invasion of microorganisms. With the help of squamous epithelium, the mucus secretions form protective covering and trap many microorganisms.

Respiratory tract: The architecture of nose prevents entry of microorganisms to a large extent. If they enter the paricles are held at mucus lining the 'epithelium' and sent to pharynx where they are coughed or swallowed. Coughing and sneezing help removal of microorganisms from respiratory tract.

Gastrointestinal tract: The gastric juice is a mixture of hydrochloric acid, enzymes and is acidic (2–3 pH). This juice kills most microorganisms and their toxins. In intestine the mucosa contain lace-like network that removes small particles by peristalsis.

Genitourinary system: Kidneys, urethra, urinary bladder are sterile under normal conditions. The flushing action of the urine eliminates so many microorganisms. The acidity of vagina makes it unfavorable for the growth of microorganisms.

Eye: The conjunctiva of eye will be moist due to tears secreted by lacrimal glands. The tears

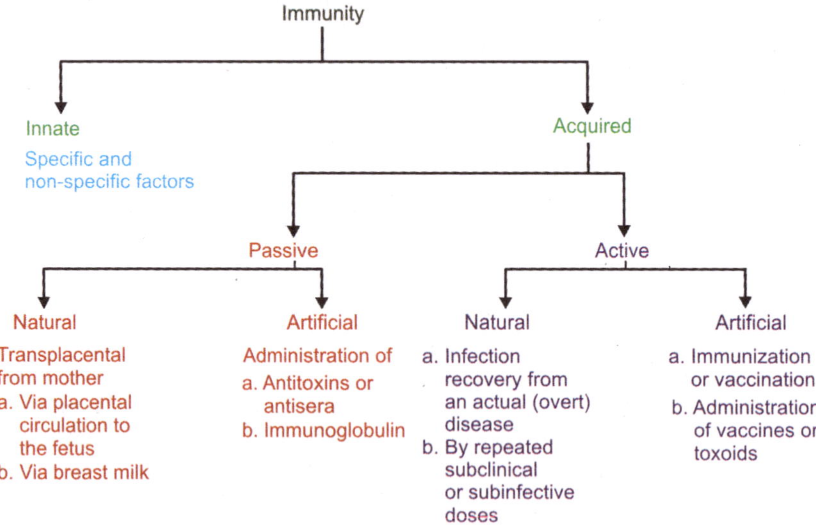

Fig. 11.1: Classification of immunity

contain lysozyme and acts on most of the microorganisms. Apart from these physical factors several other factors like age, hormones, nutrition, influence, innate immunity, inflammation, phagocytosis, complement system, interferons and fever also come under non-specific defense mechanisms.

Acquired Immunity

Acquired immunity is the resistance acquired by an individual during life time. Acquired immunity is of two types active and passive (Fig. 11.2).

Active Immunity

The resistance developed by an individual as a result of antigenic stimulus is called active immunity. It is also called adaptive immunity. Body synthesise antibodies and immunocompetent T cells in response to antigen. There are two types active immunity (Fig. 11.3). They are:

1. Naturally acquired active immunity.
2. Artificially acquired active immunity.

Naturally acquired active immunity: This immunity is acquired by natural infections by bacteria and viruses. Antibodies are produced in response to infection. In some cases the immunity may be lifelong as with small pox, measles or for few years (diphtheria, tetanus) or even lesser period (influenza, pneumonia).

Artificially acquired active immunity: It is achieved by vaccination or toxoid. Vaccines are killed or live attenuated microorganisms. Toxoids are inactive preparations of the toxins. The inactive forms of vaccines and toxoids can stimulate production of antibodies and provide long-term immunity. This is known as artificial because the antigens are intentionally introduced into host.

Passive Immunity

The resistance transmitted to recipient in 'readymade' form is known as passive immunity. There are two types of passive immunity:

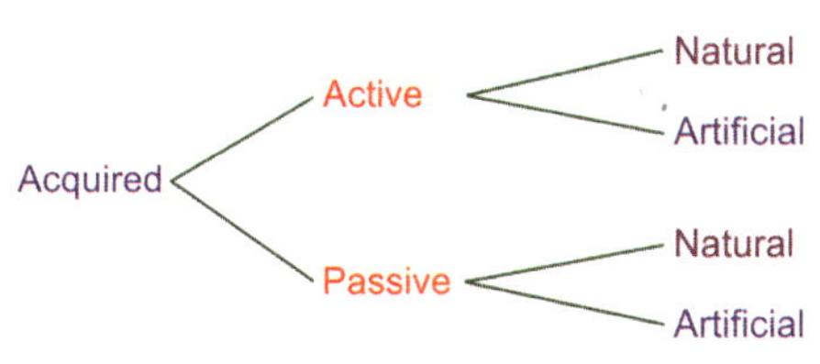

Fig. 11.2: Acquired immunity

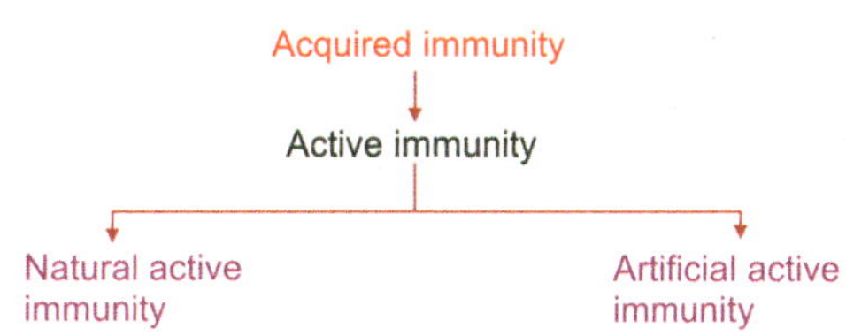

Fig. 11.3: Active immunity

1. Naturally acquired passive immunity.
2. Artificially acquired passive immunity.

Like active, in this there is no antigen stimulus instead preformed antibodies are administered.

Naturally acquired passive immunity: This occurs on transfer of antibodies immunoglobulin G (IgG) from mother to fetus and it lasts for 6 months. The maternal antibodies provide resistance to infections of streptococci, rubella, mumps, poliovirus, etc. As this immunity is developed under natural conditions it is known as natural and it is passive because recipient does not synthesize antibodies, but gets from donor.

Artificially acquired passive immunity: It is the resistance transferred to a recipient by administration of antibodies. The agents used for this purpose are hyperimmune sera of animal or human origin, convalescent sera, but this immunization should be given when necessary because in certain individuals it leads to allergic complications. Protection against snake bites and black widow spider is provided by passive immunity.

Comparison of active and passive immunity

Active immunity

1. Produced actively by host immune system.
2. Induced by infection or by immunogens.
3. Immunological memory present.
4. Not applicable in immunodeficient.
5. Long lasting and effective protection.

Passive immunity

1. Received passively. No active host participation.
2. Readymade antibody transfer.
3. No immunological memory.
4. Applicable in immunodeficient.
5. Protection short lived and less effective.

Sometimes a combination of active and passive methods of immunization is employed. This is known as combined immunization.

Local Immunity

Natural infection or the live viral vaccine administered orally or intranasally provide local immunity at the site of entry such as gut mucosa and nasal mucosa respectively.

Herd Immunity

Herd immunity refers to overall resistance in a community. When herd immunity is low, chances of epidemics increase on introduction of suitable pathogen. Eradication of epidemics, depends on herd immunity rather than individual.

ANTIGENS

Any foreign substance that can induce a detectable immune response is called antigen. Immune response means production of antibody or activation of immune cells. An antigen should possess two properties in order to establish any infection.

1. Antigenicity.
2. Immunogenicity.

The term antigenicity means the ability of a particle to be recognized by antibody.

Immunogenicity means ability of a particle to raise immune response.

Substances that are immunogenic are antigenic, but substances that are antigenic may not be immunogenic. The other name of antigens is immunogens.

Epitopes

In order to interact with antibody or immune cells, the antigen possess a recognition site. These are known as epitopes. An antigen can have many different epitopes.

Haptens

A low molecular weight compound that is not immunogenic by itself, but when coupled to another molecules (known as carrier) can produce immune response, e.g. dinitrophenol.

General Properties of Antigens

The properties, which make substance antigen are as follows.

Size

Molecular size of the antigen determines its antigenicity to a greater extent. If the molecular size is large (greater than 10,000) they show high antigenicity. If the molecular size is less (less than 5,000) they act as weak antigens, but in some cases low molecular substances like insulin and glucagons act as antigens.

Foreignness

In order to induce immune response in a host the antigen should be foreign or non-self. The animal body contains several self-antigen, but they are not recognized because during development of immune response tolerance of self-antigens takes place.

Chemical Nature

Out of the four major biomolecules, proteins act as effective antigens. When compared to carbohydrates and proteins, lipids and nucleic acid are less antigenic.

Charge

Immunogenicity is not restricted to any particular molecular charge—positive, negative and neutral substances can be immunogenic.

Conformation

Linear, branched polypeptides or carbohydrates are immunogenic. Molecules with any configuration can be immunogenic. The antibodies, which are produced against them will always be specific.

Species Specificity

Species specificity plays an important role in evolutionary relationships because tissues of all individuals in a species and in some cases closely related species contain species-specific antigens.

Iso Specificity

Isoantigens are found only in some members of a species, e.g. human erythrocyte antigens. The advantage of isoantigens is species may be grouped depending on presence of different isoantigen in members.

Auto Specificity

Auto means 'self'. They are non-antigenic, but in some cases like development of sperm where it is not treated as self because it is developed later, but not in embryonic life.

Organ Specificity

Organ-specific antigens are confined to a particular organ. Some organs like brain, kidney share specificity with that of another species.

Heterophile Specificity

The same or closely related antigens may sometimes occur in different biological species, classes and kingdoms. These are heterogenic antigens, e.g. Forssman antigen, which is a lipid carbohydrate complex, is widely distributed in many animals, birds, plants and bacteria.

ANTIBODIES

Antibodies or immunoglobulins (Ig) are glycoproteins formed by plasma cells in response to antigen and counteract with antigens with great specificity. They are found in serum and other fluids such as gastric secretions and milk. Serum containing antigen-specific antibody is called antiserum. Structure of antibody is given by GM Edelman and Porter and won Nobel Prize in 1970 in physiology and medicine for this contribution.

Structure of Immunoglobulin

Edelman and Porter treated IgG to papain and pepsin, which revealed that IgG is composed of two 50,000 molecular weight (MW) polypeptide heavy (H) chains and two 25,000 MW polypeptide light (L) chains. These are linked by disulfide bonds.

For each immunoglobulin, there are two fragment antigen-binding (Fab) sites, because they bind to antigen and one fragment crystallizable (Fc) site that crystallizes under freezing conditions (Fig. 11.4).

Heavy and Light Chains

Heavy chains possess more number of amino acids and are structurally different for each immunoglobulin class or subclass.

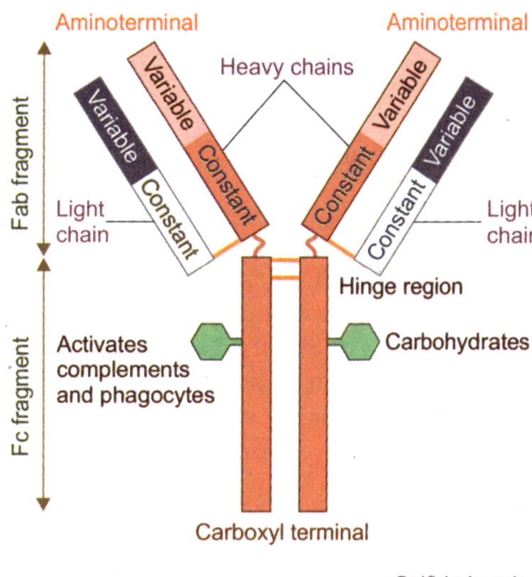

Fig. 11.4: Structure of immunoglobulin (Fc = Fragment crystallization; Fab = Fragment antigen binding).

Light chains possess lesser number of amino acids. Both H and L chains contain two different regions—constant region (C) and variable region (V). The amino acid sequences in constant region of H and L chains do not vary between antibodies of same class, but variable region of both the chains possess different amino acid sequences in different antibodies. The constant region of both H and L chains contain homologous units of 100 to 110 amino acids, each such unit is called constant domain (CH and CL respectively). Similarly, variable region of H and L chains possess variable domain (VH and VL respectively). Each light chain has a single variable domain (VL) or three and sometimes four constant domain as CH1, CH2, CH3 and CH4. Within each of both type of domains (constant and variable) disulfide bonds form a loop of approximately 60 amino acids. The antigen binding site of all antibodies is formed by cooperative interaction between variable domains of both H and L chains. The variable domains of both chains interact to form a molecular site that binds strongly, but non-covalently with the antigen. The strength of this binding is termed antigen-antibody affinity.

Classes or Types of Antibodies

The immunoglobulins are divided into five different classes:

1. Immunoglobulin G (IgG).
2. Immunoglobulin A (IgA).
3. Immunoglobulin M (IgM).
4. Immunoglobulin D (IgD).
5. Immunoglobulin E (IgE).

Immunoglobulin G

Immunoglobulin G (IgG) is termed as maternal antibody and is most abundant (80%) one. It has molecular weight of about 150,000 daltons. It is the only antibody that crosses placenta. H chain contains 440 amino acids, while L chain has 220 amino acids. There are four subclasses namely:

1. IgG1.
2. IgG2.
3. IgG3.
4. IgG4.

Immunoglobulin M

Immunoglobulin M (IgM) is the largest antibody and third most abundant (10%) in human serum. It is a pentamer, each possessing two H chains and two L chains. The monomers are held together by disulfide bonds and special J-chain (Fig. 11.5). IgM is the first immunoglobulin made.

Immunoglobulin A

Immunoglobulin A (IgA) is the second most abundant (15%) of total antibodies in humans and occurs in body fluids such as saliva, tears, breast milk and mucosal secretions from gastrointestinal, respiratory and genitourinary tracts.

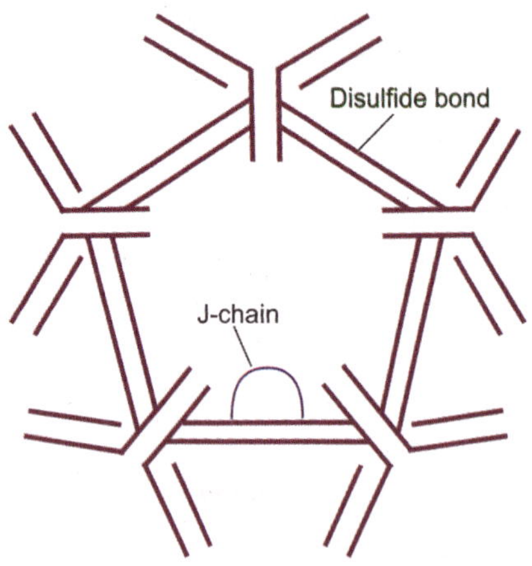

Fig. 11.5: Pentamer immunoglobulin M

Though it is a monomer initially, later it attains a secretary component and becomes dimer linked by J-chains and is known as secretary IgA.

Immunoglobulin D

Immunoglobulin D (IgD) occurs in low concentrations (only 0.2%). These are monomers and similar to IgG. IgD are short-lived. They play an important role in secondary immune response. They cannot cross placenta and occur in combination with IgM on surface of B lymphocytes.

Immunoglobulin E

Immunoglobulin E (IgE) occurs in extremely small amounts (0.002%). They mediate allergic reactions known as reagins. It shows affinity towards mast cells and is produced by linings of respiratory and intestinal tracts.

CELLS AND ORGANS OF IMMUNE SYSTEM

Immune system of an organism consists of several different organs and tissues in the body (Fig. 11.6). The organs are of two types:

1. Primary lymphoid organs—cell (lymphocytes) maturation.
2. Secondary lymphoid organs—trap antigens and make available for mature lymphocytes.

Cells of Immune System

Cells that play important role in development of immune response are known as leukocytes, of these lymphocytes are the chief cells of immune response.

Lymphoid Cells

In blood, of total white blood count 20% to 40% of cells will belong to lymphocytes and in the lymph 99 percent. Lymphocytes are classified into three types:

1. T cells.
2. B cells.
3. Null cells.

B lymphocytes: They are matured in bone marrow of mammals and in bursa of Fabricius in birds. These cells contain unique IgM receptor and are known as naive cells. When they encounter antigen, cell gets activated and divides into memory B cells and effector B cells or plasma cells.

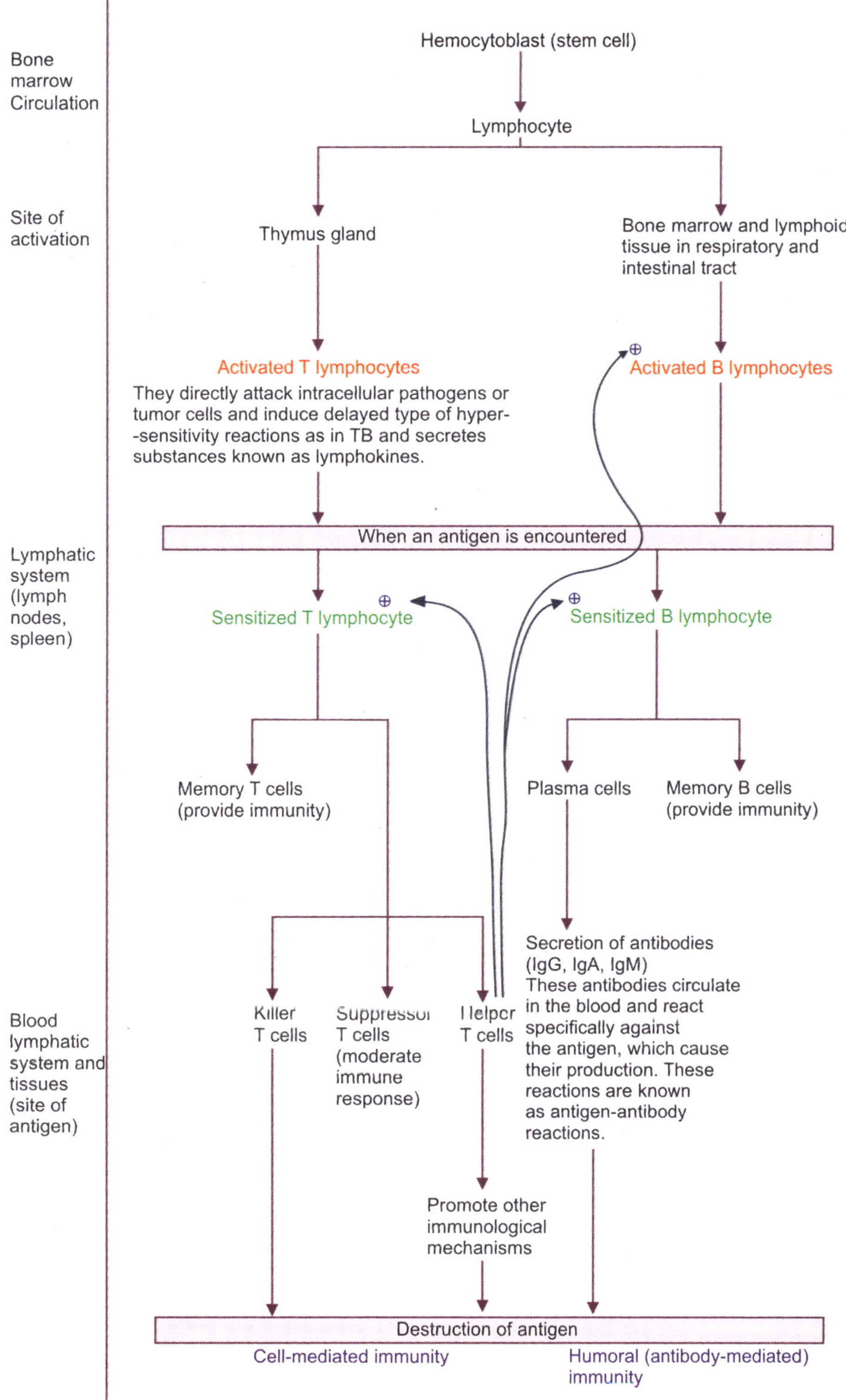

Fig. 11.6: Summary of immunity (note that helper T cells influence cell-mediated and humoral immunity) TB = Tuberculosis; Ig = Immunoglobulin.

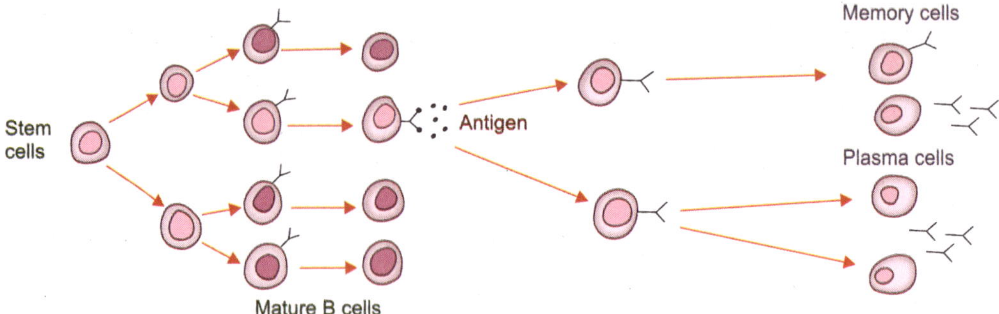

Fig. 11.7: B lymphocytes

Memory B cells continue to express membrane bound antibody where as plasma cells produce antibodies. They are responsible for humoral immunity (Fig. 11.7).

T lymphocytes: They mature in thymus. They possess antigen receptor known as T cell receptor (TCR) and these are also known as naive, which on binding with antigen divides into memory T cells and effector T cells. They are responsible for cell-mediated immunity. Apart from these there are other kinds of T cells.

- T_H cells—recognize and interact with antigen.
- T_C cells—activated under influence of cytokines.
- T_S cells—suppress humoral and cell-mediated immunity.

Null cells: These cells lack immunologic memory and specificity and are known as natural killer cells. They interact with tumor cells.

Mononuclear Phagocytes

Mononuclear phagocytes consist of monocytes in circulating fluid and macrophages in tissues. Monocytes first circulate in fluid and then differentiate into specific tissue macrophages (Fig. 11.8). For example:

Liver—Kupffer cell.
Lung—Alveolar macrophages.
Connective tissue—Histiocytes.
Bone—Osteoclasts.
Brain—Microglial cells.
Macrophages exhibit phagocytosis.

Granulocytes

On the basis of morphology and staining property, granulocytes are classified into three types (Fig. 11.9).

Neutrophils: They are predominant among white blood corpuscles and are produced in bone marrow. They have a multilobed nuclei and granulated cytoplasm that stains with both basic and acidic stains.

Eosinophils: They are mobile and show phagocytosis and are bilobed, but major role is defence against parasitic organisms.

Basophils: They are non-phagocytic and single lobed cells, they play major role in type I hypersensitivity reaction.

Mast Cells

Mast cells are produced in bone marrow. They play a major role in allergic reactions. They are found in all parts of the body.

Dendritic Cells

Dendritic cells possess long membrane and are classified on the basis of their location as:

Langerhans cells: Found in epidermal layer of skin and mucous membrane.

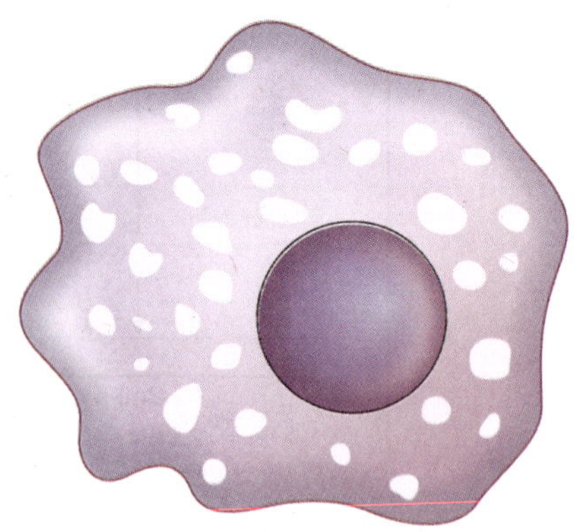

Fig. 11.8: A macrophage cell

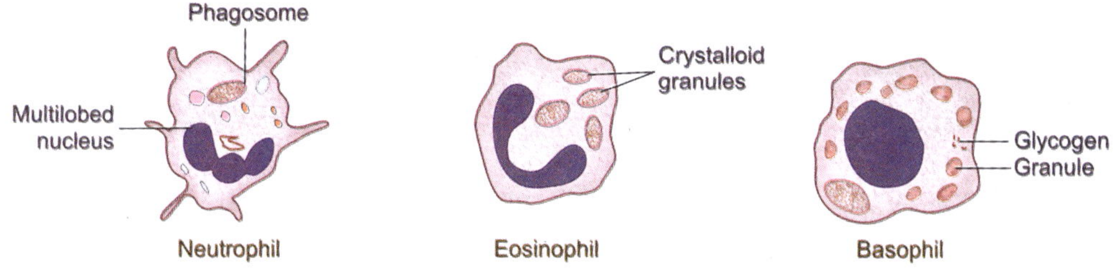

Fig. 11.9: Granulocytes

Interdigitating dendritic cells: Found in T cell areas of secondary lymphoid tissue and thymic medulla.

Interstitial cells: Found in heart, lungs, liver, kidney, blood. The circulating dendritic cells constitute about 0.1 percent of blood leukocytes and those in lymph.

Organs of Immune System

The organs of immune system are classified into:

1. Primary or cental lymphoid organs.
2. Secondary or peripheral lymphoid organs.

Primary or Central Lymphoid Organs

Thymus: It is a greyish, flat, bilobed lymphoid organ and acts as a site of development and maturation of T lymphocytes or T cells. The average weight of thymus is 10 g in infants and in old age the weight of thymus becomes 3 g. It is surrounded by capsule separated by trabeculae. Each lobule is organized into outer cortex and inner medulla (Fig. 11.10).

Bone marrow: This is the site of origin of B lymphocytes or B cells. It is equivalent to bursa of Fabricius in birds. Development of B lymphocytes begins with differentiation of lymphoid stem cells into earliest progenitor B cells, which proliferate within bone marrow.

Bursa of Fabricius: It is primary lymphoid organ in birds to produce B lymphocytes or B cells. Like thymus, bursa of Fabricius starts to shrink at puberty.

Secondary or Peripheral Lymphoid Organs

Lymph nodes: Lymph nodes are small bean-shaped clusters and contains three regions paracortex, cortex and medulla (Fig. 11.11).

Cortex is outer most region and contain lymphocytes, macrophages and dendritic cells arranged in follicles. Deeper region lying beneath cortex is paracortex and possess T lymphocytes. Medulla is inner most region with lymphoid lineage cells.

Spleen: The spleen is about 5 inches long and 200 g in weight. It traps blood-borne antigens, which contains capsule with trabeculae. It contains red pulp with erythrocytes, macrophages and white pulp with T lymphocytes.

Mucosal-associated lymphoid tissue (MALT): The group of organized lymphoid tissues lining mucous

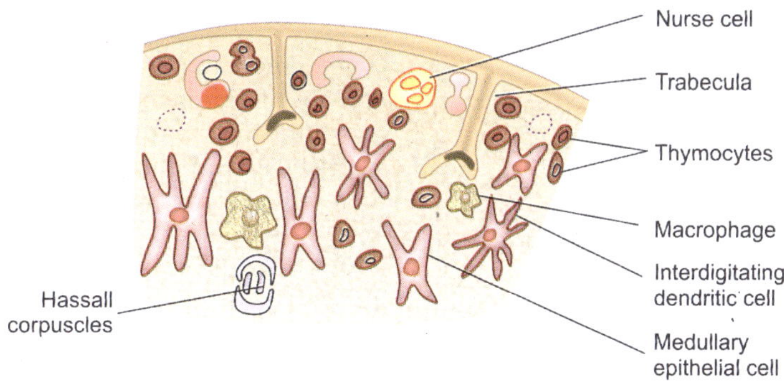

Fig. 11.10: Sectional view of thymus

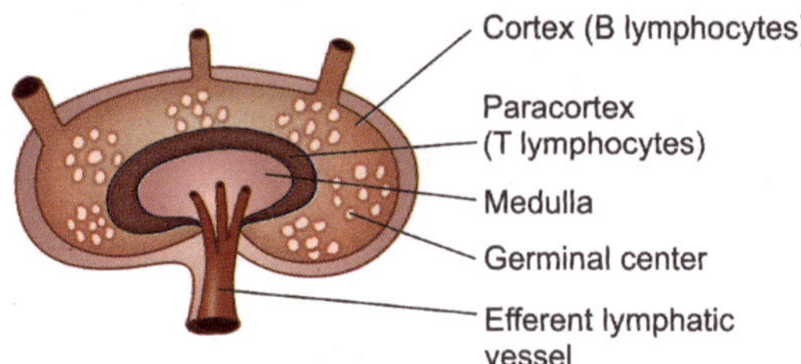

Fig. 11.11: Lymph node

membranes of alimentary, respiratory and genitourinary system are known as mucosal associated lymphoid tissue. The most studied one is the gut-associated lymphoid tissue (GALT). It contains large number of antibody producing plasma cells.

Tonsils: There are three groups of tonsils at three different locations: palatine, lingual and pharyngeal.

Palatine—occur at sides of back of mouth.

Lingual—basal region of tongue.

Pharyngeal—roof of nasopharynx.

They possess lymphocytes, macrophages, mast cells and granulocytes.

Peyer's patch: It occurs beneath lamina propria under epithelial layer of intestinal villi. It contains 30 to 40 lymphoid follicles.

Lamina propria: It occurs under epithelial layer of intestinal villi and contain large number of plasma cells, macrophages and activated T4 cells.

IMMUNE RESPONSE

The specific reactivity induced in host following antigen stimulus is known as immune response. It is of two types:

1. Humoral or antibody-mediated immunity.
2. Cell-mediated immunity.

Humoral Immunity

Humoral immunity or antibody-mediated immunity is the one where B lymphocytes synthesize antibodies in response to antigens. The B cells after antigenic stimulus convert into two different cell populations—plasma cells and memory cells. The plasma cells produce antibodies, which clump together with antigens present in circulatory systems forming antibody-antigen complex, which are taken by scavenger WBCs (Fig. 11.12).

Cellular Immunity

Cellular immunity is where T lymphocytes destroy other cells having antigens on their surface without any antibodies. When T cell matured in thymus encounter any antigen, they get differentiated into cytotoxic T lymphocyte, helper T cells and supressor cells and also release lymphokines. T cells posses T-cell receptors and respond only to major histocompatability complex (MHC), antigens and then lyse antigen. It also regulates tumor development (Fig. 11.13).

Primary and Secondary Immune Responses

Both humoral and cell-mediated responses are divided into two groups:

1. Primary.
2. Secondary.

The naive B cells and T cells that encounter antigen proliferate and differentiate into two types of plasma and memory cells. This is called primary immune response. It has lag phase where B cells proliferate and differentiate into plasma and memory cells. Following this serum antibody level increases, reaches peak at about day 14, remains at a plateaus for some time and then begins to drop off as plasma cells begin to die. The memory cells remain in G_o phase and have longer life. When antigen enters body for second time antibodies react fastly, which is known as secondary immune response.

In similar manner, recognition of an antigen MHC by T cell induces plasma memory cells. They bring primary immune response, which is relatively slower. It takes about 10 to 14 days—later if antigen enters for the second time, memory cells attacks faster than the primary response.

COMPLEMENT SYSTEM

Complement (C) is defined as a system of some non-specific proteins present in normal human and animal serum, which are activated characteristically by antigen and antibody reaction thus removing antigens. Components are designated by numeral, e.g. C1 to C9. It has the following functions:

- Lysis of cells
- Opsonization
- Activation of immune response
- Removal of immune complex.

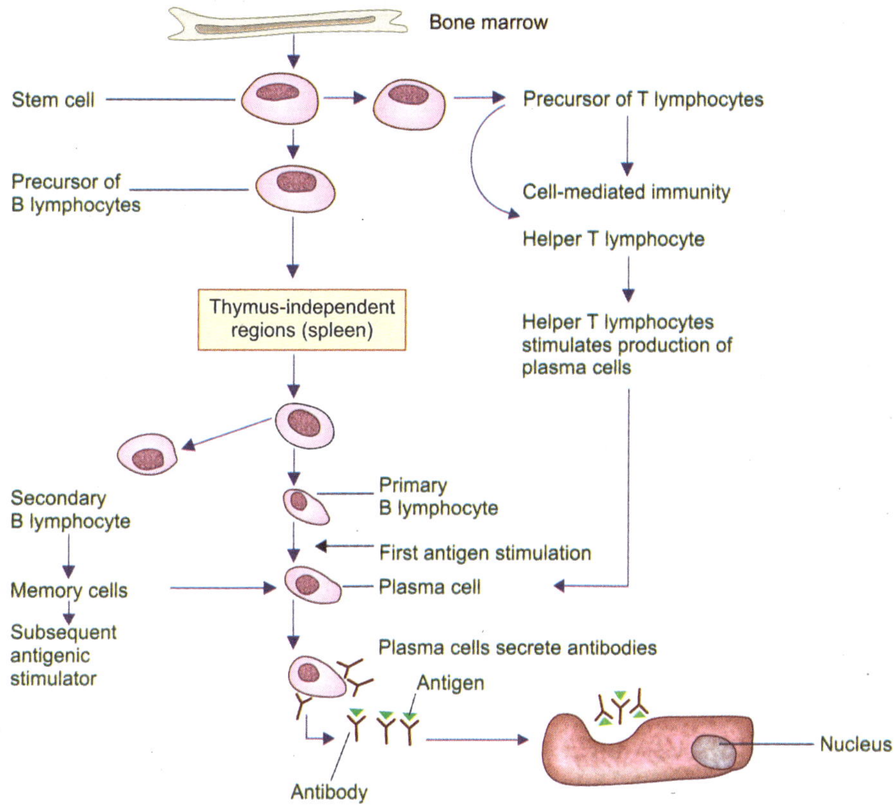

Fig. 11.12: Humoral (antibody-mediated) immunity

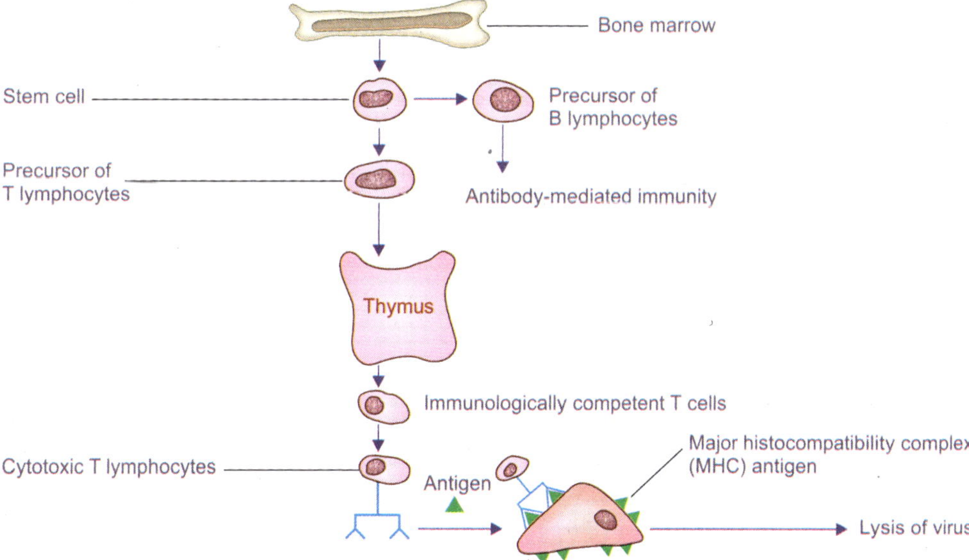

Fig. 11.13: Cellular immunity—major histocompatibility complex (MHC)

It has two pathways:
1. Classical pathway.
2. Alternative pathway.

Classical Pathway

Complement activation begins with soluble immune complex, IgM and IgG activate classical pathway complement, which binds to antigen-antibody complex that has 22 subunits. The recognition unit of C1 is C1q. Thereafter IgM and IgG activate the complex in the presence of calcium ions leading to activation of C1r and C1s. Activated C1s cleaves C4 into C4a and C4b, which binds to cell membrane along with C1.

C4b in the presence of magnesium ions cleaves C2 into C2a, which remains linked to cell bound C4b and C2b, which is released into fluid. C4b2a has enzymatic activity and referred to as classical pathway C3 convertase.

C3 convertase splits C3 into C3a, which is anaphylatoxin and C3b remains cell bound along with C4b2a to C4b2a3b, which is called C5 convertase.

The membrane attack phase begins at this stage with C5 convertase cleaving C5 into C5a (it is released) and C5b, which joins cascade C6 and C7 together. A heat-stable trimolecular complex C567 is formed, part of which binds to cell membrane and prepares it for lysis by C8 and C9, which join subsequently. Most of C567 escape and serve to amplify the reaction by absorbing unsensitised cells and rendering them susceptible to lysis by C8 and C9. In this process, holes of approximately 100 A° in diameter are produced.

Alternative Pathway

Alternative pathway is initiated by various cell surface constituents for both gram-positive and gram-negative bacteria. The serum C3 undergoes spontaneous hydrolysis at slow rate to yield C3a and C3b. The C3b binds foreign antigens, e.g. those on bacterial cells or virus particles. C3b now binds to factor B. This factor B is cleaved by D to generate Ba and Bb. Bb remains with C3b to give complex C3bBb, which act as convertase. Complex C3bBb accelerates hydrolysis of C3, so that C3b molecules deposit on antigen surface. C3b fragment associates with C3bBb to give rise to C3bBb3b complex, which acts as C5 convertase to generate C5b.

MAJOR HISTOCOMPATIBILITY COMPLEX

Major histocompatibility complex (MHC) in humans is known as human leucocytes antigen (HLA) complex.

HLA Complex

Histocompatability antigens means cell surface antigens that evoke immune response to an incompatible host resulting in allograft rejection. The genes coding them is known as HLA complex. The HLA complex is grouped into three classes.

Class I MHC

These are present on surface of all nucleated cells. They are involved in graft rejection and cell-mediated cytolysis. The cytotoxic T cells (CD_8) recognize MHC class I antigen for their action.

Class II MHC

They have limited distribution and found on surface of macrophages monocytes, activated T lymphocytes (CD_4) and B lymphocytes. They are primarily responsible for the graft versus host response.

Class III MHC

Class III genes encode C_2, C_4 complement components of classical pathway and properdin in factor B of alternative pathway.

HARMFUL EFFECTS OF IMMUNITY

1. Autoimmunity.
2. Hypersensitivity.

Autoimmunity

Autoimmunity is a condition in which immune responses occur to self-antigens resulting in structural and functional damages to the host. Autoimmunity involves both humoral and cell-mediated responses. Examples of autoimmune diseases include:

a. Autoimmune hemolytic anemia.
b. Thyrotoxicosis (Graves' disease).
c. Myasthenia gravis.
d. Rheumatoid arthritis.

Hypersensitivity

Immune system is essential for defending an individual against microorganisms. In this process, slight inflammatory reactions may occur, while removing the antigen, but the host tissue will not be damaged severly. In rare cases this inflammatory response becomes more severe and cause tissue damage such a reaction is called hypersensitivity or allergy.

Hypersensitivity can be classified into four classes (Table 11.1).

Type I Hypersensitivity (Anaphylaxis, IgE or Reagenic Dependent)

Allergens are responsible for type I hypersensitivity reactions. Allergens like other antigens stimulate production of antibodies resulting in production of antibody secreting plasma cells and memory cells. But these plasma cells secrete excessive quality of IgE. The IgE antibody has Fc receptors on mast cells and basophill cells, it sensitizes them. Such cells when react with allergens through IgE bring degranulation of cells, which brings smooth muscle contraction, vasodilation and increased vascular permeability (Fig. 11.14).

Hay fever, asthma, food allergies, erythema, etc. are the examples of Type I hypersensitive reactions.

Type II Hypersensitivity (Antibody Mediated, Cytotoxic)

Type II hypersensitivity is initiated by cell surface bounded antigens and is mediated by IgG and IgE antibodies specific to these antigens. The antibodies bind to cell surface of antigens. This either activates the complement system (Fig. 11.15) or cytotoxic T cells (antibody dependent cell-mediated cytotoxicity [ADCC]) lead-

Table 11.1: Classification of hypersensitivity

Type	Immunoglobulin involved		Cellular involvement
Antibody mediated (or immediate)			
Type I	Reagenic or anaphylaxis	IgE*	Mast cells, basophils
Type II	Cytolytic or cytotoxic	IgG† or IgM‡	RBCs§, WBCs‖, platelets
Type III	Immune complex	IgG or IgM	Host tissue
Cell mediated (or delayed)			
Type IV	Release of cytokines	None	T cells

*IgE = Immunoglobulin E; †IgG = Immunoglobulin G; ‡IgM = Immunoglobulin M; §RBCs = Red blood cells; ‖WBCs = White blood cells

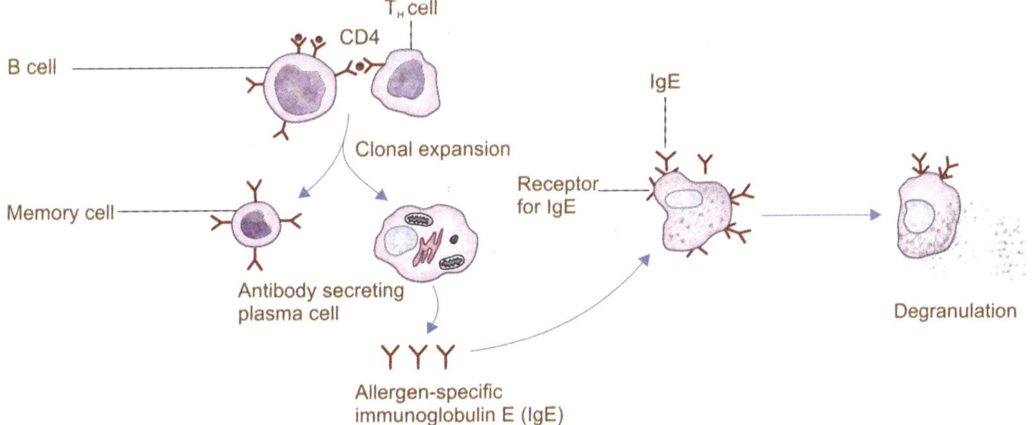

Fig. 11.14: Type I hypersensitivity (Anaphylaxis)

ing to destruction of target cells. In the case of cytotoxic T (T_C) cells, activated T_C cells secrete cytokines leading to cell death.

Blood transfusion, erythroblastosis fetalis, autoimmune hemolytic anemia are examples of type II hypersensitivity.

Type III Hypersensitivity (Antigen-antibody Complex)

Generally when antigen and antibody react, they generate immune complexes, which is cleared from the body of phagocytic cells. In some cases, large amount of immune complexes are formed, which cannot be easily cleared by phagocytic cells, resulting in tissue damage. If immune complexes activate complement system, they stimulate neutrophils and increase vascular permeability. If immune complexes attach to basement membrane of kidney and blood vessels, they interfere with phagocytosis and also cause tissue damage. Therefore, type of lesion caused depends on site of immune complexes (Fig. 11.16).

Arthus reaction and serum sickness are the best examples for type III reactions.

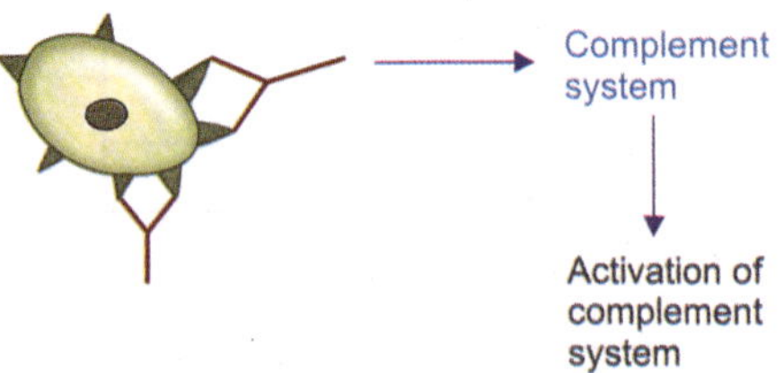

Fig. 11.15: Type II hypersensitivity (Cytotoxic)

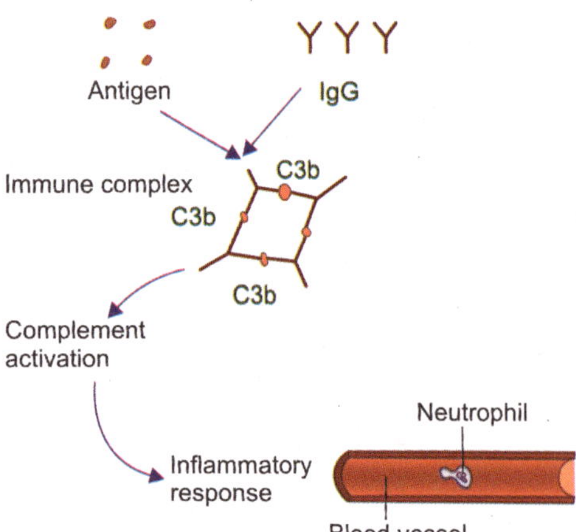

Fig. 11.16: Type III hypersensitivity (immune complex); IgG = Immunoglobulin G.

Type IV Hypersensitivity (Cell Mediated)

Type IV is initiated by soluble antigens, which activate T4 cells. The activated T4 cells release cytokines that activate macrophages or cytotoxic cells, which mediate direct cellular damage. Activated T_C cells secrete various cytokines, which act as effector molecules in this type of hypersensitivity (Fig. 11.17). Typical examples are contact dermatitis, tubercular lesions and graft rejection. This is known as delayed hypersensitivity, because it takes days to manifest from the time the subject comes in contact with the offending antigen (Fig. 11.17).

IMMUNE DEFICIENCY DISEASES

Immune deficiency diseases are conditions when defence mechanisms in the body are impaired leading to repeated infections. Deficiencies of defence mechanisms involve humoral immunity and specific mechanisms like phagocytosis and complement.

Autoimmune Diseases

Normally an immune response is mounted only against foreign (non-self) antigen, but occasionally the body fails to recognise its own tissues and attacks itself. The resulting autoimmune disorders of type II hypersensitivity include a number of relatively common conditions.

Rheumatoid Arthritis

The body produces antibodies to the synovial membranes. In most sufferers, the antibody can be detected in the blood called rheumatoid factor, it binds to the synovial membrane, leading to chronically inflamed joints that are stiff, painful and swollen.

Hashimoto Disease

The body makes antibodies to thyroglogulin, leading to destruction of thyroid hormone and hyposecretion of the thyroid.

Graves' Disease

The body makes antibodies to thyroid cells. Unlike Hashimoto disease, however, the effect of the antibodies is to stimulate the gland, with a resultant hyperthyroidism.

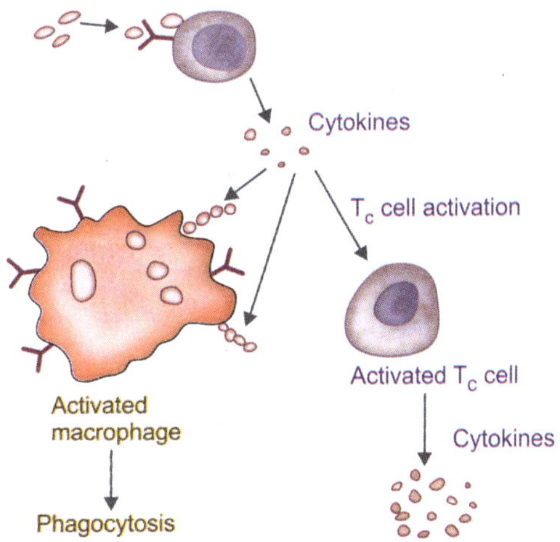

Fig. 11.17: Type IV hypersensitivity (delayed)
Tc = Cytotoxic T cells

Autoimmune Hemolytic Anemia

In this, individuals make antibodies to their own red blood cells (RBCs), leading to hemolytic anemia.

Myasthenia Gravis

Myasthenia gravis is an autoimmune condition of unknown origin, affects more women than men and usually those between 20 and 40 years. Antibodies are produced that bind to and block the acetylcholine receptors of neuromuscular junctions. The transmission of nerve impulses to muscle fibers is therefore blocked. This causes progressive and extensive muscle weakness, although the muscles themselves are normal. Extrinsic and eyelid muscles are affected first, causing ptosis (drooping of the eyelid) or diplopia (double vision), followed by those of the neck (possibly affecting chewing, swallowing and speech) and limbs. There are periods of remission, relapses being precipitated by strenuous exercise, infections or pregnancy.

Immunodeficiency

When the immune system is compromised, there is a tendency to recurrent infections, often by microbes not normally pathogenic in humans (opportunistic infections). Immunodeficiency is classified as primary (usually occurring in infancy and genetically mediated) or secondary, i.e. acquired in later life as the result of another disease, e.g. protein deficiency, acute infection, chronic renal failure, bone marrow diseases, following splenectomy or acquired immunodeficiency syndrome (AIDS).

Acquired Immunodeficiency Syndrome

Acquired immunodeficiency syndrome (AIDS) is caused by the human immunodeficiency virus (HIV), an ribonucleic acid (RNA) retrovirus, which produces the enzyme reverse transcriptase inside the cells of the infected person (host cells). This enzyme transforms viral RNA to deoxyribonucleic acid (DNA) and this new DNA called the provirus, is incorporated into the host cell DNA. The host cell then produces new copies of the virus that pass out into tissue fluid and blood and infect other host cells. When infected, host cells divide, copies of the provirus are integrated into the DNA of daughter cells, spreading the disease within the body.

Human immunodeficiency virus (HIV) has an affinity for cells that have a protein receptor called cluster of differentiation 4 (CD4) in their membrane, including T lymphocytes, monocytes, macrophages, some B lymphocytes and possibly, cells in the gastrointestinal tract and neuroglial cells in the brain. Helper T cells are the main cells involved. When infected their number is reduced, causing suppression of both antibody-mediated and cell-mediated immunity with the consequent development of widespread opportunistic infections, often by microbes of relatively low pathogenicity.

HIV has been isolated from semen, cervical secretions, lymphocytes, plasma, cerebrospinal fluid, tears, saliva, urine and breast milk. The secretions known to be especially infectious are semen, cervical secretions, blood and blood products.

Infection is spread by:
- Sexual intercourse, vaginal and anal
- Contaminated needles used:
    - During treatment of patients
    - When drug abusers share needles.
- An infected mother to her child
    - Across the placenta before birth
    - During childbirth
    - Possibly by breast milk.

The presence of antibodies to HIV indicates that the individual has been exposed to the virus, but not that a naturally acquired immunity has developed. Not all those who have antibodies in their blood develop AIDS although they may act as carriers and spread the infection to others.

A few weeks after initial infection there may be an acute influenza-like illness with no specific features, followed by a period of 2 or more years without symptoms.

Chronic HIV infection may cause persistent generalized lymphadenopathy (PGL). Some patients may then develop AIDS-related complex (ARC).

ANTIGEN-ANTIBODY REACTIONS

The antigen and antibody reactions are reversible and are highly specific. The reaction is very weak and is formed in between epitope of antigen and paratope of antibody (Fig. 11.18). Manifestation of immune reactions is given in Table 11.2.

Various types of antigen-antibody reactions are as follows.

Precipitation Reactions

Precipitation reaction takes place between soluble antigen and antibody. The reaction leads to precipitate formation and the antibody, which is responsible to form precipitate is called precipitin. In order to form a visible precipitate, the concentration of antigen and antibody should be equal in ratio. This stage is known as equivalence zone.

In laboratory, precipition reaction can be demonstrated in agarose gel on slides and test tubes by techniques such as immunodiffusion, radial immunodiffusion and immunoelectrophoresis.

Immunodiffusion

In this technique antigen-antibody diffuse radially on molten agar slide of 3 mm thickness and form a precipitin band at equilibrium.

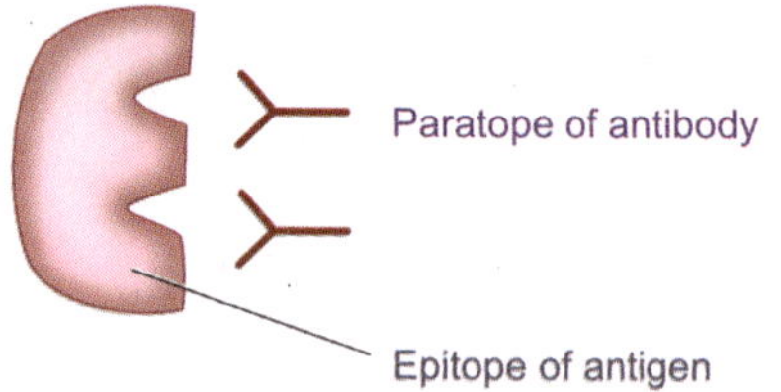

Fig. 11.18: Antigen-antibody reactions

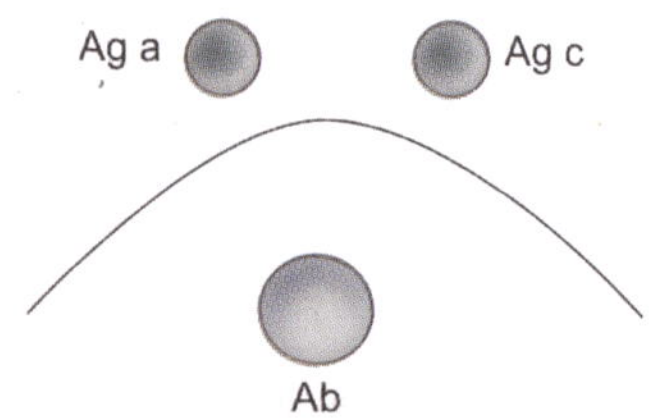

Fig. 11.19: Line of identity; Ab = Antibody; Ag = Antigen.

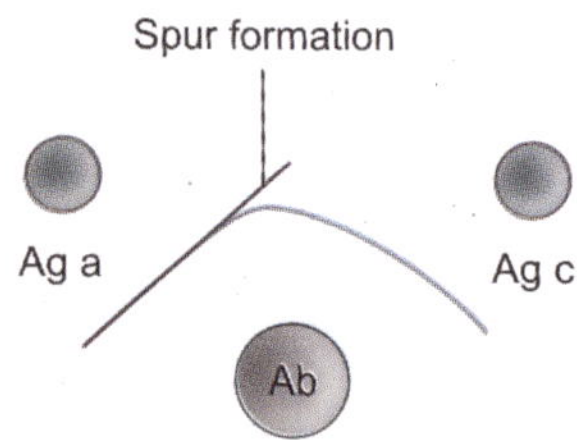

Fig. 11.20: Line of partial identity

Precipitin bands formed in this reaction can be classified into three types:

Line of identity: Band will be formed when the antigens posses identical epitopes against single antibody (Fig. 11.19).

Line of partial identity: Band is formed when antigens epitopes are partially similar a curved spur seen and is due to unique epitopes (Fig. 11.20).

Line of non-identity: Band would occur when two antigens are unrelated and do not share any epitopes (Fig. 11.21).

Table 11.2: Manifestation of immune reaction

Time required for manifestation	Chemical released	Examples
Minute	Heparin, histamine	Hay fever, food allergies, injectable antibodies (penicillin)
Variable hours to day	Complement system	Drug allergies, transfusion reaction
Variable hours to day	Immune complex	Serum sickness, Arthus' reaction
24 hour to day	Lymphokines	Contact dermatitis, tuberculosis, leprosy, kala-azar, measles and candidiasis

Radial Immunodiffusion

In this, the antibody is incorporated along with gel and antigens are added to the wells and allowed to diffuse. The precipitin ring is formed around the well, when equilibrium is reached (Fig. 11.22).

Immunoelectrophoresis

In this technique, firstly antigen is loaded in the well at one-fourth corner of a gel plate and connected to negative pole and electrophoresed after 1 hour, a trough is cut in the middle of the slide with the help of a fine blade and antiserum is loaded. The antiserum diffuses from trough and form differed bands with antigen components (Fig. 11.23).

If precipitation reactions are performed in test tubes, usually precipitate settles down the bottom of the tube. If it fails to sediment it remains

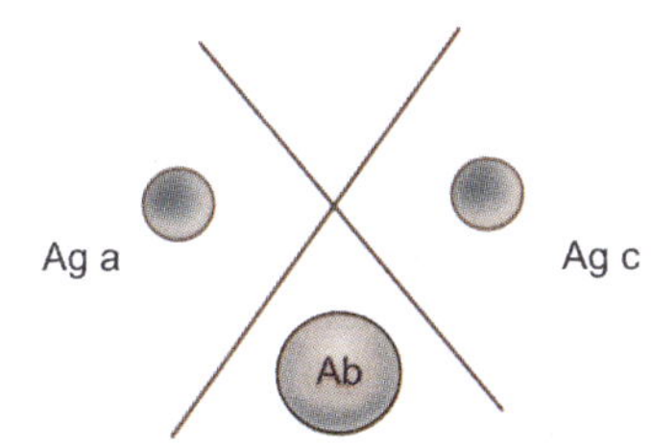

Fig. 11.21: Line of non-identity

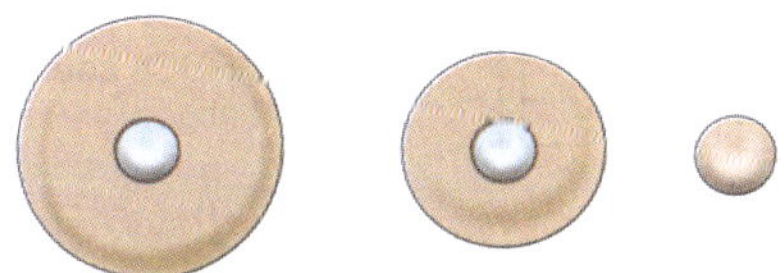

Fig. 11.22: Radial immunodiffusion

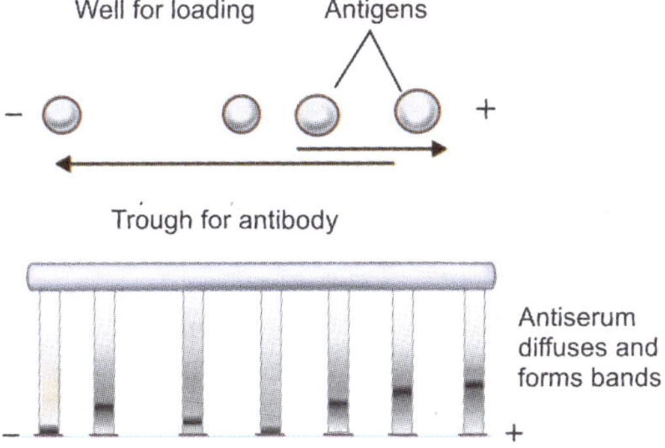

Fig. 11.23: Immunoelectrophoresis

suspended as floccules and the reaction is known as flocculation. Venereal Disease Research Laboratory (VDRL) test is the best example for flocculation test on slide.

Agglutination

Agglutination is an antigen-antibody reaction in which particulate antigen combines with its antibody in the presence of electrolytes at an optimal temperature and pH. The antibody involved in bringing about agglutination reaction is called agglutinin. As precipitation, agglutination occurs optimally when antigens and antibodies react in equivalent proportions.

Applications of agglutination reactions

Slide Agglutination

On a slide, when drop of appropriate serum or particulate antigen are mixed, agglutination takes place. Depending on concentration, clumping may occur instantly or within seconds. It is routinely used for the identification of clinical specimens, blood grouping and cross matching.

Tube Agglutination

Tube agglutination is carried out to identify the bacterial species as well as the infection rate. Generally antibodies are produced against surface antigens. In such cases serum is obtained from patient and is serially diluted (1 : 2, 1 : 4, 1 : 8, etc.) and to these equal volume suspected antigen is added. The last tube showing visible agglutination reaction will indicate the antibody titer of the patient. It is routinely employed for antibody detection in diagnosis of typhoid fever (Widal test) and typhus fever (Weil-Felix reaction).

Passive Agglutination Test

The major difference between agglutination and precipitation is nature of antigen, i.e. soluble antigen in the case of precipitation and particulate antigen in the case of agglutination. Precipitation tests can be converted into agglutination by attaching soluble antigens to surface of carrier particles. These are known as passive agglutination tests and are more sensitive.

Carrier particles such as RBC latex particles or bentonite are used. In both cases, the antigen

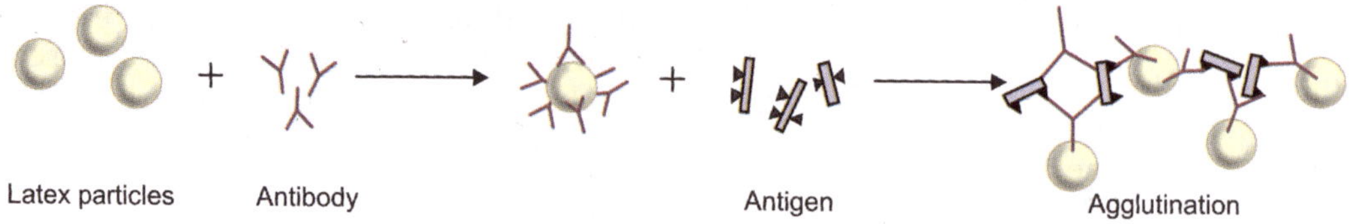

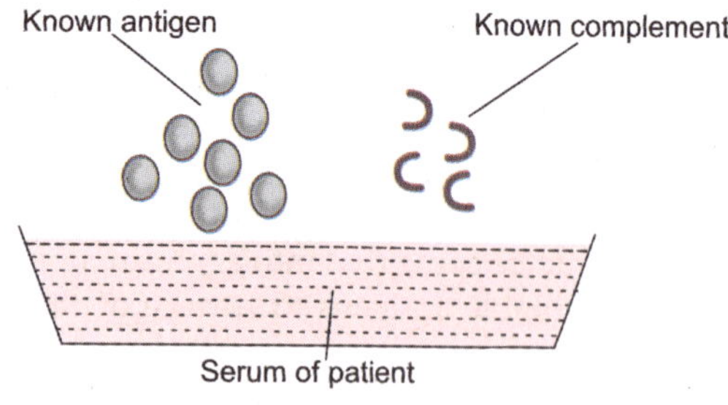

Fig. 11.24: Latex agglutination test

is coated with the respective carrier and diluted serum is added and the agglutination is observed (Fig. 11.24).

Complement Fixation Test

Complement fixation test (CFT) facilitate destruction of antigen-antibody complex by binding to Fc arm of IgG and IgM antibodies. In CFT, complement is attached to antibodies Fc fragment when antigen-antibody complex is formed. The actual test is done in two steps:

1. In the first step, patients serum to be tested for antibody or antigen is added to serum containing antigen or antibody. The mixture is incubated for antigen-antibody reaction. After some time, to this mixture known complement is added (Fig. 11.25).
2. In the second step, to the above mixture, sheep RBCs (SRBC) bound by anti-SRBC are added (Fig. 11.26).

The results can be interpreted like this. In the first step, if the antigen and antibody have formed the complex then the complement will be bound to this complex. Therefore complement will not be available for hemolysis of sensitized SRBCs when added to mixture. If in the first step, antigen-antibody complex did not occur then the complement will be freely available for sensitized SRBCs to undergo hemolysis (Fig. 11.27).

Immunofluorescence

Fluorescence is a property exhibited by certain dyes such as fluorescein and rhodamine, where in they absorb light of one wave length (UV light) and emit light at longer wave length (visible light).

For example, rhodamine absorb light in yellow green range at 515 nm and emits a deep red fluorescence at 546 nm. Immunofluorescence is of two types:

1. Direct immunofluorescence.
2. Indirect immunofluorescence.

Direct Immunofluorescence

In this method, the specific antibodies are conjugated to fluorescent substance and applied to detect unknown antigen. If the antigen is present it reacts with labeled antibodies and fluorescence can be observed under fluorescent microscope (Fig. 11.28).

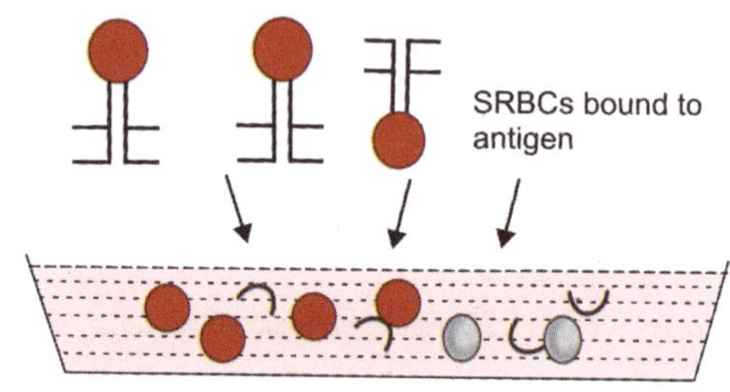

Fig. 11.26: Sheep red blood cells (SRBCs) bound by anti-SRBCs are added

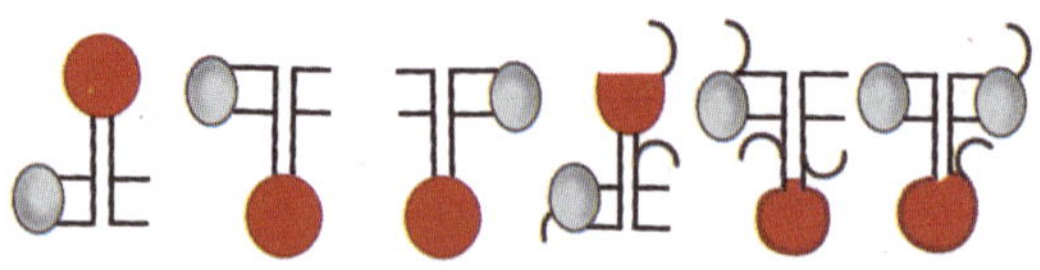

Fig. 11.25: Addition of antigen and complement to serum containing antibody

Fig. 11.27: Interpretation of complement fixation text

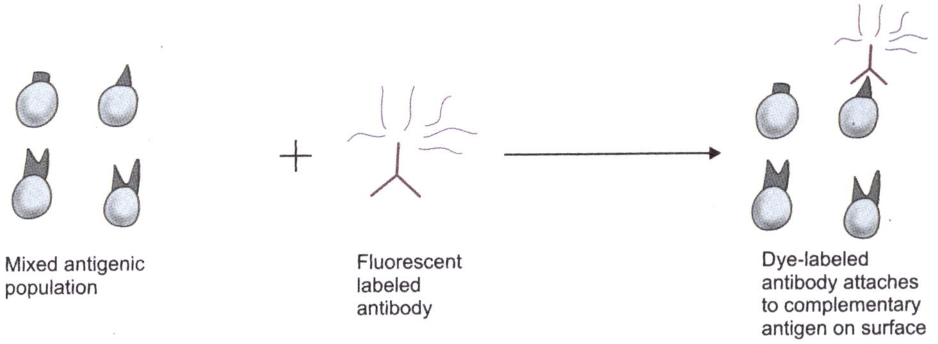

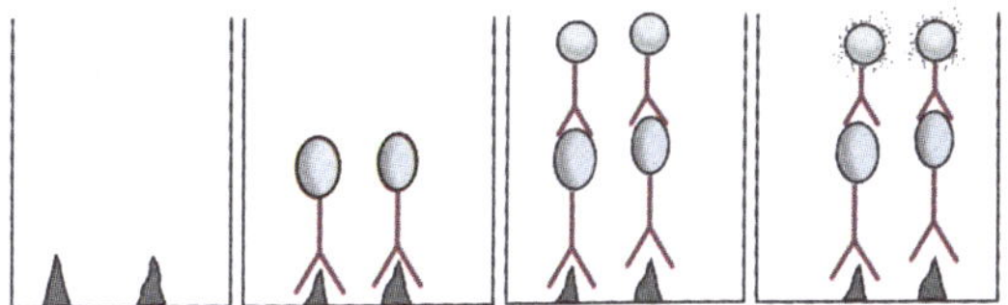

Fig. 11.28: Direct immunofluorescence

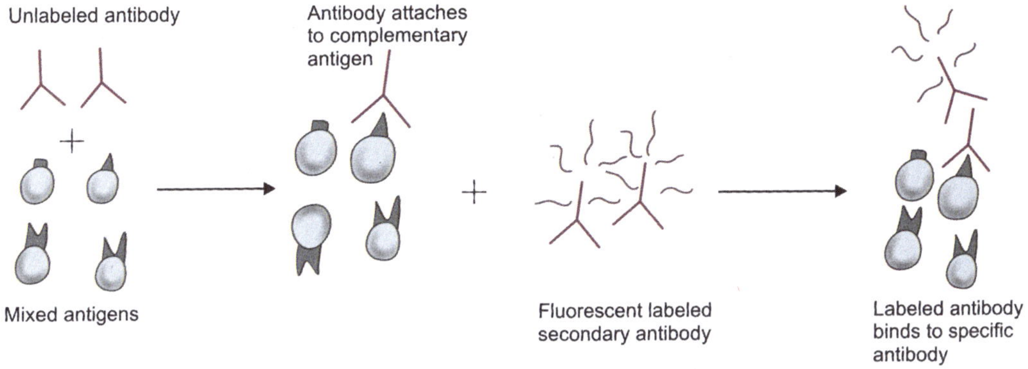

Fig. 11.29: Indirect immunofluorescence

Rabies virus and most of bacteria can be detected by this method.

Indirect Immunofluorescence

In this method, initially applied antibody is not labeled with dye. Instead secondary antibodies are applied, which are fluorescent labeled and binds to specific antibody that has already reacted with its complementary antigen present on surface of microbial cells in mixed population (Fig. 11.29).

Enzyme-linked Immunosorbent Assay Test

Enzyme-linked immunosorbent assay (ELISA) is widely used for detection of variety of antigens and antibodies. Here enzyme is used. It acts on substrate to produce color and can be done in polystyrene tubes (macro-ELISA) or polyvinyl microtiter plates (micro-ELISA). There are three methods:

1. Indirect.
2. Direct.
3. Competitive.

Indirect ELISA

The wells are coated with antigen and then sera is added. If antibody is present it binds to antigen. To detect this, goat anti-human immunoglobulin G conjugated with enzyme is added. It binds to antibody. To detect this binding substrate is added and enzyme acts on substrate to produce color in positive reaction (Fig. 11.30).

Sandwich ELISA

The wells are coated with antibody against antigen. Specimens are added. If antigen is present it binds to coated antibody. To detect this, antiserum conjugated with enzyme is added. This binds to antigen attached to coated antibody. A

Fig. 11.30: Indirect ELISA

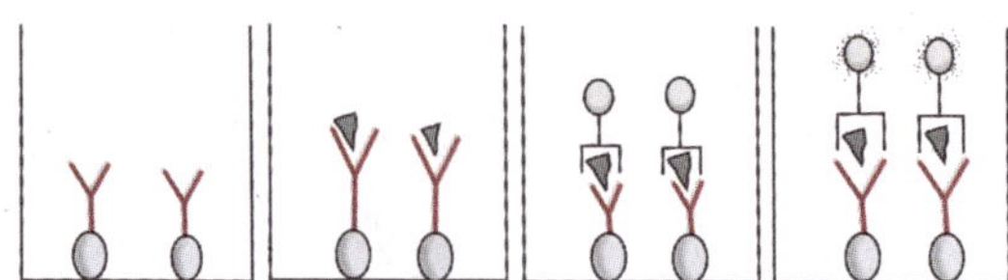

Fig. 11.31: Sandwich ELISA

substrate is added to know the binding of conjugated antiserum to antigen-antibody complex. In case of binding (positive result) an enzyme acts on substrate to produce color intensity and can be read (Fig. 11.31).

Competitive ELISA

Competitive E LISA is used for HIV virus detection. Positive result shows no color. Wells are coated with antigen and serum is added. If antibodies are present antigen-antibody reaction occurs. To detect this enzyme-labeled specific HIV antibodies are added. There is no antigen left for these antibodies to act. These antibodies remain free and washed off during washing. Substrate is added, but there is no enzyme to act to it. Therefore positive result shows no color (Fig. 11.32).

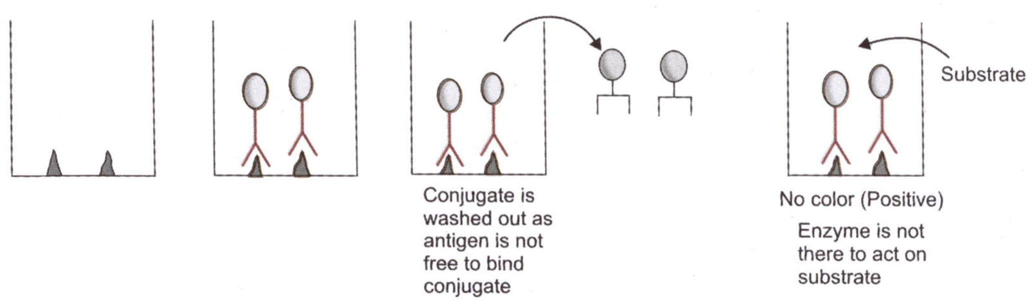

Fig. 11.32: Competitive ELISA

Immunization

IMMUNITY

Immunity can be acquired naturally or artificially and both forms may be active or passive. Active immunity means that the individual has responded to an antigen and produced his own antibodies. The lymphocytes are activated and the memory cells are formed to provide long-lasting resistance. In passive immunity, antibodies are produced by someone else. The antibodies are then destroyed unless lymphocytes are stimulated, passive immunity is short-lasting.

Antibody Production Following Immunization

When antigens, e.g. microbes are encountered for the first time, there is a primary response in which a low level of antibodies can be detected in the blood after about 10 days. Although the response may be sufficient to combat the antigen, the antibody levels then fall unless there is another encounter with the same antigen within a short period of time (2 to 4 weeks). The second encounter produces a secondary response in which there is a rapid response by memory B cells resulting in a marked increase in antibody production (Fig. 12.1). Further increases can be achieved by later encounters, but eventually a maximum is reached. This principle is used in active immunization against infective diseases like anthrax, rubella, cholera, small pox, diphtheria, tetanus, hepatitis B, tuberculosis, measles, typhoid, mumps, whooping cough and poliomyelitis.

Immunizing Agents

Immunizing agents are divided into vaccines (live attenuated, inactivated or killed vaccines) toxoids and immunoglobulins.

Vaccine is an immunological substance designed to provide specific protection against a disease. It stimulates the production of protective antibodies and other immune mechanisms. Vaccines may be prepared from live modified organisms or killed organisms, extracted cellular fractions, toxins or combination of both. More recent preparations are subunit vaccines and recombinant vaccines.

Examples of Immunizing Agents

1. Vaccines: Live attenuated vaccines—BCG (stands for Bacille Calmette-Guérin), oral polio (sabin); killed or inactivated vaccines—typhoid, cholera, rabies, polio (Salk).
2. Toxoids: Diphtheria, tetanus.
3. Immunoglobulin:
   a. Non-human immunoglobulins (antisera)——diphtheria, tetanus, gas gangrene, botulism, rabies.
   b. Human immoglobulins:
   - Human normal Ig, hepatitis A, measles, mumps
   - Human specific Ig, hepatitis B, varicella, diphtheria.

National Immunization Schedule

In 1974, the World Health Organization (WHO) officially launched a global immunization program known as expanded program on immunization (EPI) to protect all children from vaccine-preventable diseases. The Indian version of the universal immunization program was launched on November 19, 1985 and was dedicated to the memory of Smt Indira Gandhi. The national immunization schedule of India is as below:

1. For infants

   At birth: BCG and OPV '0' dose (for institutional deliveries)

   At 6 weeks   : BCG (if not given at birth)
   DPT – 1 and OPV – 1

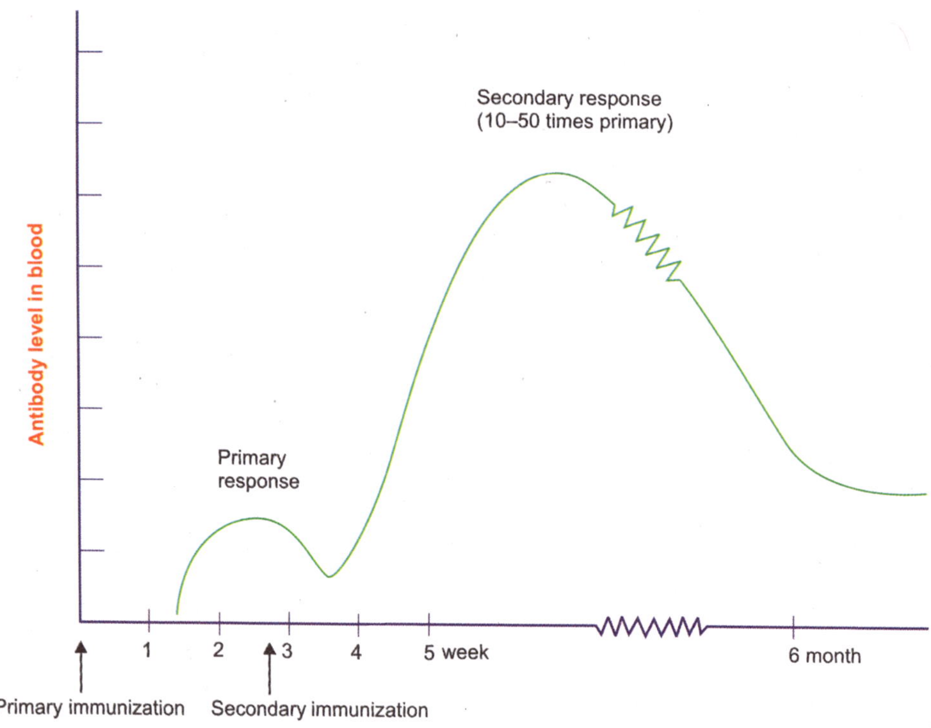

Fig. 12.1: Antibody response in immunization

At 10 weeks : DPT – 2 and OPV – 2
At 14 weeks : DPT – 3 and OPV – 3
At 9 months : Measles

2. At 16 to 24 months: DPT -1 (stands for diphtheria, pertussis, tetanus) and oral poliovirus vaccine (OPV).

3. At 5 to 6 years: DT (stands for diphtheria, tetanus); the second dose of DT to be given.

4. At 10 and at 16 years: Tetanus toxoid (TT); the second dose of TT vaccine to be given.

5. For pregnant women early in pregnancy: TT – 1 or booster, one month after TT – 1, TT – 2.

Note

1. Interval between 2 doses should not be less than 1 month.

2. Minor cough, colds and mild fever are not contraindicators to vaccination.

3. In some states, hepatitis B vaccine is given as a routine immunization.

VACCINES

Vaccination is based on the property of 'memory' of the immune system. In vaccination, a preparation of antigenic proteins of pathogens or inactivated pathogens is introduced into the body. These generate primary immune responses, B and T cells. When the vaccinated person is attacked by same pathogen, existing memory T or B cells recognize antigen quickly and remove it from the body. The term 'vaccine' is derived from Latin term 'Vacca' which means 'cow'. Edward Jenner was the first person to discover vaccine.

Vaccines can be grouped under following types:

1. Conventional vaccines.
2. Purified antigen vaccines.
3. Recombinant vaccines.

An ideal vaccine should possess the following features:

1. It should not be toxic.
2. It should have very low level of side effects.

3. It should not cause problems in individuals with an impaired immune system.
4. It should not contaminate environment.
5. It should be cheap.

Conventional Vaccines

Conventional vaccines consist of whole pathogenic organisms, which may be killed or may be live (the virulence of pathogenic organisms is reduced—attenuation). They are cheap and easy to produce, but in some cases there is a risk of disease development due to presence of active virus particle or reversion of virulence.

Purified Antigen Vaccines

Purified antigen vaccines are based on purified antigens isolated from the pathogens concerned, e.g. many bacteria produce exotoxins, the intensity decreases with storage but contain immunogenicity. They are called toxoids. Capsular polysaccharides, cell wall capsules can also be used in the production of purified antigen vaccines. Here, the risk of pathogenicity is less.

Recombinant Vaccines

Recombinant vaccines contains either protein or gene encoding a protein of a pathogen origin that is immunogenic, the vaccine is produced using recombinant DNA technology and is also called subunit vaccine.

Generally the whole protein molecule is not necessary. A small portion of the protein, i.e. polypeptide chain can be used as vaccine, e.g. foot and mouth disease vaccine.

DNA Vaccines

These are most advanced technique where the pathogenic gene itself is used as vaccines, either naked or inserted into suitable vector or after sufficient amount of protein is obtained.

BCG Vaccine

Bacille Calmette-Guérin (BCG) vaccine is used for tuberculosis (TB). This vaccine is routinely given to infants and small children in countries where TB is common. This vaccine contains a live attenuated (weakened) strain of *Mycobacterium tuberculosis*, the bacterium, which causes tuberculosis. The bacterium has been modi-

fied to produce a strain known as BCG strain, named after its discoverers. Killed vaccines (strain) cannot be used to protect against tuberculosis infections since they do not produce the necessary cellular immune response.

VACCINATION

A single dose of vaccine is administered into the skin over the upper shoulder area. Protection lasts for several years.

Polio

Poliomyelitis is caused by high infectious virus, which are known to affect only man. The virus is usually spread by contact with infected individuals via the waterborne route, though mouth-to-mouth transmission is also possible. The disease typically affects very young children, with 80% to 90% of cases occurring in children under 3 years of age.

Polio is a highly contagious disease. By the time a first case is detected in a family, all family members may have probably been infected due to the rapidity of viral spread. Viral spread is enhanced by crowding and poor sanitation.

Prevention Through Immunization

The use of the OPV was pioneered in the former Soviet Union and the approaches developed in that country led to rapid control or elimination of polio in many countries. The most prominent examples of the effectiveness of OPV is the success of the worldwide polio eradication program. Similarly Pulse Polio Program in India has gained tremendous momentum towards eradication of polio.

DTP Vaccine (Triple Antigen)

Combined DTP (diphtheria, tetanus, pertussis) vaccines have been in use worldwide since 1940s and have contributed substantially to the reduction in clinical pertussis.

Children given with 3 doses of this remarkable vaccine get good protection against three diseases namely diphtheria, tetanus and pertussis.

Diphtheria

Diphtheria is an infection that attacks the throat, mouth and nose. It is a very contagious disease (easy to get), but rare ever since the vaccine was created.

Tetanus

Tetanus is an infection caused by a bacteria found in dirt, gravel and rusty metal. It usually enters the body through a cut. Tetanus bacteria causes the muscles to spasm (move suddenly). If tetanus attacks the jaw muscles, it causes lockjaw, the inability to open and close your mouth.

Tetanus can also cause spasm of the breathing muscles, which can be fatal.

Pertussis

Pertussis also called whooping cough is caused by a bacteria that clogs the lungs with mucus (a thick, slimy substance). This can cause a severe cough that sounds like a 'whoop'. The cough can last for 2 months and allow the other bacteria, which can cause pneumonia and bronchitis (infection of lungs).

MMR Vaccination

Live attenuated virus vaccines for MMR (measles, mumps and rubella) have been combined into a single vaccine known as MMR vaccine. The MMR vaccine is effective as the single virus vaccine composed of the respective strains and has been shown to be highly effective. The immunity induced by MMR is long lasting and may be lifelong.

Why do We Need a Second Dose of MMR?

Although the first step towards the eradication of measles is to implement a primary vaccination program, WHO believes that measles eradication cannot be achieved with a single dose strategy alone.

Hence, WHO and UNICEF now jointly advise that in addition to the first dose at the age of 9 months, a second opportunity for measles immunization is essential to protect those children who were previously missed by routine services and for those children who failed to respond to their first dose of measles vaccine.

Chapter 13

Serology: Antigen-Antibody Reactions

ANTIGEN-ANTIBODY REACTIONS

Antigens and antibodies by definition, combine with each other specifically and in an observable manner. When molecules of antigen and corresponding antibody are brought together in solution, linkage is formed between 'Fab' portion of the immunoglobin molecule and antigen determinants of the antigen molecule.

The reactions between antigens and antibodies have many uses. In the body, they mediate immunity in infectious diseases or tissue injury, in some types of hypersensitivity and autoimmune diseases. In the laboratory, they help in diagnosis of infections. In epidemiological surveys, they help in the identification of infectious agents and non-infectious agents such as enzymes. In general, these reactions can be used for the detection and estimation of either antigens or antibodies. Antigen-antibody reactions *in vitro* (lab test tubes and other lab vessels) are known as serological reactions, which are classified into precipitation reactions, agglutination reactions and complement fixation tests.

When a soluble antigen combines with its corresponding antibody in presence of electrolytes, (e.g. NaCl) at a suitable temperature and pH, the antigen-antibody complex forms an insoluble precipitate. When instead of sedimenting the precipitate remains if suspended as floccules, the reaction is known as flocculation. When foccules are clumped, the reaction is known as agglutination. The principles governing agglutination and precipitation are the same.

Uses of precipitation reaction:
1. Identification of bacteria.
2. Identification of antigenic component of bacteria in infected animal tissue, e.g. *Bacillus anthracis* (Ascoli test).
3. Standardization of toxins and antitoxins.
4. Demonstration of antibody in serum, e.g. Kahn test for the diagnosis of syphilis.
5. Medicolegal serology for the detection of blood, semen, etc.

Tests Based on Antigen-antibody Reactions

1. Precipitation tests:
   a. Ring test, e.g. typing of streptococci, pneumococci.
   b. Slide test (flocculation), e.g. VDRL test for syphilis.
   c. Tube test (flocculation), e.g. Kahn test.
2. Agglutination tests:
   a. Slide test, e.g. blood grouping and cross matching.
   b. Tube test, e.g. Widal test for typhoid and paratyphoid fevers.
3. Complement fixation test:
   For example, Wassermann reaction for syphilis.

PRECIPITATION TESTS

Mechanism of Precipitation: Lattice Formation

Zone Phenomenon

The amount of precipitation formed is greatly influenced by the relative proportions of antigen and antibody. If increasing amounts of antigen are added to the same amount of antiserum in different tubes, precipitation will occur most rapidly and abundantly in one of the middle tubes, in which antigen and antibody are present in optimal or equivalent proportions. Refer Figure 13.1.

In the preceding tubes in which the antibody is in excess and in the later tubes in which the antigen is in excess, precipitation is weak or even absent.

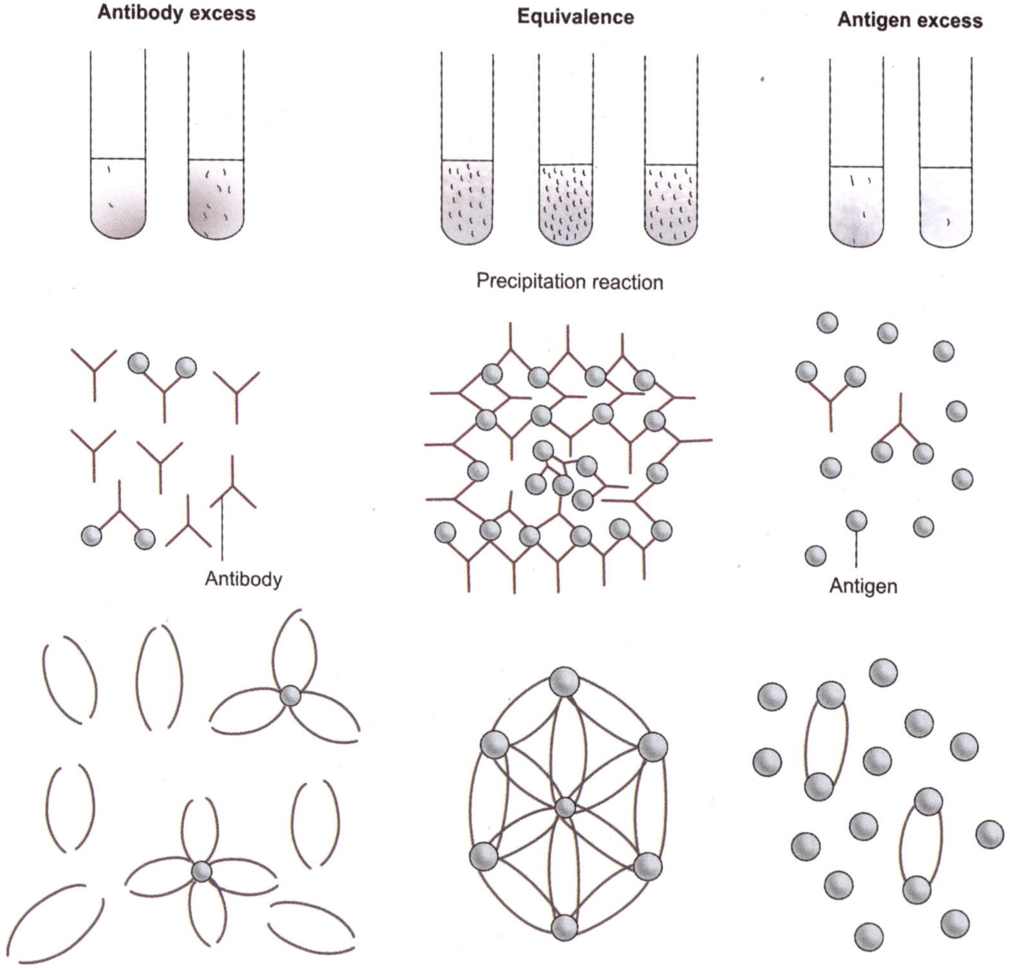

Antibody excess   Equivalence   Antigen excess

Precipitation reaction

Antibody   Antigen

Fig. 13.1: Mechanism of precipitation

If the amounts of the precipitate in the different tubes are plotted on a graph, the result will have three phases—an ascending part (prozone or zone of antibody excess), a peak (zone of equivalence) and a descending part (postzone or zone of antigen excess). This is called the zone phenomenon. Refer Figure 13.2.

Zoning occurs in agglutination and few other serological reactions also. The prozone is of importance in clinical serology as sometimes sera rich in antibody may give a false negative precipitation or agglutination result, unless several dilutions are tested.

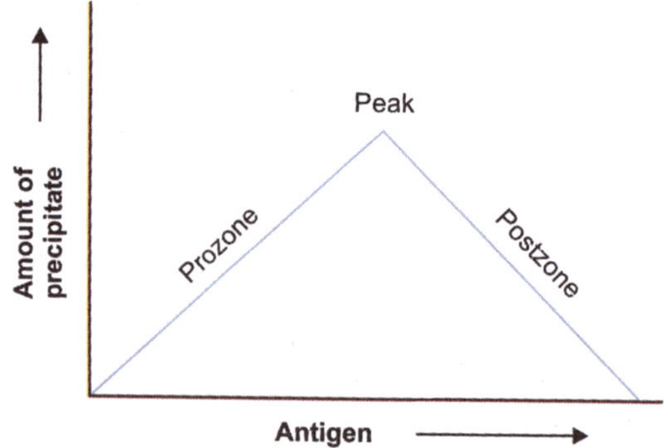

Fig. 13.2: Zone phenomenon

Measurement of Antigen and Antibody

Measurement of antigen and antibody is in terms of units of titer. The antibody titer of a serum is the highest dilution of the serum, which gives an observable reaction with the antigen in a particular test. Similarly, value of antigen can be determined against known serum.

Slide Test

Slide test consists of layering the antigen solution over a column of antiserum in a narrow tube. A precipitate forms at the junction of the two liquids, examples of ring precipitation reaction tests are the C-reactive protein test, Ascoli thermoprecipitation test and grouping of streptococci by lancified technique.

Venereal Disease Research Laboratory Test

The standard tests that are usually employed for syphilis (caused by *Treponema pallidum*) are Wassermann, Kahn and Venereal Disease Research Laboratory (VDRL) test. Wassermann is a complement fixation test, while the Kahn's test is a tube flocculation test.

The VDRL test is simple, economic and rapid, which requires only a small quantity of the serum and is as sensitive and specific as the other tests. It is the most widely used serological test for syphilis. It is also useful for monitoring the patient during treatment.

Procedure

VDRL antigen is available in the form of a kit, which contains an ampule of antigen and normal saline buffer solution for preparing the antigen emulsion.

Inactivation of Complement in the Serum

The blood samples received are serially numbered. Blood is transferred to centrifugal tubes, which are also numbered and centrifuged for 10 minutes to separate the sera. To inactivate the complement, the sera is heated to 56°C in a water bath for 30 minutes.

Preparation of the Antigen Emulsion

0.4 mL of buffered saline is taken in a glass-stoppered or screw-capped bottle. 0.5 mL of antigen solution is added to it with rotational shaking for 10 second after which 4.1 mL saline is added. The bottle is closed with the stopper and shaken from bottom to top, approximately 30 times in 10 second. The antigen is kept as such for 15 minute for its maturation, which increases its sensitivity and then it can be used for about 250 tests that day.

Qualitative VDRL test

In this, a glass slide with 12 concavities is used. 0.05 mL of the heat-inactivated serum is transferred into one of the cavities in the glass slide. One drop of antigen emulsion (1/60 mL) is added to the serum and the slide is rotated for 4 minute on a mechanincal rotator at 180 rpm. Refer Figure 13.3.

Reading

Take reading immediately after shaking under low-power objective of the microscope. The antigen looks like short rods and the agglutinated particles appear in clumps.

1. No clumping or slight roughness, uniform needles evenly distributed—non-reactive (NR).
2. Small clumps—weakly reactive (WR).
3. Medium and large clumps—reactive (R).

Quantitative Serum Test (VDRL)

Two-fold successive dilutions of the reactive serum are prepared with normal saline solution by taking 0.05 mL of serum in a special slide with depressions and subsequently diluting by addition of 0.05 mL of saline. Each dilution is treated as an individual serum and tested as described for qualitative serum test (Fig. 13.4).

The results are expressed as the highest dilution (titer), which gives a frank reaction (where precipitate is obtained).

Salmonella

Salmonella are gram-negative, motile, non-sporing, non-capsulated bacilla, morphologically indistinguishable from *Escherichia coli*. They are non-lactose fermenters, but ferment many other

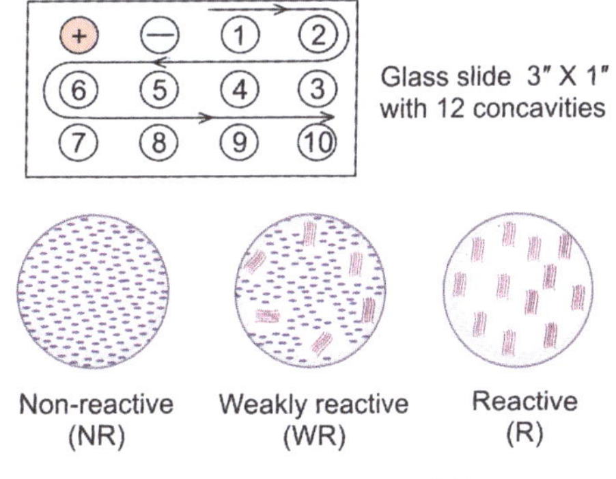

Fig. 13.3: Agglutination in VDRL test

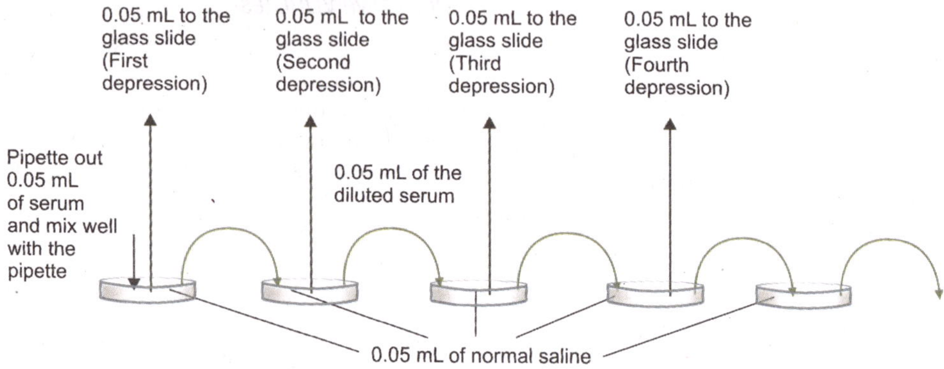

Fig. 13.4: Quantitative VDRL test (VDRL = Venereal Disease Research Laboratory)

sugars, most species producing acid and gas. On the basis of pathogenecity, *Salmonella* may be divided into:

1. Enteric fever group: Comprises organisms capable of producing enteric fever in man viz *Salmonella typhi (S. typhi)* and *Salmonella paratyphi (S. paratyphi)* bacilli. These species are found only in the intestinal tract of man.
2. The food poisoning group: They are essentially parasites of animals from whom man is occasionally infected.

AGGLUTINATION REACTIONS

When a particulate antigen is mixed with its antibody in the presence of electrolytes at a suitable temperature and pH, the particles are clumped or agglutinated.

Unlike precipitation, in agglutination reactions, the antigen is a part of the surface of some particulate material such as an erythrocyte, bacterium or an inorganic particle, e.g. polystyrene latex, which has been coated with antigen. Antibody added to suspensions of such particles combines with surface antigens and links them together to form a clearly visible aggregate called agglutins.

Agglutination is more sensitive than precipitation for the detection of antibodies. The same principles govern both agglutination and precipitation. Agglutination occurs optimally when antigens and antibodies react in equivalent proportions. The zone phenomenon may be seen when either an antibody or an antigen is in excess. 'Incomplete' or 'monovalent' antibodies do not cause agglutination though they might combine with the antigen. They might act as 'blocking' antibodies, inhibiting agglutination by the complete antibody subsequently.

Applications of Agglutination Reactions

When a drop of appropriate antiserum is added to a smooth uniform suspension of a particulate antigen in a drop of saline on a slide or tube, agglutination takes place. A positive result is indicated by the clumping together of particles and the clearing of drop mixing the antigen and antiserum with a loop or by gently rocking the slide, facilitates the reaction. Depending on the titer of the serum, agglutination may occur instantly or within seconds.

Clumping occurring after a minute may be due to drying of the fluid and should be disregarded. It is essential to have on the same slide, a control consisting of the antigen suspension in saline, without the antiserum to ensure that the antigen is not autoagglutinable. Agglutination is usually visible to the naked eye, but may require confirmation under a microscope. Slide agglutination is a routine procedure for the identification of many bacterial isolates from clinical specimens. It is also the method used for blood grouping and cross matching.

Tube Agglutination

Tube agglutination is a standard quantitative method of measurement of antibodies. When a fixed volume of a particular antigen suspension is added to an equal volume of serial dilutions of antiserum in test tubes, the agglutination of the serum can be estimated. Tube agglutination test is routinely employed for the serological diagnosis of typhoid, paratyphoid, brucellosis and typhus fevers.

Diagnosis of Enteric Fever

Enteric fever is a septicemic disease caused by *S. typhi, S. paratyphi* A, B or C, through unhygienic food and drinks. The pathogenesis of enteric fever is as shown in the Figure 13.5.

Laboratory diagnosis by three parameters:

1. Isolation of causative agent.
2. Detection of microbial antigen.
3. Titration of antibody against causative agent.

Clinical Diagnosis—Widal Test

1. A clinical suspension—from the signs and symptoms.
2. Blood culture in the early stage (first 2 to 5 days of fever).
3. Widal test after 5 to 7 days of fever. When high fever is present without symptoms of cold or sore throat, typhoid may be suspected. Widal test is a serological test to detect the antibody in the patient's blood. Two types of antigens are used—the 'H' or flagellar antigen and the 'O' or somatic antigen of the *S. typhi*.

Procedure

1. Seven small test tubes in four rows are taken, in which two rows are of round bottom tubes for somatic antigen (O) and two of conical bottom tubes for flagellar antigen (H).
2. 0.4 mL of normal saline is added to each tube from numbers two to seven leaving the first tube in each row without saline.
3. 1 : 15 dilutions of the patient's serum is prepared by adding 0.5 mL serum to 7 mL of normal saline. 0.4 mL of this diluted serum is added to tubes 1 and 2 in each row. Tube 2 now has 0.8 mL serum diluted to 1 : 30.

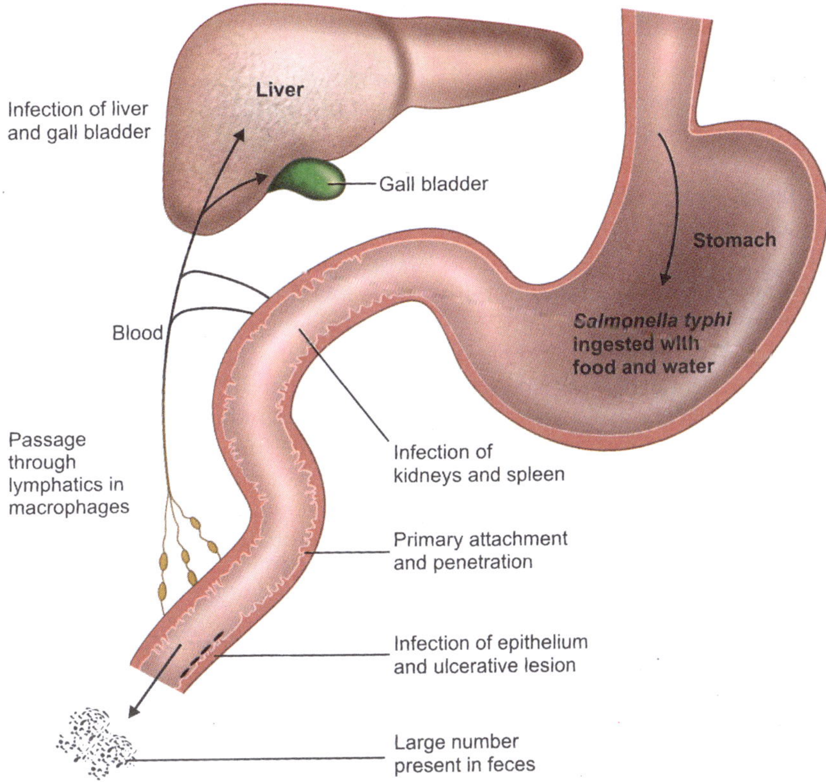

Fig. 13.5: Pathogenesis of enteric fever

4. Mixture in tube 2 is now thoroughly mixed and then 0.4 mL is transferred to tube 3 and the process is repeated till tube 6 from which 0.4 mL is discarded. Tube 7 contains only saline.
5. With a fresh pipette, 0.4 mL of bacterial antigen is added to each tube than making serum dilution in tubes 1 to 6 from 30 to 960.

Incubation

Incubation for H antigen is done for 2 hours at 37°C in water bath and read after keeping the tubes at 40°C overnight.

Reading of the Result

For H agglutination, large flakes are seen with naked eye. For 'O' agglutination, small granules are seen with a magnifying glass. The titer of patient's serum for each *Salmonella* suspension is read as the highest dilution of the serum giving visible agglutination, e.g. if the highest dilution giving visible agglutination is 1 : 240, the titer shall be 240 for that antibody.

Interpretation

The result of the Widal test should be interpreted keeping the following points in mind:
a. The antibody titer depends on the stage of the disease. Antibodies normally appear by the end of the 1st week of illness. Hence the samples taken earlier may give false (negative) result.
b. The titer will increase readily till 3rd or 4th week after which it declines gradually.
c. Demonstrating a rise in the titer of the antibodies by testing two or more serum samples is more meaningful.
d. Patients treated with chloramphenicol or other antibodies to which the organisms is sensitive, usually show poor antibody response.
e. Patients immunized with vaccine against typhoid show high titer.

COMPLEMENT FIXATION TEST

Complement takes part in many immunological reactions and is absorbed during the combination of antigens with their antibodies. The ability of antigen-antibody complexes to 'fix' complement is made use of in the complement fixation test (CFT).

CFT is a very sensitive test and is capable of detecting as little as 0.04 µg of antibody and 0.1 µg of antigen. It is used in the serological diagnosis of various diseases:
1. Bacterial diseases, e.g. gonorrhea, brucellosis.
2. Spirochetal diseases, e.g. syphilis (Wassermann reaction).
3. Rickettsial diseases, e.g. typhus fever.
4. Viral diseases, e.g. lymphogranuloma venereum (sexually transmitted disease [STD]).
5. Parasitic diseases, e.g. kala azar, amebiasis.

Wassermann Reaction

Complement fixation test (CFT) was formerly used as a routine serological diagnostic test for syphilis. The test consists of two steps. In the first, the inactivated serum of the patient is incubated at 37°C for 1 hour with the Wassermann antigen and a fixed amount (2 units) of guinea pigs complement. If the serum contains syphilis antibody, the complement will be utilized during the antigen-antibody interaction. If the serum does not contain the antibody, no antigen-antibody reaction occurs and therefore the complement will not be fixed and so will be left intact.

Testing for complement (Table 13.1) in the postincubation mixture will therefore indicate whether the serum had antibodies or not. This constitutes the second step in the test. This second step consists of adding sensitized cells (sheep erythrocytes coated with 4 MHD, i.e. minimum hemolytic dose), hemolysin and incubating at 37°C for 30 minutes. Lysis of the erythrocytes indicates that complement was not fixed in the first step and therefore, the serum did not have the antibody (negative CFT). If the complement was used up, then no hemolysis and therefore the serum contained the antibody (positive CFT).

Antiglobulin or Coomb Test

Coomb test is used in erythroblastosis fetalis, for the detection of incomplete antibodies (non-agglutinating anti-Rh antibody) for *Brucella*, *Shigella* and *Salmonella* antigen. This is a test to detect the presence of incomplete anti-Rh antibodies in the maternal blood (that coat and damage red blood cells [RBCs] of the fetus) and used to anticipate the hemolyte disease of the new born.

Table 13.1: Testing for complement

SI No	Reaction	Complement positive test	Result
1	Antigen + test serum (contains antibody) + hemolytic system	Complement fixed	No hemolysis Positive test
2	Antigen + test serum (no antibody) + hemolytic system	Complement not fixed	Hemolysis Negative test

Erythroblastosis Fetalis

Erythroblastosis fetalis is a severe hemolytic disease that develops when an Rh negative mother carries an Rh positive child and the mother produces anti-Rh antibodies. These antibodies cross the placenta and cause the destruction of the fetal RBCs. Depending on the amount of the antibodies produced, the fetus may abort or be born with a hemolytic disease. This disease is rarely associated with the first Rh negative incompatible pregnancy, but subsequent pregnancies increase the risk of this problem and is prevented by giving the mother an injection of Rh antibody.

Principle

When sera containing incomplete anti-Rh antibodies are mixed with Rh positive red cells, the antibody globulin coats the surface of erythrocytes, though they are not agglutinated. When such erythrocytes coated with the antibody globulin are washed free of all unmatched proteins and treated with a rabbit antiserum against human gammaglobulin (antiglobulin or Coomb serum) the cells are agglutinated. This is the principle of Coomb test. Refer Figure 13.6.

Enzyme-linked Immunosorbent Assay

Enzyme-linked immunosorbent assay test (ELISA) is now the most widely employed technique for detection of antigens, antibodies, hormones, toxins and viruses.

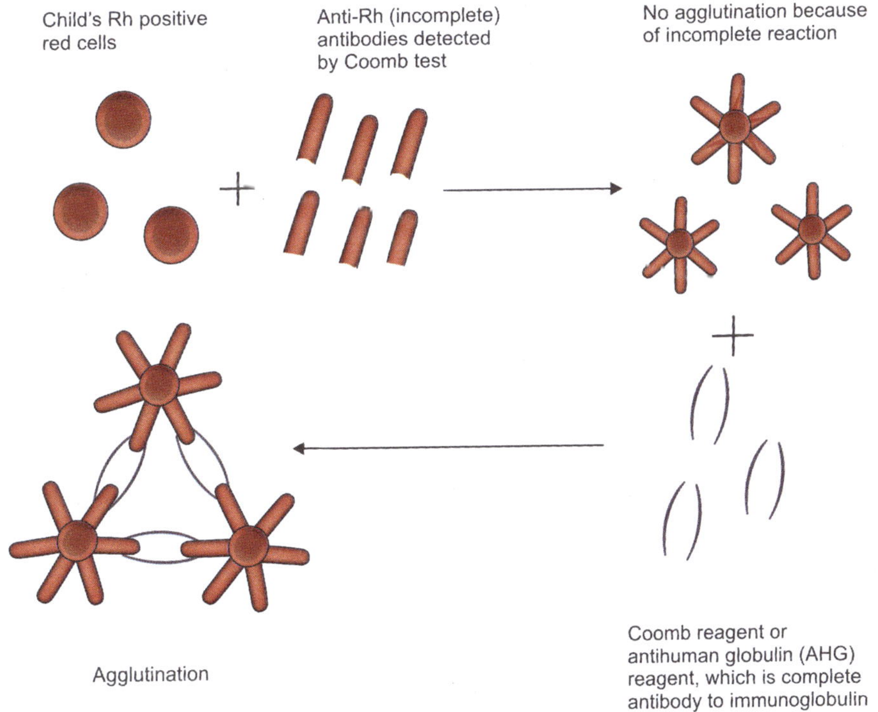

Fig. 13.6: Antiglobulin or Coomb test

Antibodies are conjugated with enzyme by addition of gluteraldehyde so that resulting antibody molecule has both immunological and enzyme activities and quantified by their ability to degrade a suitable substrate. The commonly used enzymes are alkaline phosphatase and horse raddish peroxidase. Their respective substrates are p-nitrophenyl phosphate and O-phenyldiamine dihydrochloride (OPD). Enzymatic activity results in a color change, which can be assessed visibly or quantified in a simple spectrophotometer.

ELISA can be performed with sensitized carrier surfaces in the form of polystyrene tubes (macro-ELISA) or polyvinyl microtiter plates (micro-ELISA).

Several variations of ELISA techniques are now available with the aim to provide simple diagnostics for clinical and bedside utilities. These include card and dipstick methods. Simplicity and sensitivity are the highlights of ELISA. Refer Figure 13.7.

1. Microassay plate coated with HIV antigen.
2. Test serum added and incubated. Anti HIV antibody if present in the serum will attach to HIV antigen.
3. After washing, add goat antihuman immunoglobulin antibody conjugated with horse

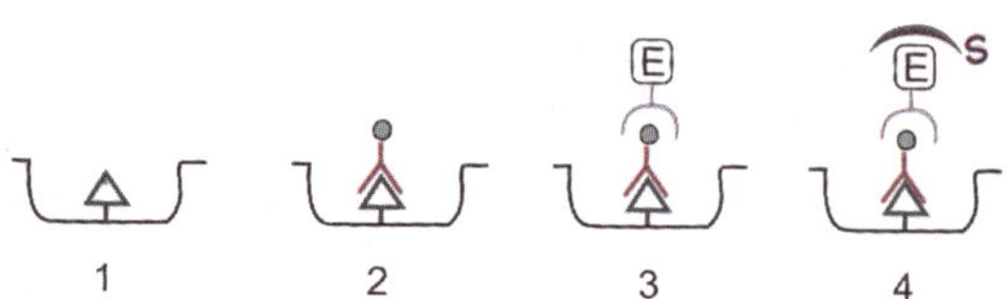

Fig. 13.7: Enzyme-linked immunosorbent assay

serum peroxidase enzyme. The conjugate will attach to the anti-HIV antibody in a positive test.
4. After washing add substract OPD. Yellow color will develop in a positive test.

Procedure

Purified, inactivated HIV antigen is absorbed on to microassay plate and walls, excess of antigen is removed by washing. Test material is then added, patient's serum unbound to antibody is removed by washing. Now enzyme (alkaline phosphatase) linked antihuman gammaglobulin (known) is added. Again excess is removed by washing. This mixture is incubated at 37°C. Finally corresponding enzyme substrate (p-nitrophenyl phosphate) is added, which may be hydrolysed by enzyme, yielding a yellow product. The optical density of the yellow product is measured in a spectrophotometer.

Virology

VIRUS

Definition

Virus is a Latin word meaning poison. They are unicellular, ultramicroscopic particles containing RNA or DNA, which replicate (not by binary fission) inside living cells, pass through filters that retain bacteria and are covered by a protein coat.

Viruses are infectious agents so small that they can be seen only by electron microscope. They are 10 to 100 times smaller than most bacteria. They are referred to as obligate intracellular parasites and contain either DNA or RNA, but never both. They look for cellular organization and for enzymes necessary for nucleic acid and protein synthesis. They have no metabolic activity outside the cell and hence referred as 'virions' (extracellular infectious virus particle).

Characteristic Properties

Their general properties are:
1. Smallest infectious agent.
2. Do not possess cellular organization.
3. Obligate intracellular parasites due to lack of enzymes and so depend on the synthetic machinery of host cells.
4. Contains one type of nucleic acid, either DNA or RNA, but never both.
5. The nucleic acid is enclosed in a protein shell.
6. Fail to grow on artificial media.
7. Limited host range.
8. Multiply by a complex process called replication and not binary fission.
9. Unaffected by antibiotics.
10. Sensitive to interferon.

Other properties:

Viruses are heat labile (destroyed by heat) and are inactivated at 50°C to 60°C within minutes but are stable at low temepature. They are preserved at -40°C or better at -70°C. For prolonged storage of viral vaccine, lyophilization or deep freezing (rapid drying in the frozen state under vaccum) is necessary. Disinfectants like phenol or cresol are not very effective. Formaldehyde, β-propiolactone (BPL), Cl_2, I_2 and H_2O_2 are very effective. Hypochlorite solution and gluteraldehyde are the best disinfectants for infected specimens. They are too small to be seen with an ordinary microscope. Their shape and size are demonstrated by the electron microscope.

Antibiotics are not effective as viruses are resistant to their action. The purpose of administration of antibodies in certain viral infections is to control secondary bacterial infections.

Recently, few antiviral drugs have been introduced, e.g. Acilvir, Iodoxurudine and Vidarabine, which are useful in the treatment of herpes simplex infections. Zidovirudine is useful in acquired immunodeficiency syndrome (AIDS).

MORPHOLOGY

Viruses are composed of nucleic acids and proteins (Fig. 14.1). The genome consists of a single nucleic acid and stores all vital information required by the virus for its replication. The genome is surrounded by a shell or a coat made of proteins and is called capsid. The genome and capsid are collectively designated as nucleocapsid.

Most viruses have an additional covering of lipid around their nucleocapsid, which is known as viral envelope. The complete viral particle is also known as virion.

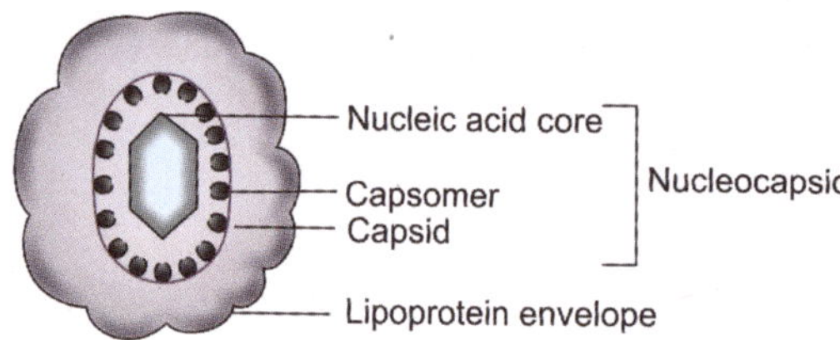

Fig. 14.1: Virus

Size

Virions range in size from 20 to 350 nm, the largest virus is poxvirus (300 nm) and the smallest is parvo (20 nm). Generally, electron microscope is used but some viruses like pox can be seen under light microscope when suitably stained, such particles are known as elementary bodies.

Shape

The shape varies in different groups of viruses. Most animal viruses are spherical, some are irregular and pleomorphic. Shape of different viral groups is as follows:

- Bullet shape—Rabies virus
- Brick shape—Poxvirus
- Rod shape—Tobacco mosiac virus.

Structure

Viruses are composed of central core of nucleic acid, capsid and an envelope.

Capsid: Capsid is a protein coat, which protects nucleic acids from nucleases and is composed of large number of capsomers.

Nucleic acid: The viral genome contains all the genetic information and is composed of nucleic acid. They contain either DNA or RNA but never both. DNA or RNA is either double stranded or single stranded.

  Double-stranded DNA—Poxviridae, etc.

  Single-stranded DNA—Parvoviridae.

  Double-stranded RNA—Reoviridae.

 Single-stranded RNA—Orthomyxoviridae, etc.

Envelope: Certain viruses contain envelope and are lipoprotein aqueous in nature. The lipid is largely from host whereas, protein is from virus. Some have projections called peplomers.

Symmetry

The way capsomers of the viruses are arranged is known as symmetry. Viruses exhibit three kinds of symmetry:

1. Icosahedral symmetry.
2. Helical symmetry.
3. Complex symmetry.

Icosahedral symmetry: An icosahedron is a polygon with 12 vertices or corners and 20 facets or sides. Each facet is in a shape of equilateral triangle (Fig. 14.2). For example, adenovirus.

Helical symmetry: In this type, nucleic acid core is covered by a capsid consisting of closely-packed capsomers arranged in regular helix (Fig. 14.3). For example, herpes virus.

Complex symmetry: These are the viruses with complex or uncertain symmetry (Fig. 14.4), e.g. tailed bacteriophages C viruses, which attack bacteria.

Cultivation of Viruses

As they are obligate intracellular parasites they can not be grown on culture medium.

 Three methods are employed:

1. Inoculation into animals.
2. Inoculation into embryonated eggs.
3. Tissue culture.

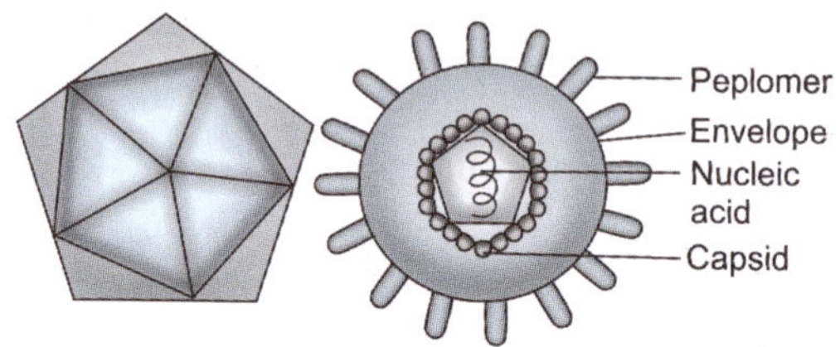

Fig. 14.2: Icosahedral symmetry in viruses

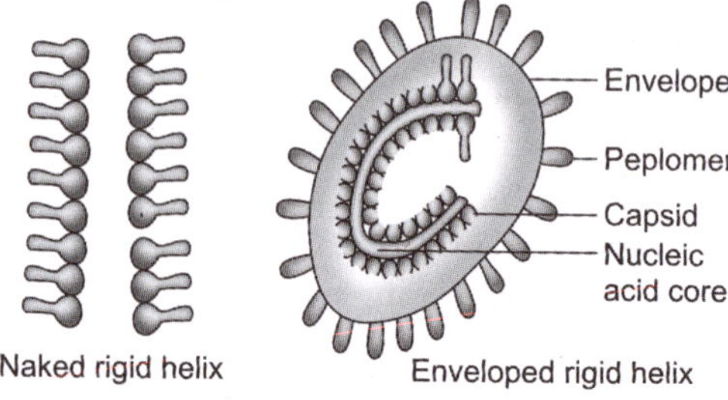

Fig. 14.3: Helical symmetry in viruses

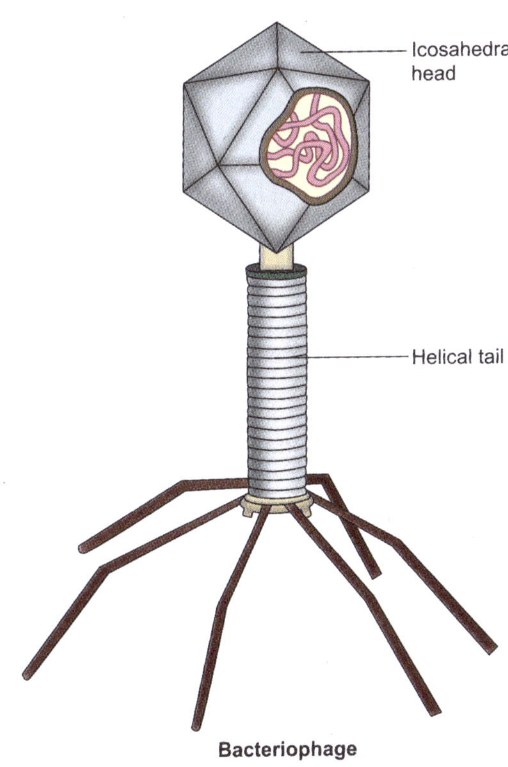

Fig. 14.4: Complex symmetry in viruses

Inoculation into Animals

Mice, guinea pigs, rabbits and primates are used for this purpose. Several routes like intracerebral, subcutaneous, intraperitoneal, intranasal are used. Growth of the virus is indicated by death, lesions, etc.

Inoculation into Embryonated Eggs

Fertile chicken eggs incubated for 5 to 12 days can be inoculated through shell aseptically (Fig. 14.5). The opening may be sealed with paraffin wax. Several methods of inoculations are found. Example:

Vaccinia virus—chorioallantoic membrane (CAM).

Yolk sac—some viruses, *Chlamydia*, *Rickettsia*.

Amniotic sac—influenza.

Growth is indicated by lesions known as pocks, each virus shows individual pock morphology.

Cell Cultures/Tissue Cultures

Tissue cultures are the method of choice and on the basis of origin, cell cultures are of three types:

a. Primary cell culture.
b. Diploid cell lines.
c. Continous cell lines.

Primary cell lines: Derived from normal tissue of animal and human. They can be cultured for limited number of times.

Diploid cell lines: These are derived from primary cell cultures established from a particular type of tissue (kidney, lung) and can undergo 50 to 100 divisions.

Continuous cell lines: They are capable of infinite number of doubling, usually from cancerous tissue.

Tissue culture involves obtaining living cells derived from kidney of monkey or human amnion, which are processed under sterile conditions and suspended in a solution of salt, sugar, sera and antibodies needed for their survival and growth. The cells in tissue culture not only remain alive but also repeatedly divide to produce sheets of shells on the walls of the containers used.

When viruses containing infectious specimens are introduced into such tissue culture system, the viruses invade and multiply inside the cells. Virus growth and multiplication produce

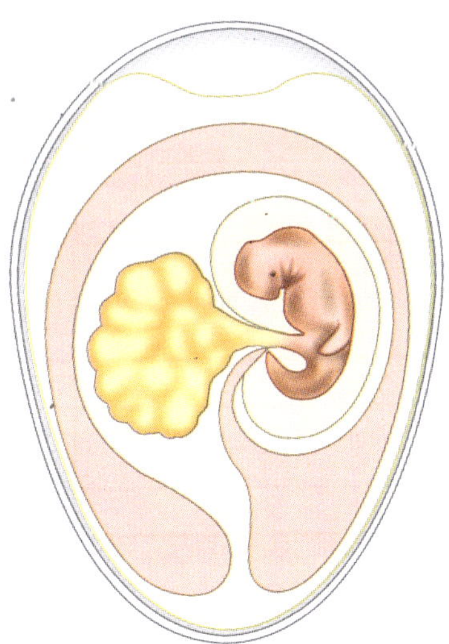

Fig. 14.5: Embryonated egg

changes in the morphological appearance of these cells known as cytopathic effect (CPE), which can be seen under an ordinary microscope.

Cytopathic Effect

Many viruses kill the cells in which they grow and bring about certain detectable changes in the morphology of host cells. All these effects are collectively called cytopathic effect. Some viruses however, do not produce CPE.

CPE can be visualized under the microscope in both stained and unstained preparation. CPE may include rounding of cells, syncytium formation (rounding and aggregation of cells into grape-like clusters) and production of inclusive bodies, which are intracytoplasmic or intranuclear aggregate of viral replication and can be seen only after staining.

Growth of virus is indicated by the cytopathic effect (CPE).

CLASSIFICATION OF VIRUSES

Human viruses can be broadly classified on the basis of two sets of criteria. The first set partains to clinical criteria and classifies viruses as respiratory viruses, enteric viruses on the basis of certain epidemiological features such as arboviruses.

Nowadays, viruses are classified into two groups depending on the type of nucleic acids they possess, those containing RNA are called riboviruses and those containing DNA are called deoxyriboviruses. RNA virus are further divided into nine groups and DNA viruses into five groups. Refer Table 14.1 and 14.2.

VIROIDS

The term was introduced by Diener, they are infectious agents with protein-free, low molecular weight RNA, resistant to heat and organic solvents but sensitive to nucleases.

Table 14.1: DNA viruses

Category	Virus	Diseases
Poxvirus	Variola virus	Small pox (now extinct)
Herpes virus	Herpes simplex type 1 and type 2	Herpetic stomatitis, cold sores, genital herpes (STD), chickenpox glandular fever, Burkitt lymphoma (tumor of the jaw)
Adenovirus	Adenovirus	Respiratory, eye and gastrointestinal diseases
Hepadnaviruses	Hepatitis B virus (HBV)	Serum hepatitis
Papovaviruses	Papillomavirus	Wurtz and human skin cancer

Table 14.2: RNA viruses

Category	Virus	Diseases
Picornaviruses	Polioviruses, enteroviruses, rhinoviruses	Poliomyelitis, hepatitis A infections (HAV), common cold
Togaviruses commonly called arboviruses-transmitted by blood-sucking mosquitoes (Arbo=arthropod borne)	*Alphavirus* (arbovirus group A), *Flavivirus*	Encephalitis, Japanese encephalitis (JE), brain fever, dengue fever/yellow fever
Orthomyxovirus	Influenza virus	Influenza
Paramyxovirus	Parainfluenza virus, respiratory syncytial virus	Croup, respiratory infections, bronchitis, measles, mumps
Rhabdovirus (Rhabdo = rod)	Rabies virus	Rabies (hydrophobia), zoonoses
Reovirus	*Rotavirus*	Infantile gastroenteritis diarrhea, virus causing respiratory infection
Retrovirus	Human immunodeficiency virus (HIV) type I (HIV–1) and type II (HIV–2)	Acquired immune deficiency syndrome (AIDS)

PRION

Prions are infectious proteins without nucleic acid and are resistant to physical and chemical agents. They are resistant to heat, UV rays and nucleases. They cause diseases like Kuru, Creutzfeldt-Jakob disease, bovine spongi-form encephalopathy and scrapie disease in sheep and goats.

DNA VIRUSES

Poxviruses

Poxviruses are the largest viruses and can be seen under light microscope. Poxviruses are characterized by skin lesions. The most important of these skin lesions was smallpox, caused by variola virus.

Variola and Vaccinia

The variola virus is the causative agent of smallpox, which has been eradicated. Vaccinia virus is used as the vaccine for smallpox disease. Vaccinia and variola are similar in their properties. The only variation is vaccinia virus is an artificial virus.

Morphology

Shape : It is a brick-shaped virus.
Size   : The virion measures about 300 × 200 × 100 nm and can be seen under light microscope.

Cultivation

Both viruses grow on CAM of 11 to 13 days old chick embryo producing pocks in 48 to 72 hours. Pocks are small, shiny, white, non-hemorrhagic in case of variola, whereas in vaccinia they are large, irregular, flat, grayish and in some cases hemorrhagic (Fig. 14.6).

Monkey kidney cells, HeLa cells can also be used. CPEs are produced in 24 to 48 hours by vaccinia and slowly by variola.

Pathogenesis

Smallpox has been eradicated. The source of infection is patient. Virus enters body through inhalation and undergoes initial multiplication

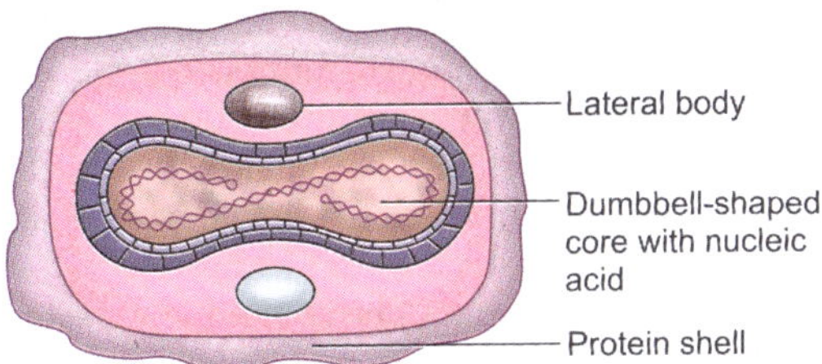

Fig. 14.6: Vaccinia virus

in local lymphoid tissue. Further multiplication takes place in reticuloendothelial cells. Lesions are caused.

Laboratory Diagnosis

Detection of virus is done by isolation of virus from blood due to distinctive morphology of virion. Rapid diagnosis is possible by electron microscopy.

Prophylaxis

Smallpox vaccine was used. It was a compulsory vaccine. Freeze-dried vaccine and the technique of vaccination eradicated the disease.

Herpesviruses

Herpesviridae family contains hundred species of enveloped DNA viruses that affect humans and animals.

Morphology

Herpesviruses are icosahedral enveloped viruses and contain double stranded genome. The envelope contains spikes.

Herpes Simplex

The herpes simplex virus (HSV) occurs only in humans. There are two types of herpes simplex virus—HSV type I and HSV type 2. HSV type I is usually isolated from lesions in and around the mouth and is transmitted by direct contact or by droplets or carriers. HSV type 2 is responsible for genital tract infections transmitted venereally.

Cultivation

The virus grows in a variety of primary and continous cell cultures, CAM of chick embryo.

Pathogenesis

Herpes simplex is the most common viral infection in humans. Sources of infection are saliva, skin lesions or droplets. Genital infection occurs by close contact and venereally. They are more frequent in HIV-infected and immunodeficient subjects. HSV–1 causes above the waist lesions and HSV-2 cause below the waist lesions.

Clinical Manifestation of Herpes

1. Cutaneous infection—cheeks, chin, mouth, forehead are affected.
2. Mucosal—buccal mucosa, pharyngitis.
3. Ophthalmic—causes corneal blindness, keratoconjunctivitis.
4. Nervous system—encephalitis.
5. Visceral—dysphagia, substernal pain and weight loss.
6. Genital—penis, urethra are affected.
7. Congenital—multiorgan involvement.

Laboratory Diagnosis

The diagnosis is made as follows:

Microscopy: It may be demonstrated in smears or sections from lesions by fluorescent antibody technique. It can also be detected by electron microscopy.

Virus isolation: Primary human embryonic kidney, human amnion, human diploid fibroblasts are preferred.

Serology: Enzyme-linked immunosorbent assay (ELISA), complement fixation tests are generally used.

Chemotherapy: Idoxuridine, acyclovir, valacyclovir, famciclovir are more effective.

Varicella Zoster Virus

Varicella zoster virus (VSV) is similar to herpes simplex virus. Varicella (chickenpox) and herpes zoster are different manifestations of same virus. Chickenpox is a primary infection, whereas herpes zoster is reactivation of latent virus when immunity has fallen.

Varicella (Chickenpox)

Chickenpox is one of the most common childhood infections. The source of chicken pox is the patient. Rash appears on the trunk and progresses through macule, papule, vesicle, pustule and scab. Chickenpox in pregnancy can be dangerous for mother and baby.

Herpes Zoster

Herpes zoster is common in old age or after 50 years. The virus remains latent in sensory ganglia in persons who had chickenpox. When the immunity falls, the virus reactivates and inflammation of nerve leads to neuritic pain that often leads to skin lesions.

Laboratory Diagnosis

The steps involved are:

Direct microscopy: Electron microscopy of vesicle fluid may demonstrate virus with typical herpes morphology. Another method is examination of early vesicles, which show multinucleated giant cells and inclusion bodies.

Virus isolation: Human fibroblasts, human amnion, HeLa cells, Vero cells are used.

Serology: Varicella-zoster specific immunoglobulin M (IgM) antibody in patient's serum can be detected by ELISA.

Treatment

Acyclovir and vidarabine are effective.

Cytomegaloviruses

Cytomegaloviruses (CMV) are formerly known as salivary gland viruses. They show latency. They are the largest virus being 150 to 200 nm in size.

Pathogenesis

Cytomegalovirus (CMV)-related disease is rare, but infection is common. CMV can be transmitted from mother to fetus, which remains latent at birth or lead to cytomegalic inclusion disease in infants.

The other clinical disease is intrauterine infection, which leads to fetal death and may be acquired during sexual intercourse. CMV is an important pathogen.

Laboratory Diagnosis

Urine/saliva or body fluids are generally taken as samples. Urine or saliva samples are centrifuged to demonstrate large intranuclear 'owl's eye' inclusions.

Isolation: Human fibroblast cultures are used to grow virus.

Serology: Enzyme-linked immunosorbent assay (ELISA), complement fixation test are generally performed to demonstrate IgM antibody.

Treatment

Ganciclovir is the generally preferred drug. No vaccine is available.

Epstein-Barr Virus

Epstein-Barr virus (EBV) is ubiquitous in all human populations. Oral contact, kissing appears to be predominant modes of transmission.

Pathogenesis

Epstein-Barr virus shows affinity for lymphoid tissue. They show the following clinical manifestations:

1. Infectious mononucleosis.
2. EBV-associated malignancies.
   a. Burkitt lymphoma.
   b. Nasopharyngeal carcinoma.
   c. Lymphomas in immune-deficient persons.

Laboratory Diagnosis

Blood generally examined. Initial phase leukopenia is generally observed. Later stages show abnormal mononuclear cells.

Paul-Bunnell Test: This is the standard test and generally IgM antibodies are demonstrated by inactivated serum (56°C for 30 minute) in doubling dilutions mixed with equal volumes of 1 percent suspension of sheep erythrocytes and tubes are examined for agglutination.

Similar type of antibodies may occur after infections of sera and even sometimes in normal individuals. To confirm these antibodies, absorption of agglutinins with guinea pig kidney cells and ox red cells are necessary. Forssman antibody induced by injection of horse serum is removed by treatment with guinea pig kidney cells and ox red cells. Antibodies in infectious mononucleosis are removed by ox red cells whereas normally occurring agglutinins are removed by guinea pig kidney cells.

Adenoviruses

Adenoviruses belong to family adenoviridae. They are non-enveloped, double-stranded DNA virus and infect humans, animals and birds.

Morphology

Adenoviruses are 70 to 75 nm in size and exhibit icosahedral symmetry with spikes. Refer Figure 14.7.

Pathogenesis

Adenovirus causes infections of respiratory tract, eye, bladder and intestine. The following syndromes have been recognized:

1. Pharyngitis.
2. Pneumonia.
3. Acute respiratory disease.
4. Pharyngoconjunctival fever.
5. Diarrhea.

Laboratory Diagnosis

Mircroscopy: Electron microscopy is used for detecting samples such as throat, conjunctival swab, urine, anal swab, genital secretions and biopsy.

Isolation: Tissue cultures are generally used, e.g. HeLa, HEp–2.

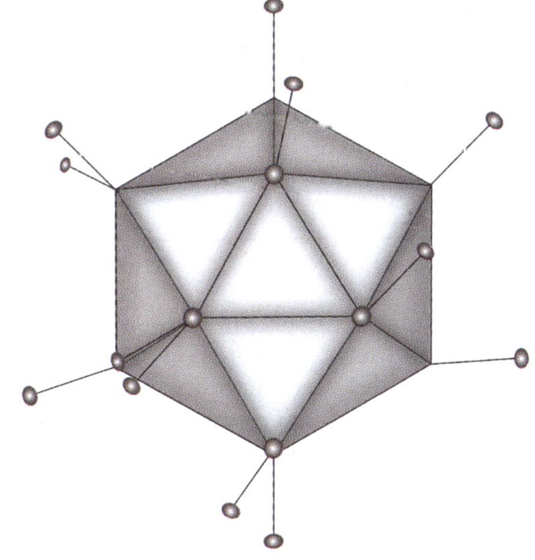

Fig. 14.7: Adenovirus

Serology: Immunofluorescence for viral antigen detection is useful.

Prophylaxis: Killed and live vaccines have been used with some success.

Parvoviruses

Parvoviruses are very small (20 nm) and contain single-stranded DNA genome. Parvovirus B 19 is present world wide. It usually causes respiratory infection with erythematous maculopapular rash and arthralgia. It occurs usually in children of 5 to 10 years age and has been called the fifth disease, as it was the fifth in the old list of six exanthematous fevers of children.

Transmission appears to be through respiratory system and blood. Infection leads to viremia followed by antibody response.

Papovaviruses

Papovaviruses are small, non-enveloped icosahedral DNA tumor viruses. Most of the tumors are benign, but some such as rabbit papilloma are malignant. There are two genera:

1. *Papillomavirus.*
2. *Polyomavirus.*

Papillomaviruses

Papillomaviruses are species specific and infect squamous epithelia and mucous membranes, inducing different types of warts and cervical cancer. These infections are transmitted by indirect or direct contact including sexual contact.

Polyomaviruses

Polyomaviruses produce variety of malignant tumors in animals and hence the name polyoma.

RNA VIRUSES

Picornaviruses

Picornaviridae consists of large number of very small RNA viruses. They are non-enveloped, 27 to 30 nm in size. Enteroviruses and rhinoviruses are the two important groups. Refer Table 14.3.

Poliovirus

Morphology

Shape: The virion is a spherical particle.
Size: It measures about 27 nm in diameter.

Symmetry: It exhibits icosahedral symmetry.
Genome: It contains single-stranded RNA.

Table 14.3: Important groups of very small RNA viruses

Groups	Common virus	Target organ/tissue
Enteroviruses	Poliovirus, Coxsackie virus	Infects enteric tract
Rhinoviruses	Human rhinovirus; type A, B, C	Infects nasal mucosa

Cultivation

Monkeys may be infected by intracerebral or intraspinal inoculation. It also grows in primary monkey kidney cultures.

Pathogenesis

The mode of infections is through ingestion by fecal-oral route. It multiplies in epithelial cells of alimentary canal and lymphatic tissue, then spreads to lymph nodes and to bloodstream and then to spinal cord and brain. Damage is in the anterior horns of spinal cord causing flaccid paralysis.

Laboratory Diagnosis

Blood, cerebrospinal fluid (CSF), throat swab and feces are the generally collected samples.

Microscopy: Virus can be demonstrated by electron microscopy or by immune electron microscopy.

Isolation: Tissue cultures (primary monkey kidney cells are employed). Growth is indicated by CPE in 2 to 3 days.

Serology: Generally, neutralization and complement fixation tests are employed.

Prophylaxis: Two types of vaccines can be administered, Salk and Sabin vaccine.

Slak vaccine (killed polio vaccine): It was developed by Salk. Vaccine is formalin inactivated. Preparation of three types of poliovirus grown in monkey kidney tissue culture. It is given by injection and hence known as injectable poliovaccine (IPV). Three doses given 4 to 6 weeks apart followed by booster six months later. It induces IgM and IgG, but do not stimulate IgA in intestine.

Sabin vaccine (live polio vaccine): It was developed by Koprowski, Cox and Sabin. Sabin vaccine strains were developed by plaque selection in monkey kidney tissue culture. It is administered orally and is therefore known as oral polio vaccine (OPV). It is given in trivalent form. It can be given to young infants in three doses at 4 to 8 weeks intervals. It stimulates IgM, IgG and IgA (in intestines).

Rhinoviruses

Common cold is the most common infectious disease in humans. The virus attaches to nasal epithelial cells, enters and replicates. Damages cilia and cells. Local inflammation and cytokines are responsible for common cold.

Orthomyxoviruses

Influenza viruses are included in this group and it causes acute respiratory tract infection.

Morphology

Shape: It is spherical in shape.
Size: It varies with a diameter of 80 to 120 nm.
Symmetry: It exhibits helical symmetry.
Genome: It contains single-stranded RNA segmented into 8 pieces.
Envelope: Capsid is surrounded by envelope, which is lipoproteinaceous in nature. It contains two spikes (peplomers): hemagglutinin spikes (triangular) and neuraminidase (mushroom-shaped) respectively. Refer Figure 14.8.

Antigen Structure

Influenza viruses are classified into three types A,B,C based on their antigenic structures. This variation is due to hemagglutination and neuraminidase spikes. These three antigens are subdivided into 3A (H_1, H_2, H_3) and 2NA (N_1, N_2) types.

Antigen Variation

Influenza viruses has the ability to undergo antigenic variation, which may be antigenic drift or antigenic shift.
Antigenic drift: It is due of mutation and selection leading to minor changes in hemagglutinin or neuraminidase or both.
Antigenic shift: It is an abrupt drastic discontinous variation in antigens (HA or NA) and results in new subtype unrelated antigenically to previous strains.

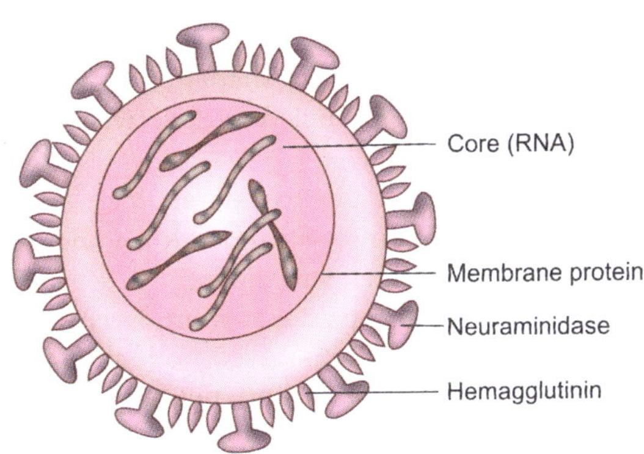

Fig. 14.8: Influenza virus

Cultivation

Influenza viruses grows well in amniotic cavity of chick embryos, primary monkey kidney or human embryo kidney cells.

Pathogenesis

Influenza viruses enters through respiratory tract. Incubation period is 1 to 3 days. Severity varies from mild coryza to fatal pneumonia.

Laboratory Diagnosis

The steps involved in the diagnosis of virus are:
Demonstration of the virus antigen: Influenzal antigen is detected by immunofluorescence.
Isolation of the virus: Throat garglings are collected using broth saline or buffered salt solution. The material immediately is either inoculated into the amniotic cavity of 11 to 13 days old egg or monkey kidney cell culture. Positive samples can be detected by hemagglutination or hemadsorption.
Serology: Complement fixation and hemagglutination tests are employed.

Treatment

Amantadine or rimantadine are used.

Paramyxoviruses

Paramyxoviruses resemble orthomyxoviruses in morphology, but are larger and more pleomorphic. They belong to the family paramyxoviridae.

Morphology

Shape: They are spherical in shape.
Size: The size of the particle varies between 100 to 300 nm in diameter.
Symmetry: They exhibit helical symmetry.
Genome: It is linear single-stranded RNA and do not exhibit any antigen variation.
Envelope: The nucleocapsid is surrounded by lipid envelope and contains glycoprotiens, hemagglutinin (longer spike) and neuraminidase. Mumps, measles and parainfluenza exhibit almost similar morphology.

The important viruses of family paramyxoviridae are:

1. Parainfluenza viruses: Parainfluenzal viruses are responsible for about 10 percent of respiratory infections in children. In infants and young children, they produce respiratory tract disease such as laryngotracheobronchitis or croup. Viruses can be isolated and detected by monkey kidney cell cultures, ELISA.

2. Mumps virus: Children are commonly affected by this virus and characterized by enlargement of parotid gland. Infection is transmitted by direct contact, airborne droplets or with saliva and urine. One attack of mumps confers lasting immunity.

3. Measles virus (rubeola): It is highly infectious childhood disease and enters through respiratory tract or conjuctiva and multiplies in lymph nodes. It is characterized by conjunctivitis, koplik spots on buccal mucosa. After 2 to 4 days, virus spreads and causes maculopapular rash on neck and rest of the body. The rash fades and patient recovers by 10 to 14 days. The simple diagnostic test is immunofluorescence. Neutralization and complement fixation can also be done. For measles and mumps disease, a triple vaccine is given called MMR (measles, mumps, rubella) vaccine and is administered by subcutaneous injection.

4. Respiratory syncytial virus (RSV): It belongs to genus *Pneumovirus* of family paramyxoviridae. Infants are more prone to this disease. It begins with rhinorrhea, cough, wheezing and cause bronchiolitis and pneumonitis. It is transmitted with contaminated hands. Refer Figure 14.9.

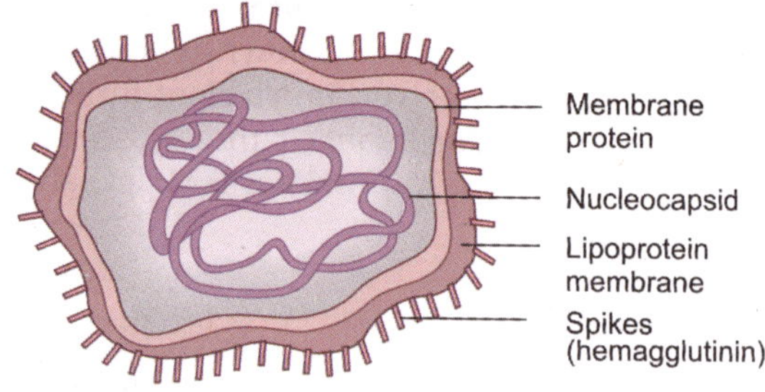

Fig. 14.9: Measles virus

Rhabdoviruses

Rhabdoviruses are included in the family rhabdoviridae. Refer Figure 14.10

Morphology

Shape: It is a bullet-shaped virus ('Rhabdo' means rod).
Size: The size of virus is about 75 × 180 nm.
Symmetry: Capsid exhibits helical symmetry.
Envelope: The capsid is surrounded by a lipoprotein envelope and carries glycoprotein spikes.
Genome: It contains single-stranded unsegmented RNA.

Cultivation

Rhabdoviruses can be grown in chick embryo yolk sac, primary and continous cell cultures (growth will be less).

Pathogenesis

In humans, rabies is caused by bite of rabid dogs (mad dogs). Saliva of the animal is deposited in the wound. It multiplies in muscles, connective tissue and nerves at site for 48 to 72 hours. The disease is classified into four stages — prodrome, acute encephalitic phase, coma and death. The main feature is difficulty in drinking with in tense

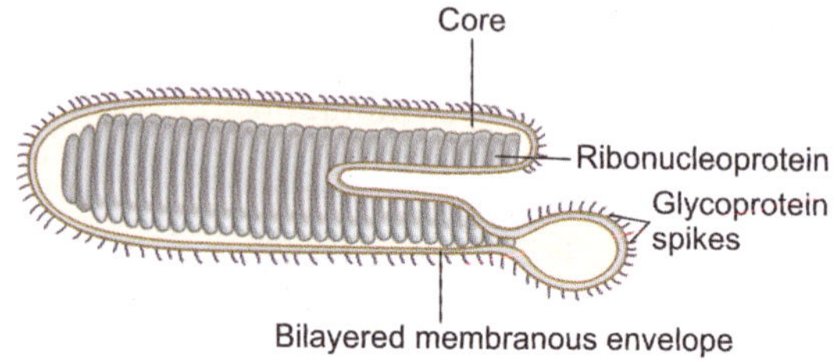

Fig. 14.10: Rhabdovirus

thirst. Attempts to drink, bring pain of pharynx and larynx and patients develop hydrophobia. The other characteristic feature is formation of negri bodies in neurons, cerebellum, hippocampus.

Laboratory Diagnosis

Specimens like corneal smears, skin biopsy (face or neck) or saliva antemortem and brain postmortem are preferred.

Serology: Immunofluorescence is the commonly used method where antirabies serum is tagged with fluorescein isothiocyanate.

Isolation of virus: By intracerebral inoculation in mice and demonstration of negri bodies can also be done. Negri bodies consists of fibrillar matrix and rabies virus particles.

Prophylaxis

Prophylaxis include local treatment, antirabic vaccines and hyperimmune serum.

Local treatment: Animal bites deposit virus in the wounds. So it should be immediately scrubbed with soap and water and wound must be treated with quaternary ammonium compounds, tincture of iodine or alcohol. Use of antitetanus and antibiotic prevent sepsis.

Antirabic vaccines

Neural vaccines and non-neural vaccines are the two different types of vaccines available.

Neural vaccines – The Semple, βPL, infant brain vaccines, fall into this category.

a. Semple vaccine: It is developed by Semple. It is prepared by suspending 5 percent of sheep brain infected with fixed amount of virus and inactivated with phenol at 37°C.

b. Beta-propiolactone (βPL) vaccine: This is the major antirabic vaccine. As it is more antigenic, smaller doses are sufficient. The only difference between Semple and βPL vaccines is that here inactivating agent used is βPL.

c. Infant brain vaccine: Due to presence of myelin protein, brain tissue vaccines cannot be prepared. But in newborn animals, it is scanty or absent so vaccines were developed using infant mouse, rat or rabbit brain.

Non-neural vaccines – It includes:

1. Duck egg vaccine: It is prepared from a fixed virus adapted for growth in duck eggs and inactivated with βPL. Disadvantage is that it shows poor immunogencity.

2. Tissue culture vaccines: Human diploid cell (HDC) vaccine is the first cell culture vaccine, it is prepared by purifying and concentrating fixed rabies virus grown on human diploid cells and inactivated with βPL. But it is very expensive. Purified chick embryo cell culture vaccines (PCEC), purified vero cell vaccine (PVC) are also available. Subunit vaccines are still in experimental stage.

Hyperimmune serum: Human antirabies immunoglobulin (20 IU per kg body weight) is reserved for high-risk cases. It is safest antirabies antiserum.

Vaccination schedule: Vaccination depends on the rabid dog, if it is observed and found healthy then vaccination may be discontinued. If not, course should be started.

Neural vaccines: Dosage depends on the degree of risk. The immunity lasts for only 6 months. The vaccine is administered subcutaneously on the anterior abdominal wall.

Cell culture vaccines: HDC, PCEC, PVC have same dosage schedule and is same for both adults and children. The vaccine is given intramuscular and subcutaneous in the deltoid region or in children on the anterolateral aspect of the thigh. Five injections are required. One on the day of bite to be followed on the 3rd, 7th, 14th and 28th days.

Rabies (Hydrophobia)

Rhabdoviruses (rabies virus) are transmitted from animal to animals by bite. It infects the salivary gland and brain. The brain disease makes the animal irritable and it bites indiscriminately. While it bites, the virus in the saliva is inoculated into the wound. Infected dogs are the common source of infection for humans. Rabies virus reaches the brain and causes an illness commonly called rabies or hydrophobia (fear of water). The patient gets pharyngeal spasms upon drinking water. These spasms are very painful. As the disease progresses, even the sight of water causes spasms.

Human saliva is often free of rabies virus and human-to-human transmission is very rare. However, persons at increased risk of infection like veterinary, medical and nursing personnel may take prophylactic (pre-exposure) immunization. Pet dogs, cats, cattle, etc. should also be protected by immunization. Modern cell culture vaccine is used for immunization and is now available in India. The conventional sheep brain vaccine was banned by World Health Organization (WHO) in 1994.

Only five injections are required by modern cell culture vaccine as against 10 by the conventional sheep brain vaccine. The first dose should be taken on the day of the bite followed up on the 3rd, 7th, 14th and 28th days.

Arboviruses

Arboviruses are viruses of veretebrates and transmitted by hematophagous insect vectors. They mulitiply in blood-sucking insects and are transmitted by bite to vertebrate hosts.

Rubella Virus

Rubella or German measles is pleomorphic and characterized by macular rash and lymphadenopathy.

Morphology

Shape: It is spherical particle.
Size: It is 50 to 100 nm in diameter.
Genome: It possess single-stranded RNA.
Envelope: It is surrounded by envelope possessing hemagglutinin peplomers.

Cultivation

The virus can be grown in primary cell cultures and continuous cell lines.

Pathogenesis

Infection is acquired by inhalation or congenitally.

Inhalation infections are disseminated throughout body by bloodstream. Patient develops fever, rash appears first on face and then spreads to trunk and legs.

Congenital infections are common during first trimester. The common malformations are cardiac defects, cataract, deafness.

Laboratory Diagnosis

Blood sample is generally preferred. Virus is cultivated in rabbit kidney or Vero cells. Serological tests like ELISA are performed.

Prophylaxis

Rubella infection confers lasting immunity. Live attenuated vaccines have been developed. The vaccine now in use is RA 27/3 strain. The vaccine is given in combination with measles and mumps as MMR vaccine.

HEPATITIS VIRUSES

Hepatitis refers to primary infection of liver and consists of types A, B, C, D, E and G.

Viral Hepatitis

Viral hepatitis refers specifically to primary infection of the liver by one of the etiologically associated but different hepatotropic viruses as below:

1. Hepatitis type A—infective hepatitis, incubation hepatitis or epidemic jaundice.
2. Hepatitis type B—serum hepatitis or transfusion hepatitis.
3. Hepatitis type C.
4. Hepatitis type D.
5. Hepatitis type E—epidemic prone, enterically transmitted.
6. Hepatitis type G.

Clinical manifestation of these types are similar.

Methods of transmission are as below:
1. Hepatitis A and C—fecal-oral route.
2. Hepatitis B:
    a. Contaminated blood and blood products.
    b. Contaminated (unsterile) syringes and needles.
    c. Unsafe sex.
    d. Perinatal.
    e. Intimate physical contact between children or between mother and child.
3. Hepatitis C and D:
    a. Contaminated blood and blood products.
    b. Unsterile (contaminated) syringes and needles.

Hepatitis A (Epidemic jaundice)

Hepatitis A does not cause chronic liver disease. HAV is excreted in the feces and spreads primarily by fecal-oral route. The virus is common in places with poor standards of hygiene and sanitation. It has a relatively long incubation period and is infectious. The infected individual can pass on the disease to others even before the symptoms develop. In children under 2 years it is often unrecognized. Direct contact with an infected person or indirect contamination of food, water, hands and cooking utensils may result in the virus being ingested causing infection. The severity of infection is age related with symptoms being more common in very young and adolescent. Hepatitis A can relapse in 20 percent of the cases.

Symptoms

Symptoms include vomiting, jaundice (yellowness of eyes, skin and urine), diarrhea, pale stools, abdominal pain, malaise, fatigue, chills and fever.

Hepatitis A and hepatitis B are two different forms of viral hepatitis caused by two different viruses. HAV is a RNA virus, while HBV is DNA virus. Hepatitis A is transmitted mainly through food and water, while hepatitis B is transmitted through blood, sexual contact or from mother to the new born. Jaundice, the yellowness of the eye, is an early symptom of both hepatitis A and hepatitis B, hepatitis A is the largest single cause of jaundice.

There is separate vaccination for hepatitis A and hepatitis B. Efforts are on to develop a single vaccine as a protection from both. There is no vaccination for hepatitis C.

Hepatitis B (Serum Hepatitis)

Hepatitis B is a viral infection of the liver caused by HBV including liver failure (cirrhosis) and liver cancer. In India, 3% to 5% of population are carriers of HBV and 6,000 people die every year from hepatitis B related liver diseases.

How is HBV Spread?

Hepatitis B virus is found in blood and certain body fluids of infected people (fluids such as serum, semen, vaginal secretion and saliva). The mode of transmission is similar to HIV (AIDS).

HBV is much more infectious than HIV, only 0.00004 mL of blood is needed to transmit HBV while 0.1 mL is needed to transmit HIV. HBV can spread by:

1. Unprotected sex.
2. Sharing of syringes by drug addicts.
3. From mother to child during birth.
4. Contact with blood or open sores of an infected person.
5. Human bites.
6. Sharing items such as razors, tooth brushes or clothes.
7. Prechewing food for babies or sharing chewing gum.
8. Using unsterilised needles in ear or body— piercing, tattooing or acupuncture
9. Using the same immunization needle on more than one person.

Symptoms

1. Extreme tiredness, pain in joints.
2. Loss of appetitis, nausea, fever.
3. Dark colored urine.
4. Bloated tender belly.
5. Yellowish tinged skin and eyes. Only about half of the infected people show any symptoms. Others are carriers.

An effective vaccine has been developed to prevent hepatitis B, which is based on the surface antigen of the virus—hepatitis B surface antigen (HBsAg) positive or reactive means that the persons infected with HBV can potentially pass it to others who are in close daily contact. Patients who remain HBsAg positive and are aymptomatic are termed as HBsAg carriers.

Prevention

Following groups of people are recommended to undergo active immunization with hepatitis B vaccine:

1. Healthcare workers handling blood and blood products.
2. Medical and paramedical workers in dialysis units or hemophilic centers.
3. Individuals receiving prolonged inpatient treatment.
4. Immune deficient individuals.
5. Patients with malignancies.

6. Spouses and sexual contacts of patients with acute hepatitis B or carriers of HBV.
7. Prostitutes and promiscuous male homosexuals.

Hepatitis C

By contact with infected blood and other body fluids leading to inflammation of liver.

Symptoms

The only symptom is fatigue in early stages. People may not know any other symtoms for decades. Later on, cirrhosis (liver failure) a serious liver disease, muscle and joint pain, kidney diseases, antoimmune disorders develop.

Diagnosis

Diagnosis is by blood test. There is no vaccine against hepatitis C.

At risk: Anyone who had blood transfusion. Healthcare workers, users of illegal drugs, people getting tattoos and long term hemodialysis patients. There is no vaccine against hepatitis C.

Hepatitis D: Delta Antigen

Hepatitis D virus is defective virus and depends on HBV for replication. It is spherical 36 to 38 nm in diameter and is surrounded by HBsAg envelope. It can cause infection only in the presence of HBV. It can be detected by ELISA and RIA. No specific prophylaxis exists but immunization with hepatitis B is effective because delta antigen cant infect persons immune to HBV.

Hepatitis E Virus

Hepatitis E virus is spherical, non-enveloped and 27 to 38 nm in diameter and possess single-stranded RNA genome surrounded by icosahedral capsid. It is associated with ingestion of fecally contaminated water. It can be detected by ELISA, PCR, Immunoelectron microscopy. It can be prevented by sanitation of chlorinated water.

Type A Hepatitis

Type A affects mainly children and young adults. It is 27 nm non-enveloped RNA virus and belongs to picornaviridae family.

Hepatitis A virus (HAV) causes infection through fecal-oral route and multiplies in intestinal epithelium and reaches liver by hematogenous spread and cause jaundice.

Diagnosis is usually done by ELISA. Sanitary practices should be improved to prevent disease. No specific antiviral drug is available.

Type B Hepatitis

Morphology

Hepatitis B virus is a 42 nm DNA virus with outer envelope and an inner core 27 nm in diameter enclosing viral genome and a DNA polymerase. Refer Figure 14.11.

The DNA has a plus strand and a minus strand and contain DNA polymerase at one end. Replication takes place in hepatocytes. DNA is synthesized from RNA by reverse transcriptions.

Pathogenesis

Transmission: Hepatitis B virus is transmitted from infected to healthy individual by parental, perinatal and sexual means. It contains three phases.

Preicteric phase: It is also called prodromal phase. During this phase, patient develops weakness malaise, anorexia, nausea, vomiting and pain.

Icteric phase: This phase occurs after 2 days to 2 weeks. During this phase patient develops jaundice, pale stools and dark urine.

Convalescent phase: Malaise and fatigue lasting for several weeks develop during this phase, which is quite long.

Laboratory Diagnosis

Hepatitis B surface antigen (HBsAg) is most commonly used test for diagnosing acute HBV infections or detecting carriers.

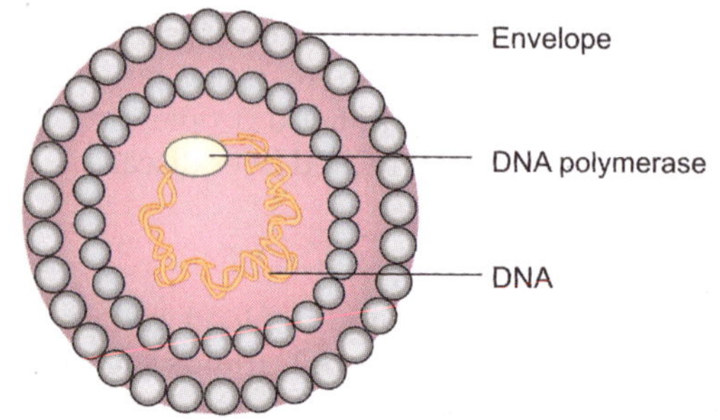

Fig. 14.11: Hepatitis virus

HBV are believed to be highly infectious whereas HCV is not detectable in serum and can be demonstrated by immunofluorescence. ELISA, radioimmunoassay (RIA) are highly sensitive.

Prophylaxis

Practices like promiscuous sex, injectable drug abuse, direct and indirect blood contact should be avoided.

Universal immunization prevent the diseases. Hyperimmune hepatitis B immunoglobulin (HBIg) is prepared from human volunteers with high titre anti-HBS and administered in a dose of 300 to 500 IU soon after exposure to infection, constitutes passive immunization. Active immunization containing 'S' gene of HBV is also effective.

No specific treatment is available, lamivudine, famciclovir are more effective.

Type C Hepatitis

Hepatitis C virus is 50 to 60 nm with single strand. Maternal neonatal transmission has also been reported. Clinical infection is less severe and can be detected by polymerase chain reaction (PCR).

RETROVIRUSES

Human Immunodeficiency Virus

Human immunodeficiency virus (HIV) causes acquired immunodeficiency syndrome (AIDS) (Fig. 14.12). HIV is divided into two major types HIV–1 and HIV–2.

Morphology

HIV–1 is of 100 nm in diameter containing a protein envelope to which glycoprotein are attached. The envelope encloses the icosahedral capsid core that contains two identical macromolecules of ssRNA as genetic material. Each of two RNA genome is made of 9749 nucleotides.

The three dimensional structure of viral envelope is made up of two proteins gp120 and gp41. gp120 is connected with gp41 through chemical connections and constitute the target of neutralizing antibodies. The central mass possess two helix of RNA molecules in the folded form to which reverse transcriptase is attached.

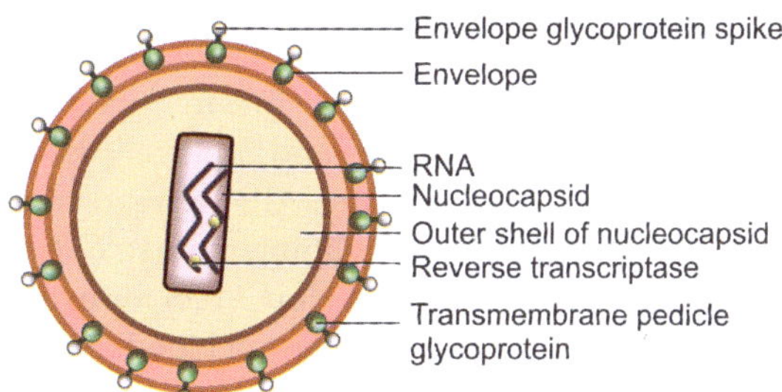

Fig. 14.12: Retrovirus—HIV

Mechanism of Infection

HIV–1 infection first occurs in macrophages. The gp120 binds to CD4 and then with CCR 5 thus forming site where HIV–1 fuses host cell membrane allowing insertion of viral nucleocapsid. The net result is destruction of T cells. Due to this opportunistic infections appear in the body.

Laboratory Diagnosis

Reverse-transcription polymerase chain reaction (RT-PCR) test is developed. Techniques like ELISA, western blot techniques can also be employed.

Acquired Immunodeficiency Syndrome

Acquired immunodeficiency syndrome (AIDS) is a disease of the immune system, in which the body's natural defences against infection breaks down due to an infection caused by a virus known as HIV (HIV–1 and HIV–2), ultimately leading to the death of the individual.

HIV is a RNA retrovirus in the *Lentivirus* genus. These viruses cause 'slow infection'. The virus remains silent and symptoms appear many years after the infection.

After entry into the blood, HIV invade and destroy T4 (CD4) helper cells, a subset of T lymphocytes leading to their destruction and depletion. This results in impaired cell-mediated immunity.

Transmission of AIDS

Sexual intercourse: Homosexual, heterosexual or bisexual contact. During sexual activity (vaginal and or oral sex) exchange of body fluids occur. Infection is effected as HIV is present in blood, semen, vaginal secretion and breast milk. 80 percent of the transmission is through sex, 7 percent through blood transfusion, 9 percent via blood infected needles and 3 percent from mother to child. World wide, AIDS spreads primarily through heterosexual intercourse (70%–75%) and three women develop AIDS for every two men. The HIV survives best in blood tissues and some body fluids such as semen and vaginal fluids. HIV cannot survive in air, water or on things that people touch (fomite).

Blood: Blood transfusions, sharing of needles as in drug addicts, accidental contamination by inadequately sterilized syringes, surgical and dental instruments.

Congenital (vertical): Infected mother can transmit to her child either through placental circulation or perinatally or postnatally through breast feeding.

Symptoms

Usually, incubation period is long (5–10 years as an average). The initial reactions is silent, years later progressive.

1. Weight loss (slim disease).
2. Prolonged and persistant fever.
3. Chronic diarrhea.
4. Persistent lymphadenopathy (lymph gland enlargement).
5. Opportunistic secondary infections due to fungi, protozoa, bacteria and viruses.
6. CNS is affected leading to neurological and psychological disturbances causing dementia.
7. Certain types of cancers—Kaposi's sarcoma appears as purplish nodules over the chest and abdomen.

Diagnosis

Serological tests for specific antibodies to HIV antigen by:
1. ELISA.
2. Western blot.

Prophylaxis

1. *Screening:* Before blood transfusion and organ transplantation the donors should be tested by serological tests.

2. *Health education (sex education):* To practice safe sex, avoid multiple partners, use of barrier contraceptives (condoms).
3. No effective vaccine has been found.

High-risk Groups

1. Male homosexual and their partners.
2. Intravenous drug addicts.
3. Transfusion recipients.
4. Hemophiliacs.

Prevention

The following methods are recommended:
Sexual contact: The use of condoms, sex education.
Sharing of needles: Contaminated syringes should not be shared.
Screening of individuals within risk groups.
Therapy: Zidovudine, Zalicitabine, Stavudine, abacavir.

What is HIV positive?

HIV positive means that a retrovirus has been proved positive by any of the direct or indirect methods of laboratory investigations.

Any HIV positive case, even if there is no overt signs and symptoms of the disease is classified as AIDS group II as per international classification laid down by the Center for Disease Control (CDC). The center has also classified 'syndrome' into various groups and subgroups according to clinical presentations.

How Effective are Antiretroviral Drugs?

Antiretroviral drugs reduce virus in blood. The white blood count (WBC) goes up and helps fight opportunistic infection like TB, malaria and meningitis, which are most common in HIV patients.

DISEASES CAUSED BY VIRUSES TRANSMITTED BY MOSQUITO

Japanese Encephalitis

Culex mosquito transmits Japanese encephalitis (JE) virus. It infects animals, birds and man. Among many infected individuals, a fever develop encephalitis. Others develop immunity. From the clinical features of patients, one cannot distinguish between JE and other forms of encephalitis. The name 'Japanese' came from the fact that this virus was first identified in Japan.

Dengue Fever

Aedes mosquito transmits dengue virus, which causes a syndrome of high fever, severe body aches, particularly of the back around large joints and in the periorbital region and in some, a fine generalized erythematous skin rash. The rash may occur in palms and it may be accompanied by itching. Early reporting and treatment is essential. Remove water from coolers and small containers at least once a week. Observe weekly dry day. Use aerosol during the day. All suspected cases of fever with bleeding should be thoroughly investigated for platelet count. Use larvivorous fishes in large mosquito breeding containers. Do not wear clothes that expose arms and legs. Do not use Aspirin. Do not keep water in the open container.

Chikungunya Fever

Chikungunya fever is a vector-borne viral disease transmitted to human beings by the bite of infected *Aedes, Culex* mosquitoes including the daybiting *Aedes aegypti* and *Aedes albopictus* species, incubation period is 2 to 3 days with a range of 1 to 12 days.

Clinical Manifestation

Fever, severe arthralgia with chills, headache, photophobia, anorexia, nausea, vomiting and abdominal pains. Migrating polyarthritis mainly affects small joints of hands, wrist, ankle and feet, lesser involvement in larger joints. Maculopapular rashes seen mainly seen in trunk and limbs.

Diagnosis

Increased AST, increased C-reactive proteins, IgM-capture ELISA.

Preventive Measures

There is no vaccine, according to WHO, the main preventive measures is to stop proliferation of mosquito by reducing their breeding ground, wearing long sleeved shirts, mosquito nets, staying in screened indoor. Insect repellant containing up to 50 percent DEET (N, N-diethyl-meta-toluamide).

VIRUS INFECTIONS TRANSMITTED BY DROPLET INFECTION

H1N1 Flu (Swine Flu)

Symptoms

In adults, fever, cough, sore throat, running nose, breath lesser, chest pain, drowsiness, fall in blood pressure, sputum mixed with blood, bluish discoloration of nails. In children, influenza like illness, high and persistent fever, inability to feed well, convulsions, shortness of breath, difficulty in breathing, etc.

Precaution

1. Wash your hands frequently with soap and water. Alcohol-based hand cleansers are also effective.
2. Avoid touching your eyes, nose or mouth as far as possible.
3. Avoid close contact with sick people.
4. Maintain high levels of personal hygiene.
5. Stay home when you are sick. Take medicine strictly as per doctor's advice.
6. Cover your nose and mouth with a handkerchief when you cough or sneeze.
7. Keep your body fit and strong by exercising.
8. Avoid smoking and alcohol intake.
9. Drink 8 to 10 glasses of water every day to flush out toxins from your system.
10. Avoid crowded areas as far as possible.

A person with H1N1 flu symptoms should go to the designated hospital for check-up. Only severe cases will be admitted. If the patient is detected with H1N1 flu, but shows mild symptoms, he/she will be given the option of being treated at home.

Common Cold

Since there are more than twenty types of cold viruses, an individual may get repeated attacks of cold. A person with cold broadcasts viruses while coughing or sneezing. Covering nose and mouth by a handkerchief reduces the chance of infecting others.

Sore throat, bronchitis, bronchiolitis, croup and pneumonia are commonly caused by many viruses. They include adenoviruses, parainfluenza viruses, influenza viruses and respiratory syncytial viruses.

Measles

All children get measles virus infection and most of them develop clinical measles characterized by fever, generalized maculopapular skin rash, cough, stuffy running nose, conjuctival redness and Koplik spot. Measles vaccine is now used to prevent measles and its complications. A disease of older children and young adults called subacute sclerosing panencephalitis is late sequala of measles virus infection.

German Measles or Rubella

Rubella is another exanthematous fever, occasionally confused with measles. The disease is important because of severe congenital (teratogenic infection) malformations in the child if the mother contracts this infection during the first trimester of pregnancy. The salient features of this virus are as below:

Member of the genus *Rubivirus*, family togaviridae:

- RNA virus with envelope
- Nucleocapsid is 30 nm in diameter
- Stable at 4°C, pH = 6 to 8
- Sensitive to lipid solvents, UV rays
- Four types of antigens
- Does not produce CPE in cell lines.

Clinical Features

Clinical features are atypical, mainly rash and lymphadenopathy with fever. It enters the body by inhalation. Replication of virus occurs in cervical lymph nodes. Incubation period is 2 to 8 weeks. Arthritis is a common complication especially in females.

If rubella infection occurs in early pregnancy, the fetus may die, otherwise congenital malformation is common in first trimester. The commonest malformations are cardiac defect, cataract and deafness. The other features in babies of congenital rubella are hepatosplenomegaly, thrombocytopenic purpura, myocarditis and bone lesions. Rubella virus is found in all excretion of congenitally-infected infants. That is the reason why infected babies cause infection to staff in nurseries.

Diagnosis

Can be established by virus isolation from blood (early stage) and throat swab. However, serological diagnosis is made by hemagglutination, inhibition, neutralization, complement fixation, immunofluoresence of platelets and aggregation tests. In congenital rubella, diagnosis is made by demonstrating IgM.

Prevention

Vaccine is now available as a component of MMR vaccine, where it is available along with vaccines of measles and mumps. New vaccine is RA 27/3. The safe period of giving vaccine to young girls is 12 months prior to puberty.

Chickenpox or Varicella

Varicella virus is transmitted by droplet infections. The resultant infection manifests as an illness characterized by a vesicular rash. After recovery, the virus may remain dormant in the body for many more years and then cause another illness called herpes zoster. Children may get chickenpox after contact with a patient with herpes zoster.

VIRUS INFECTIONS TRANSMITTED BY FECAL-ORAL ROUTE

Poliomyelitis

Poliovirus type 1, 2 and 3 may cause this disease. While the vast majority get infected without ill effects, one in 100 to 300 develop a neurological disease—either limp paralysis, bulbar paralysis (paralysis of the medulla oblongata) or a combination of both. Disease is due to the infection and destruction of motor nerve cells of the spinal cord or the cranial nerve nuclei. One of the predisposing factors causing an increased chance of paralysis is the intramuscular infection during an abdominal infection. Such a disease is called provocative poliomyelitis.

Two types of vaccines are now available to prevent poliomyelitis. They are inactivated or killed vaccine given by injection (Salk) and the live-attenuated vaccine given orally (Sabin).

Polio Vaccine

Oral polio vaccine (Sabin) is prepared with three types of attenuated polioviruses. Potency of this vaccine should be maintained by cold chains. Three doses are administered. Interval between two doses should be 4 to 6 weeks. The parents are instructed not to give anything by mouth to the children 30 minutes before and after administration of polio vaccine. It is necessary to give polio vaccine to children who had suffered from poliomyelitis to protect them from the other two viruses—against which they may not possess immunity.

Pulse Polio Immunization

Pulse polio immunizations (PPIs) are when polio vaccine is given to all the children of India—0 to 5 years of age on a single day regardless of their previous immunization. Government of India conducted the first round of PPI consisting of two immunization days—6 weeks apart—9 December 1995 and 20 January 1996. The first PPI targeted all children under 3 years. Later on, as per WHO recommendations it was decided to increase the age from under 3 to under 5 years.

So far, 30 rounds of PPIs have been conducted (up to January 2011). Polio should have been eradicated by now but the vaccine in some places was not adequately protected by cold chain and had become ineffective. This year the program may be stopped and polio is almost eradicated in India.

Rotavirus Diarrhea

One of the commonest causes of gastroenteritis in infants and young children is a newly identified vcirus called *Rotavirus.*

Mycology

INTRODUCTION

Study of fungi is called mycology. Fungi are eukaryotic, saprophytic, obligate or facultatively aerobic organisms. They possess cell walls made up of chitin, mannan and polysaccharides. Fungi may be unicellular (yeasts) or multicellular (molds) and divide asexually or sexually.

Human fungal infections are broadly of two types, namely superficial and deep seated (systemic). A third type of fungal infection is opportunistic, which occurs in debilitating persons (Fig. 15.1).

SUPERFICIAL MYCOSES

Superficial mycoses are of two types:
1. Surface infections.
2. Cutaneous infections.

Surface Infections

Fungi live on dead layers and have no contact with living tissue. Example include, tinea versicolor and tinea nigra.

Cutaneous Infections

Dermatophytosis

Dermatophytes are filamentous fungus, which infect skin, hair and nails. They cause dermatophytosis popularly called tinea or ring worm.

They have been classified into three genera:
i. *Trichophyton*—skin, hair and nails are infected.
ii. *Microsporum*—hair and skin are infected.
iii. *Epidermophyton*—attacks skin and nails but not hair. Refer Figure 15.2.

Laboratory diagnosis—Are as follows:

Specimen—Skin, hair and nail are collected.

Direct microscopy—10 percent KOH is used to observe fungal hyphae, lactophenol cotton blue preparation can also be used.

Culture—Sabouraud dextrose agar (SDA) with bacterial antibodies is used.

Treatment: Oral griseofulvin is the drug of choice.

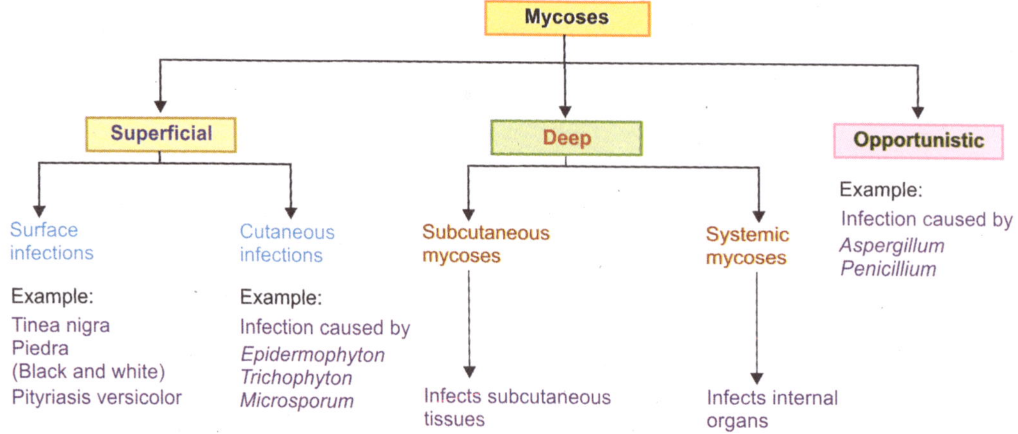

Fig. 15.1: Classification of human fungal infections

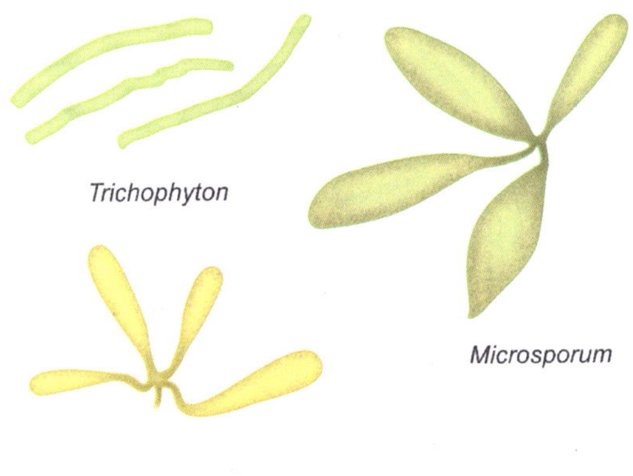

Fig. 15.2: Three genera of dermatophytes.

DEEP MYCOSES

Deep mycotic infections may be classified as subcutaneous and systemic mycoses.

Subcutaneous Mycoses

Mycetoma

Mycetoma affects foot and other parts of body as seen in Madurai district of Tamil Nadu. It is referred as 'Madura foot'. It enters through trauma and releases fluid from abscess, which contains granules. Sulfonamides are generally used.

Sporotrichosis

Sporotrichosis is disease of skin and subcutaneous tissue and enters through thorn pricks or some injuries. Causative agent is *Sporothrix* (Fig. 15.3).

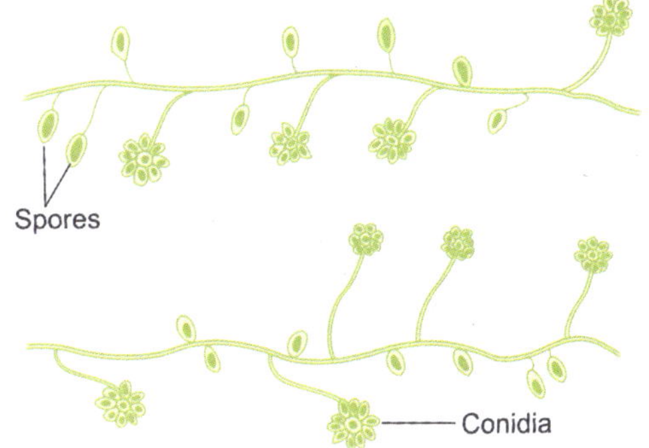

Fig. 15.3: *Sporothrix*

Rhinosporidiosis

Rhinosporidiosis is confined to nose, mouth or eye and causative agent is *Rhinosporidium*. Most infections occur in males who have frequent contact with stagnant water and aquatic life.

Systemic Mycoses

Cryptococcosis

Crytococcosis is caused by yeast *Cryptococcus neoformans* abundant in feces of pigeons and other birds. Infection is acquired by inhalation. It contains a capsule, which may be demonstrated by Indian ink or nigrosin staining.

Skin, lymph nodes, bones and other organs may be involved. It causes three types of diseases pneumonitis, meningitis and cutaneous cryptococcosis.

Usually, SDA plates are used for culture. Cells can be observed under microscopy by either gram staining technique or lactophenol cotton blue. Refer Figure 15.4.

Histoplasmosis

Histoplasmosis is caused by *Histoplasma capsulatum* and affects reticuloendothelial system. It is present in soil enriched with excreta of birds or bats. As it involves reticuloendothelial system it results in lymphadenopathy, hepatosplenomegaly, fever, anemia. It is dimorphic, i.e. it exists as both yeast and mycelial forms.

Blastomycosis

Blastomycosis is caused by a dimorphic fungus, *Blastomyces dermatitidis*. Infection is caused due to inhalation of spores in soil. Refer Figure 15.5.

It infects lungs and other tissues like skin, bone and genitourinary tract.

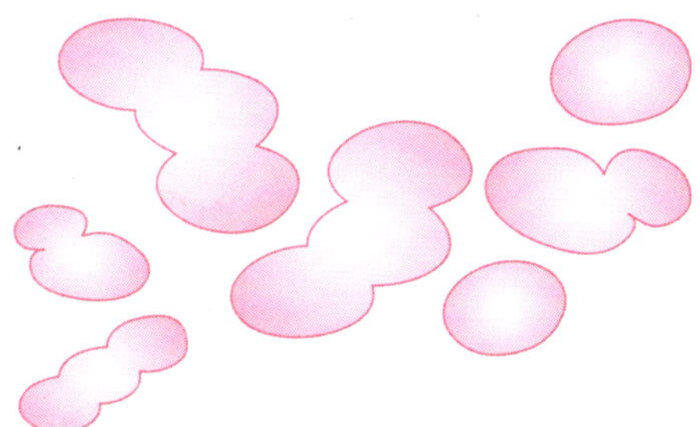

Fig. 15.4: *Cryptococcus neoformans*

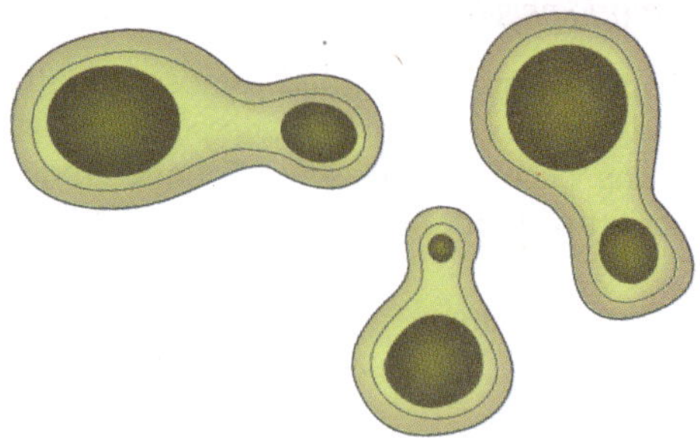

Fig. 15.5: *Blastomyces dermatitidis*

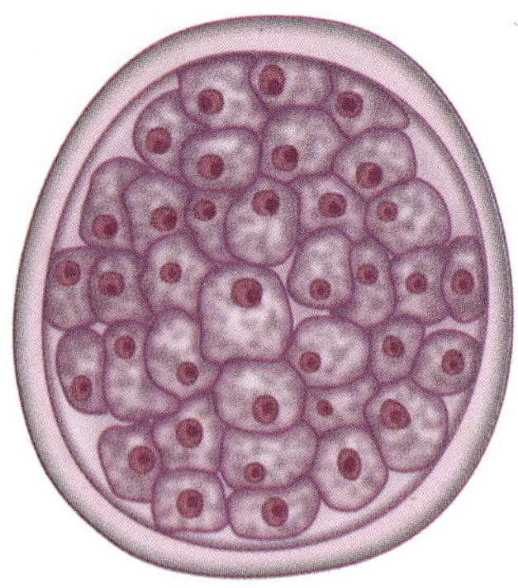

Fig. 15.7: Appearence of spherules of *Coccidioides immitis*

Paracoccidioidomycosis

Paracoccidioidomycosis is caused by dimorphic *Paracoccidioides brasiliensis*, a dimorphic fungus. It involves lungs, mucosa, skin and lymphatic system. Infection is by inhalation of spores. It causes ulcers of buccal and nasal mucosa. Refer Figure 15.6.

Coccidioidomycosis

Coccidioides immitis, a dimorphic fungus is the causative agent. Disease is caused due to inhalation of dust containing fungal spores. It causes pulmonary diseases like influenza fever to severe pneumonia. Refer Figure 15.7.

Mucormycosis

Rhizopus, Mucor causes this disease in diabetes and other debilitating diseases. Primary infection occur in lungs invading arteries. The fungi can be grown on sabouraud medium without cycloheximide. Refer Figure 15.8.

OPPORTUNISTIC MYCOSES

Some saprophytic fungi usually do not produce disease but may cause infection under special

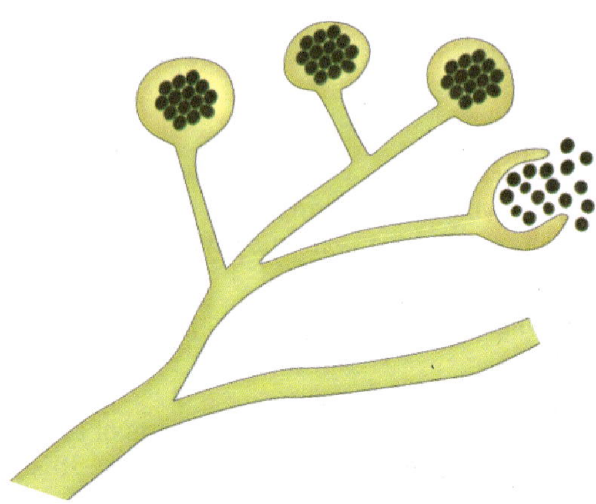

Fig. 15.8: *Mucor*

conditions such as immunocompromised individuals. *Aspergillus, Penicillium, Mucor, Rhizopus* species grow on everything. Aspergillosis and mucormycosis are important opportunistic systemic mycoses. *Aspergillus* produces conidiospores at tips of hyphae.

Aspergillosis

Aspergilli are ubiquitous in nature. *Aspergillus fumigatus (A. fumigatus)* is the main opportunistic pathogen. It occurs as following clinical types:

1. Pulmonary aspergillosis.
2. *Aspergillus* asthma.
3. Bronchopulmonar aspergillosis.
4. Aspergilloma.

Disseminated Aspergillosis

Aspergillosis is caused by inhalation of *Aspergillus* spores.

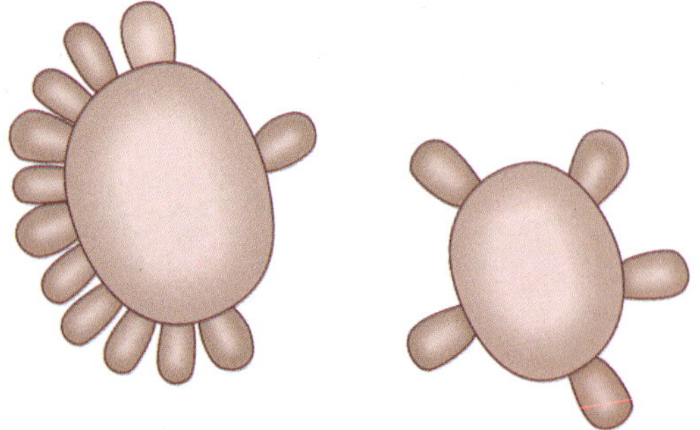

Fig. 15.6: *Paracoccidioides brasiliensis*

For culture of *A. fumigatus*, SDA without cycloheximide are used. Lactophenol cotton blue preparation from colonies shows branching and septate hyphae. *A. flavus* produce a mycotoxin called 'aflatoxin'.

Penicilliosis

Penicillium species causes opportunistic human infections. Refer Figure 15.9.

It causes penicilliosis, keratitis, otomycosis and deep infections. They grow rapidly on SDA.

P. marneffei has been reported as opportunistic pathogen especially in HIV-infected individuals. *Penicillium* produces an important antibiotic.

Athlete's Foot

Athlete's foot is a fungal infection of the skin. It usually occurs between the toes or on the soles of the feet. Fungus most commonly affects the feet because shoes ensure a warm, dark and humid environment, which encourages fungus growth. Damp areas around swimming pools, locker areas and showers are breeding grounds for these fungi. Since infection was common among athletes who used these facilities, the term 'athlete's foot' became popular.

Symptoms of Athlete's Foot

1. Red, scaly rash between the toes.
2. Itching and burning in the affected areas.
3. After itching, the areas become raw and weepy.

4. Common in adolescent children, especially boys.
5. Bad smelly feet.

Prevention

1. Do not allow the child to walk barefoot around damp areas.
2. Sun dry the child's shoes between uses.
3. Change his socks daily or more often, if needed.
4. Wash his feet daily and after play.
5. Dry his feet carefully especially between his toes.
6. Cotton socks are preferred, since they absorb sweat.

Candidiasis or Candidosis

Candidosis an infection of the skin, mucosa and rarely of internal organs is caused by a yeast-like fungus *Candida albicans* and occasionally by other *Candida* species.

Candida albicans is an ovoid or spherical budding cell, which produces pseudomycelia both in culture and in tissues. *Candida* species are normal inhabitants of the skin and mucosa. Candidosis is an opportunistic endogenous infection, the common predisposing factor being diabetes.

Cutaneous candidosis may be intertriginous or paronychia. The former is an erythematous scaling or moist lesion with sharply demarcated borders, where papular lesions are most prominent. The sites affected are those where the skin is macerated by perspiration—groin, perineum, axillae and inframammary fold. Paronychia and onychia are seen in operations that lead to frequent immersion of hands in water.

Common mucosal lesions are vaginitis characterized by an acidic discharge and found frequently in pregnancy and oral thrush found commonly in bottle fed infants, aged and debilitated. Creamy white patches appear on the tongue or buccal mucosa, that leave a red oozing surface on removal.

Intestinal candidosis is a frequent sequel to oral antibiotic therapy and may present as diarrhea not responding to treatment.

Bronchopulmonary candidosis is seen as a rare complication of persisting pulmonary or systemic disease. Systemic infections such as

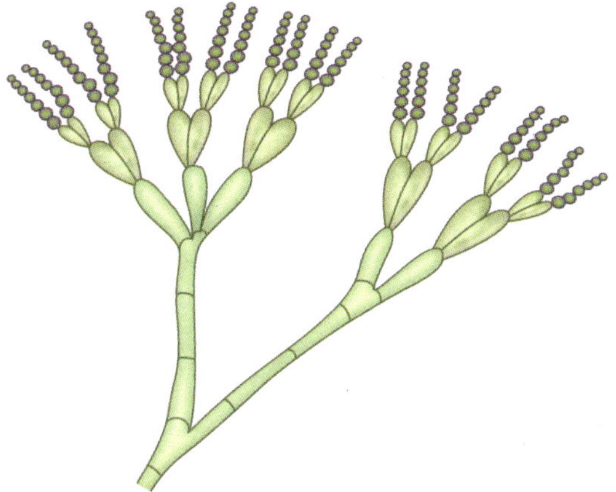

Fig. 15.9: Penicillium

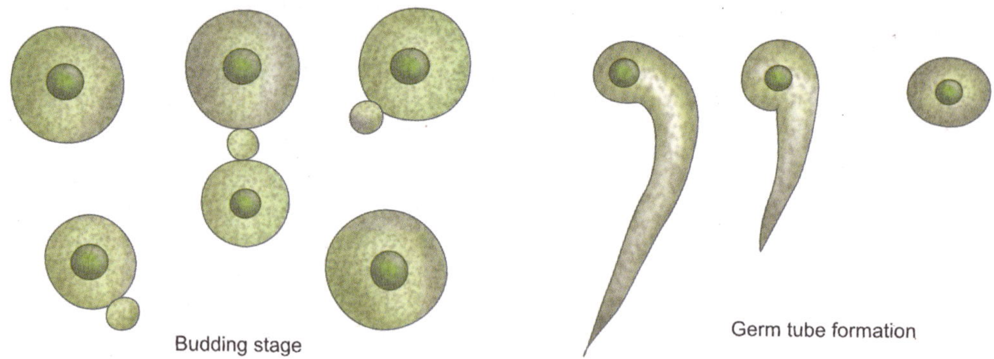

Fig. 15.10: *Candida albicans*

septicemia, endocarditis and meningitis may occur as terminal complications in severe generalized diseases such as leukemia and in patients on prolonged immunosuppression.

Candida granuloma and chronic mucocutaneous candidosis are serious manifestations seen in immune deficiencies.

Laboratory Diagnosis

Diagnosis is by microscopy and culture.

Collection of infected material: Skin or nail scrapings, mucous patches from mouth, vagina or anus, sputum, blood, cerebrospinal fluid (CSF) or feces may be collected for laboratory diagnosis. The materials must be collected in sterile containers or as smears on slides.

Microscopic examination: Skin and nail scrappings are mounted in 10 percent KOH with a coverslip and heated gently. Sputum or mucous material should be pressed as a thin film with a coverslip on a slide. Wet films or gram-stained smear from lesions or exudates show *Candida*. Since have *Candida* in normal skin or muscle as well, only their abundant presence is of significance.

Culture: Demonstration of mycelial forms indicates colonization and tissue invasion. The clinical material is cultured in Sabouraud's glucose agar at room temperature and at 37°C. The growth appears in 3 to 4 days as cream-colored, pasty, smooth colonies and has a yeasty odor.

Germ tube formation: This can be ascertained by inoculating 0.5 mL of rabbit, fetal calf or human serum with a small quantity of young test serum. The suspension is incubated at 37°C for 3 hours and a drop of it is examined with the microscope. Germ tubes are seen as long tube-like projections from yeast cells. Refer to the Figure 15.10.

Parasitology

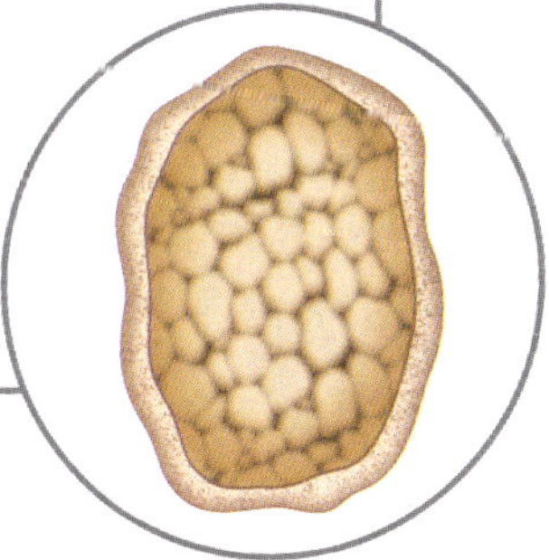

Introduction to Medical Parasitology—Amebiasis

MEDICAL PARASITOLOGY

Medical parasitology deals with the parasites, which infect man and diseases produced by them.

Parasite

An organism, which is dependent on another organism for its survival. It obtains nourishment and shelter from the organisms on which it thrives. Parasite are broadly classified into protozoa and helminths, the details are given in Figure 16.1.

Obligate Parasite

A parasite, which is completely dependent on the host.

Pathogen

A parasite, which is able to produce disease in the host.

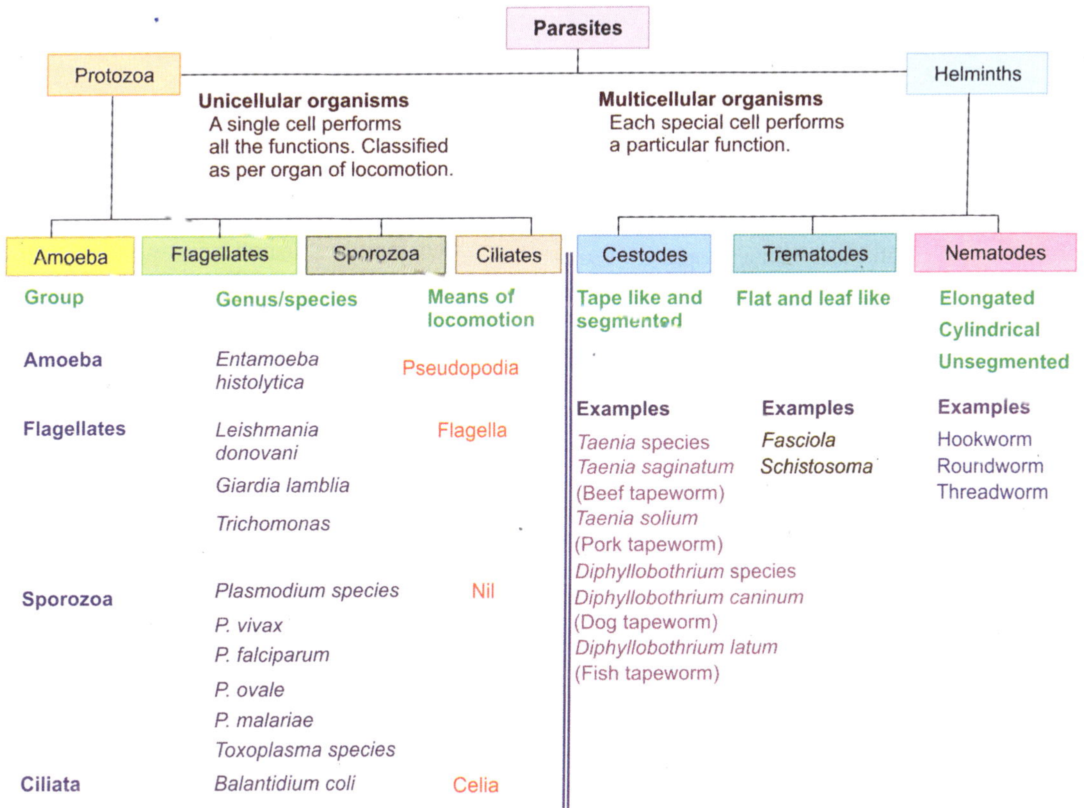

Fig. 16.1: Classification of parasites

Host

An organism, which harbors the parasite and is usually larger than the parasite.

Intermediate Host

A host in which the intermediate stage of the parasite develops. The species in which the larval stage of the parasite lives or asexual multiplication takes place.

Definitive Host

A host in which sexual reproduction takes place or the adult form of the parasite resides.

Man is the definitive host in most human parasite infection (e.g. filarial, roundworm, hookworm), but it is in the intermediate host in malaria and hydatid disease.

The vertebrate species in which the parasite passes its life cycle and which may act as a source of infection for man is called reservoir host. Intermediate hosts in which metazoan parasite undergoes multiplication is called amplifier hosts. Parasitic infections man acquires from animals are called zoonoses.

PROTOZOA: AMOEBA

Amoeba are structurally simple protozoa, which have no fixed shape. The cytoplasm is bound by a unit membrane and can be differentiated into an outer ectoplasm and an inner endoplasm. Pseudopodia are formed by the ectoplasm thrusting out, being followed by the endoplasm flowing into it to produce blunt projections. Pseudopodial process appears and disappear, producing quick changes in the shape of the cell. Pseudopodia are employed for locomotion and engulfment of food by phagocytosis.

Amoeba may be free living or parasite. The parasite amoeba inhabit the alimentary canal. Parasite amoeba belongs to the genus *Entamoeba*, e.g. *E. histolytica, E. coli*.

Entamoeba Histolytica

Entamoeba histolytica is an important human pathogen causing amebic dysentery, as well as hepatic amebiasis and other extraintestinal lesions. *E. coli* is a common commensal in the colon and it may be mistaken for *E. histolytica*.

The infection with *E. histolytica* is known as amebiasis, which is defined as the presence of *E. histolytica* in the body with or without clinical manifestation of the disease. It may manifest as diarrhea, dysentery or in any of its extra complications especially hepatic or pulmonary amebiasis.

Morphology

Three phases have been recognized, trophozoite (active), precystic (intermediate) and cystic (inactive).

Trophozoite

Trophozoite stage is also known as growing stage, feeding stage or active vegetative stage (Fig. 16.2A). It is irregular in shape and varies in size from 10 to 40 nm. Trophozoites have the following:

1. Ectoplasm.
2. Endoplasm.
3. Ingested red blood cells (RBCs).
4. Pseudopodia.
5. Nuclei.
6. Chromatoidal bars.
7. Glycogen mass.

A fixed shape is lacking because of constantly changing position. In wet microscopic preparations made from freshly passed stool, trophozoites are actively motile. They move by pseudopodia, which are cytoplasmic protrusions that may be formed on any point on the surface of the organism. The pseudopodium is quickly thrust out and may vary in form from short, blunt and broad to long and fingerlike.

The cytoplasm is differentiated into a thin outer layer of clear transparent, refractive ectoplasm and an inner granular endoplasm. There is only one nucleus, which is 4 to 6 nm in size, spherical in shape and placed eccentrically.

Precystic stage

Precystic stage is colorless, round or oval and smaller than trophozoite, but larger than cyst. It ranges between 10 to 20 nm in size (Fig. 16.2B). The endoplasm is free of RBCs and other food particles. Pseudopodial action in sluggish and there is no progressive movement. The structure of the nucleus is the same as in trophozoite.

Cyst

During encystment, the parasite becomes rounded and is surrounded by a smooth refractile non-staining wall, which is about 0.5 nm. The nucleus retains the characteristics of the trophozoite. Early in the development, the cyloplasm of the cyst shows 1 to 4 chromatoidal bars, which are refractile, oblong bodies with rounded ends, which stain black with iron hematoxylin stain and a glycogen mass, which stains brown with iodine. The cyst is initially unicellular (Fig. 16.2C), but by binary fission soon develops into a binuclear (Fig. 16.2D) and quadrinuclear body (Fig. 16.2E). As the cyst matures, both the glycogen mass and the chromatoidal bars generally disappears. The cyst containing 1 to 4 nuclei are passed in feces.

Life Cycle

The life cycle of *E. histolytica* is essentially completed in a single host. The main source of infection is the cyst-passing chronic patient or asymptomatic carrier (Fig. 16.3). Acutely ill patients do not act as reservoir since, they excrete non-infective trophozoites. On ingestion, the quadrinucleate cyst passes unharmed through the stomach and encysts in the cecum where the pH is alkaline. The resistant cell wall is lysed by the action of the intestinal trypsin and a single trophozoite with four nuclei called metacyst is

liberated. The trophozoite divides by binary fission to give rise to eight daughter trophozoites. The daughter trophozoites are actively motile and migrate to ileocecal region. The optimum habitat for the metacystic trophozoites is the submucous tissue of the large intestine where they grow and multiply by binary fission. Some develop into precystic forms and cysts, which are passed in feces to repeat the cycle. The entire life cycle is completed in one host, the man.

During growth *E. histolytica* secretes a proteolytic enzyme, which brings about destruction and necrosis of tissues leading to ulcers. A large number of trophozoites are excreted along with blood and mucus in the feces. This condition is called amebic dysentery. Sometimes the trophozoites enter into deeper layers and may gain entry into the liver. In the liver they multiply and produce amebic hepatitis and amebic liver abscess. The difference between amebic dysentery and bacillary dysentery is given in the Table 16.1.

Infection with *E. histolytica* does not necessarily lead to disease. In most cases, it remains within the lumen of the large intestine feeding on colonic contents and mucus as a commensal without causing any ill effects. Such persons become carriers or asymptomatic cyst passers as

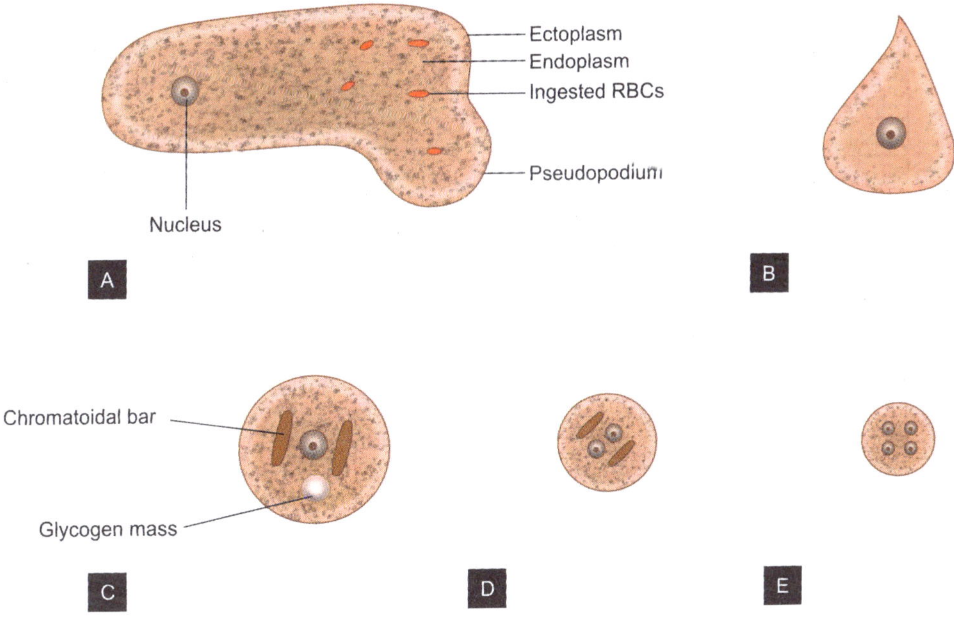

Fig. 16.2: Stages of *Entamoeba histolytica*. **A.** Trophozoite; **B.** Precystic stage; **C.** Uninucleate; **D.** Binucleate; **E.** Mature quadrinucleate cyst.

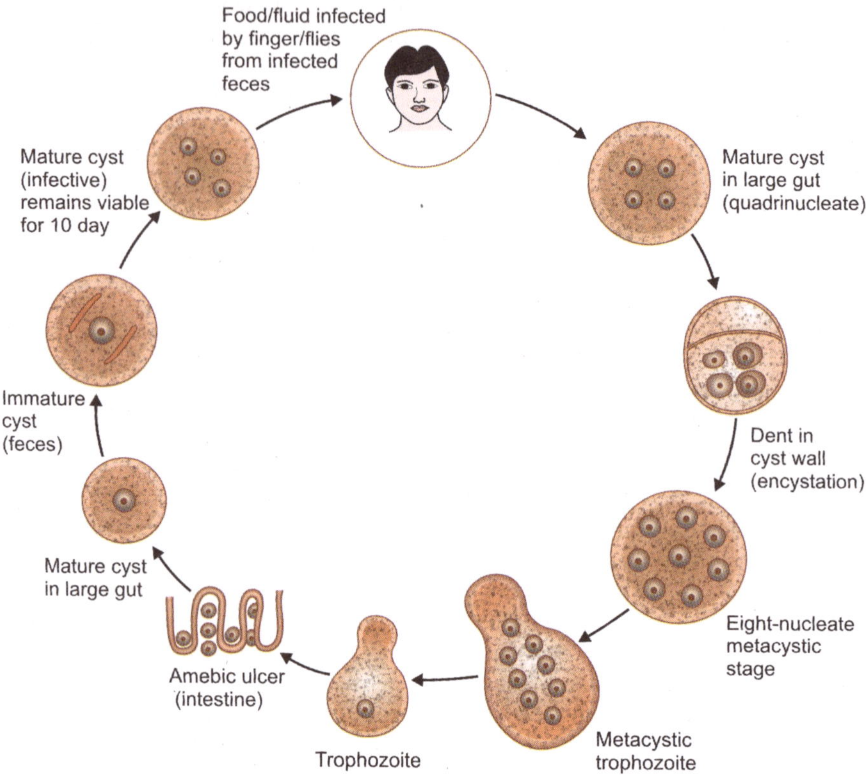

Fig. 16.3: Life cycle of *Entamoeba histolytica*

Table 16.1: Difference between amebic dysentery and bacillary dysentery

Features	Amebic dysentery	Bacillary dysentery
Number	6 to 8 per day	> 10 per day (*Shigella*)
Amount	Relatively copious	Small
Appearance	Feces with stratum of blood and mucus seen over the surface	Consists of blood and mucus, hardly any fecal matter
Color and consistency	Dark red (altered blood) liquid is formed, not adherent to container	Bright red (fresh blood)
Odor	Offensive	
Chemical action	Acidic	Alkaline
Microscopic examination		
Pus cells	Scanty	Numerous
Red blood cells	In clumps, discolored	Discrete
Eosinophils	Present	Absent or rare
Macrophages	Absent	Present, showing ingested erythrocytes (RBCs)
Charcot-Leyden crystals	Present	Absent
E. histolytica	Trophozoites present	Absent
Bacteria	Numerous and motile	Scanty, non-motile

their stools contain cysts. They are responsible for the maintenance and spread of infection in the community. The infection may get spontaneously activated and clinical disease ensures. Such latency and reactivation are characteristic of amebiasis.

Laboratory Diagnosis

Laboratory diagnosis depends on the demonstration of *E. histolytica* in the material obtained from any particular lesion such as stools, pus, from hepatic abcess and sputum.

Intestine amebiasis

Stool examination: In acute amebic dysentery stool or colonic scrapings from ulcers are examined by naked eye and microscopic examination.

Normal saline preparation is useful for demonstration of actively motile trophozoites, while iodine preparation is required for the study of cysts or dead trophozoites.

Kala-azar, The Black Sickness

INDIAN LEISHMANIASIS

Leishmania, the flagellated protozoan causes kala-azar. All members of this group pass their life cycle in two hosts, the mammalian host and the insect vector female sandfly. In man and other mammalian hosts, they multiply within macrophages in which they occur extensively in the amastigote form (LD bodies—named after discoverers Leishman and Donovan, both of them reported on the organism simultaneously, Leishman from London in May 1903 and Donvan from Madras in July 1903) having an ovoid body containing a nucleus and a kinetoplast (blepharoplast plus basal body [Fig. 17.1]).

When stained with Giemsa or Wright stain, the cytoplasm appears pale blue and nucleus appears red.

Promastigote Form

Promastigote form is present in the digestive tract of the sandfly and in cultures. The mature form is spindle shaped and measures 15 to 20 nm × 1.2 nm, the nucleus is centrally located.

A delicate flagellum equal to or longer than the body length projects from the front. Using Leishman stain, the cytoplasm appears blue, nucleus pink or violet and the kinetoplast bright red.

Life Cycle

Natural transmission from man-to-man occurs by the bite of sandfly. After a blood meal, the flagellate develops in the gut of the insect to infective forms that migrate forward to pharynx, buccal cavity and mouth parts of the sandfly producing partial or complete blockage of the mouth. The parasites are dislodged by the efforts of the blocked sandfly to ingest blood. Transmission may also take place by contamination of the bite wound and by contact.

When promastigote forms gain entry to man, they lose their flagella, assume the amastigote form and multiply mainly within the mononu-

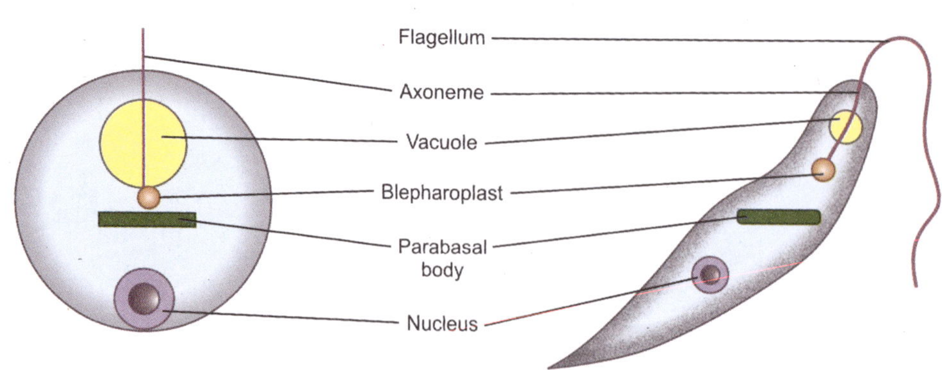

Fig. 17.1: Leishmania

clear cells and polymorphs. When the cells rupture, free parasites invade other cells and are phagocytosed.

Clinical Features

The incubation period is usually 3 to 6 months and may exceed 1 to 2 years. The clinical features of kala-azar are:
- Irregular fever
- Progressive enlargement of spleen and liver
- Anemia
- Loss of weight
- Dry skin and brittle hair (cutaneous leishmaniasis, cutaneous sore)
- Pigmentation of skin.

Laboratory Diagnosis

Depends upon demonstration or isolation of the parasite from blood or biopsy material and demonstration of *Leishmania* antibodies in the serum.

Demonstration of LD bodies (amastigote form) in specimens, blood, spleen, bone marrow or liver.

Malarial Parasites

Malaria is the most important parasitic disease of mankind. It accounts for 300 million cases and 2 million deaths annually, the large majority of them is in sub-Saharan Africa. Once prevalent over most of the world, it is now confined to the tropical and subtropical areas of Asia, Africa and South and Central America.

CAUSATIVE AGENTS

Malaria is a protozoan infection. There are four species of *Plasmodium*, which can cause malaria in human beings. They are:

- *Plasmodium vivax* (65% of cases in India)
- *Plasmodium falciparum* (also prevalent in India)
- *Plasmodium malariae* (causes cerebral malaria)
- *Plasmodium ovale*.

The international center for genetic engineering and biotechnology (ICGEB) in New Delhi has developed a vaccine against *P. vivax*.

LIFE CYCLE

The development of the parasite involves two hosts, one in man (intermediate host) and another in mosquito (definitive host). Asexual development of the parasite occurs in man and sexual development in mosquito (Fig. 18.1).

Human Cycle (Schizogony)

Man is the intermediate host. Sporozoite is the infective form of malarial parasite. These sporozoites are present in the salivary gland of the female *Anopheles* mosquito. Man gets infection by the bite of infected mosquito and sporozoites are introduced directly into blood circulation. The human cycle starts and it comprises of the following stages:

1. Pre-erythrocytic schizogony.
2. Erythrocytic schizogony.
3. Gametogony.
4. Exoerythrocytic schizogony.

Pre-erythrocytic Schizogony

Before starting erythrocytic schizogony in blood, sporozoite undergoes a developmental phase inside liver cells, called pre-erythrocytic schizogony. The sporozites (elongated and spindle shaped) become rounded inside the liver parenchymal cells. They undergo multiple nuclear division and develop into schizont. Size of the schizont varies in different species and it contains 20,000 to 50,000 merozoites (from schizo—split, gone—generation). The pre-erythrocytic cycle lasts for 8 days in *P. vivax*, 6 days in *P. falciparum*, 13 to 16 days in *P. malariae* and 9 days in *P. ovale*. After completion of this cycle, liver cells rupture and release merozoites into the blood stream.

Erythrocytic Schizogony

The merozoites released from pre-erythrocytic schizogony penetrate red blood cells (RBCs). They pass through the stages of trophozoite, schizont and merozoite (mero—part, zoon—animal). Depending on the species of malarial parasite there may be 6 to 12 merozoites in the RBCs. The RBCs rupture to release merozoites, which attack new RBCs and continue their erythrocytic schizogony repeating the cycle.

In *P. falciparum* infection, erythrocytic schizonts develop into male and female gametocytes known as microgametocytes. They develop in the RBCs. These are sexual forms and are found in the peripheral blood. The microgametocytes

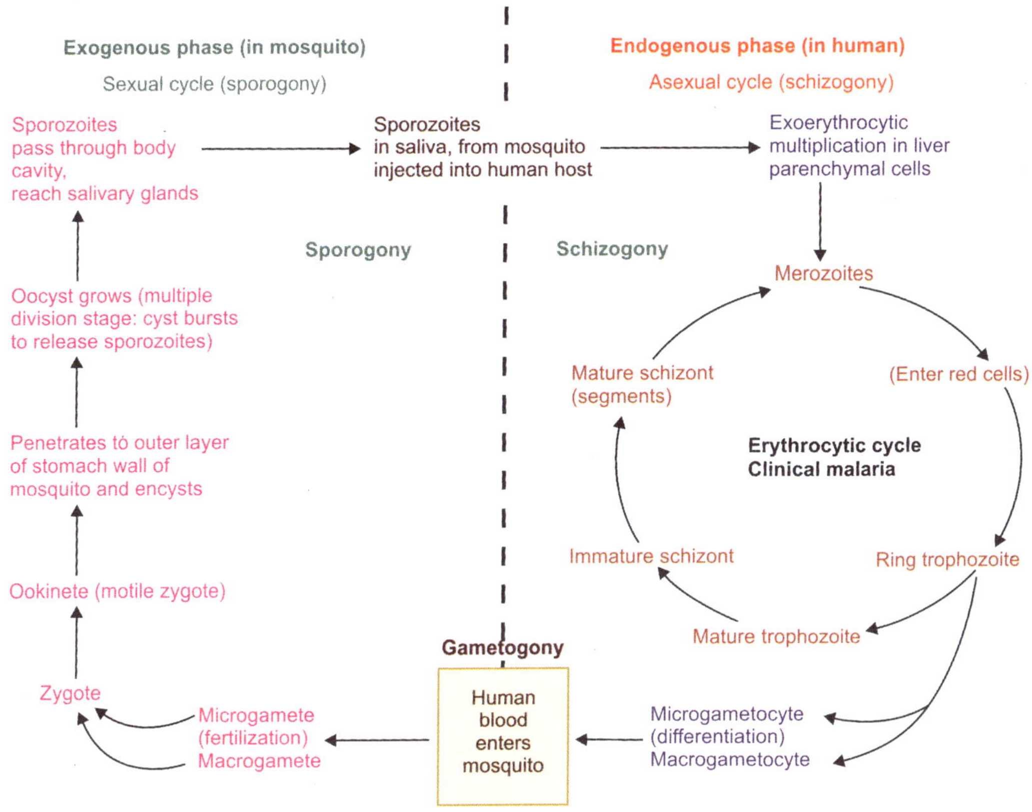

Fig. 18.1: Life cycle of malarial parasites

of all the four species are similar in size, cytoplasm stains blue and the nucleus is large and diffuse (Fig. 18.2). In contrast, the macrogametocytes are larger, the cytoplasm stains deep blue and the nucleus is small and compact.

Exoerythrocytic Schizogony

The exoerythrocytic schizogony resembles the pre-erythrocytic cycle. Some sporozoites on entering into liver cells do not undergo asexual multiplication, but enter a resting (dormant) phase. The resting stage is known as hypnozoite. After some period (usually 2 years) hypnozoites reactivate to become schizont and release merozoites. These merozoites attack RBCs and are responsible for relapse of malaria. Erythrocytic schizogony is absent in *P. falciparum* infection, therefore relapses do not occur in malaria caused by *P. falciparum*.

Mosquito Cycle (Sporogony)

The sexual cycle of malarial parasite actually starts in the human host by the formation of gametocytes, which are then transferred to mosquito for further development.

A female *Anopheles* mosquito during its blood meal from the patient, ingest both the sexual and asexual forms of the parasite, only the natural sexual forms are capable of further development in the mosquito and the rest die immediately.

In this midgut of the mosquito one microgametocyte develop into four to eight thread-like filamentous structures named microgamete. From one macrogametocyte only one macrogamete is formed. Fertilization occurs when a macrogamete penetrates into an opposite macrogamete. The fertilized macrogamete is known as zygote. The zygote lengthens and matures into an ookinete. The ookinete develops into an

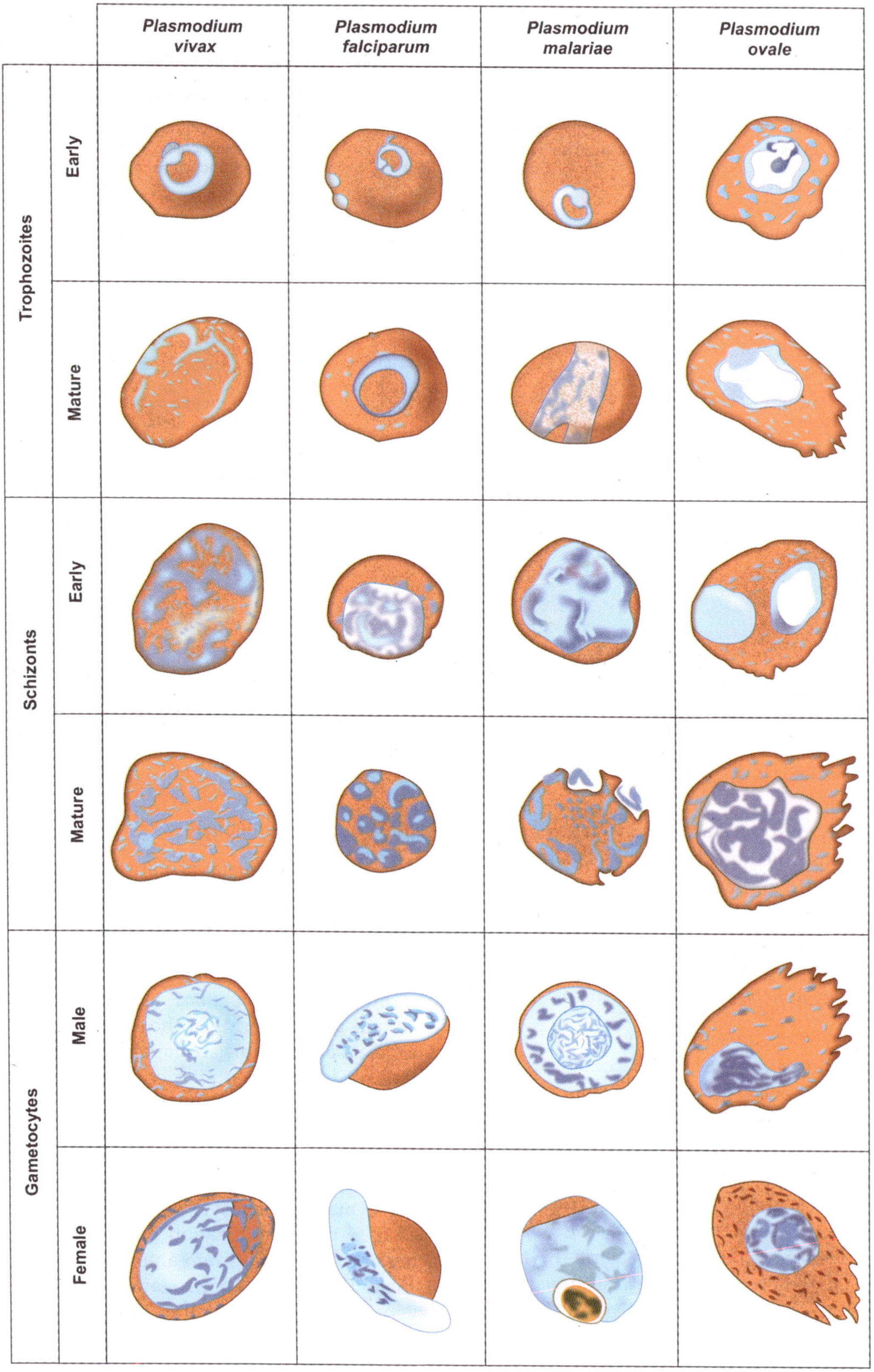

		Plasmodium vivax	*Plasmodium falciparum*	*Plasmodium malariae*	*Plasmodium ovale*
Trophozoites	Early				
	Mature				
Schizonts	Early				
	Mature				
Gametocytes	Male				
	Female				

Fig. 18.2: Malarial parasites—Erythrocytic stages of the four species of Plasmodium (Giemsa stain, magn. x 2,000)

oocyst. As oocyst matures, it increases in size and a large number of sporozoites (a few hundred to thousands) develop inside it. The number of oocysts in the stomach wall varies from a few to more than 100. The oocyst ruptures and releases sporozoites in the body cavity of the mosquito. The sporozoites are distributed into various organs and tissues of the mosquito. However, they have a special predilection for salivary glands. The mosquito is now capable of transmitting infection to man.

PERNICIOUS MALARIA

Pernicious malaria is life-threatening complication that somehow occurs in acute falciparum malaria. It is due to heavy parasitization. Various manifestation of pernicious anemia are grouped as cerebral malaria, algid malaria or septicemic malaria.

Cerebral Malaria

Cerebral malaria is characterized by hyperpyrexia, coma and paralysis, brain is congested.

Algid Malaria

Algid malaria is characterized by cold, clammy skin leading to peripheral circulatory failure.

Blackwater Fever

Blackwater fever is a manifestation of infection with *P. falciparum* occurring in those people who have been previously infected and have had inadequate dose of quinine. It is characterized by intravascular hemolysis, fever and hemoglobinuria.

Immunity

Immunity is species specific, stage specific and strain specific and lasts only till malaria parasite infection remains active. This type of immunity is known as premonition immunity.

LABORATORY DIAGNOSIS— MICROSCOPIC EXAMINATION

Thick and thin smears of the blood are prepared on the same slide or different slides. Thin smears are best for detection of species of *Plasmodium*. Thick smears are used for detection of more cases.

Blood for smear should be collected, a few hours after the height of the febrile paroxysm because the parasites are most abundant during this period. Blood is collected by pricking a finger prior to start of antimalarial therapy. For thick smear, take a drop of blood on the slide and spread it on an area of 1 sq cm. For thin smear take one drop of blood at one corner of the slide and spread with another slide so that talc formation occurs at the other end. Both, the thick and thin peripheral blood are stained with Leishman stain and examined under oil immersion objective of the microscope. Characteristic of stained malaria parasites inside RBCs are:

1. Cytoplasmic body, which is stained blue.
2. Nucleus (chromatin), which is stained red.
3. Presence of central unstained portion (vacuole) in the early stages of infection.
4. Presence of pigment in vacuole and protoplasma.
5. Presence of granules.
6. Red blood cells (RBCs) enlarged in *P. vivax* infection.
7. Multiple invasions of RBCs in *P. falciparum* infection.
8. Late stages of *P. falciparum* not seen in peripheral blood.
9. Gametocytes of *P. vivax*, *P. malariae* and *P. ovale* are round, while those of *P. falciparum* are crescent shaped.

Filariasis

WUCHERERIA BANCROFTI

As an Etiological Agent

There are eight species of parasites that can cause filariasis. Lymphatic filariasis is caused by *Wuchereria bancrofti* (filum = thread, helminth = nematode). The largest number of filariasis cases occurs in India.

Habitat

Adult worms are found in the lymphatic vessels and lymph nodes of man. Microfilariae are found in the blood.

Morphology

Adult worms are long hair-like transparent creamy white structures (Fig. 19.1). The male measures 35 to 40 mm × 0.1 mm and the female around 90 to 100 mm × 0.25 mm. The female is viviparous (bringing out live offsprings and not eggs) and liberates sheathed microfilariae into lymphs from where they find their way into blood. Males and females remain coiled together

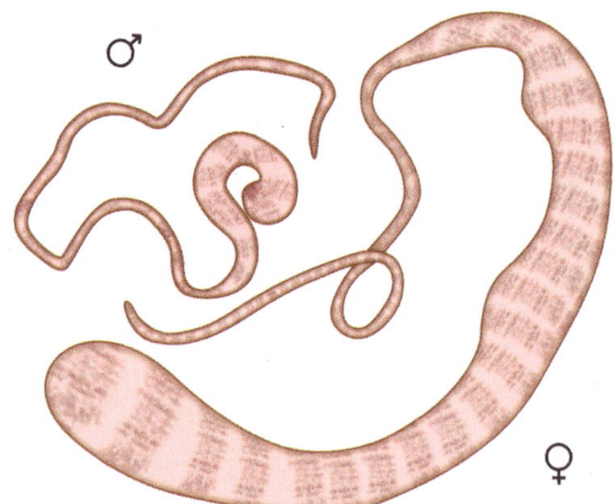

Fig. 19.1: Wuchereria bancrofti

usually, in the abdominal and inguinal lymphatics and in the testicular tissues. Adults live for 10 to 15 years.

Sheathed Microfilariae

The microfilariae has colorless, translucent body with a blunt head and pointed tail measuring 250 to 300 µm in length and 6 to 10 µm in thickness (Fig. 19.2).

It is actively motile and can move forward and backward within the sheath, which is much longer than the embryo (microfilariae).

When stained with Leishman or Romanowsky stain, the structural details can be made out as follows:

1. Along the central axis of the microfilariae can be seen a column of granules, which are called somatic cells or nuclei.
2. At the head end is a clear space devoid of granules called cephalic space. In *W. bancrofti* the cephalic space is as long as it is broad. With vital stains, a stylet can be demonstrated projecting from the cephalic space.
3. In the anterior half of the microfilariae, is an oblique area devoid of granules called the nerve ring.
4. Approximately midway along the length of the microfilariae is the anterior V-spot, which represents the rudimentary excretory system.
5. The posterior V-spot (tail spot) represents the cloaca or anal pore.
6. The genital cells (G-cells) are situated anterior to the anal pore.
7. The tail tip is devoid of nuclei (granules).

The microfilariae circulate in the blood stream. In India, China and many other Asian countries, they show a nocturnal periodicity

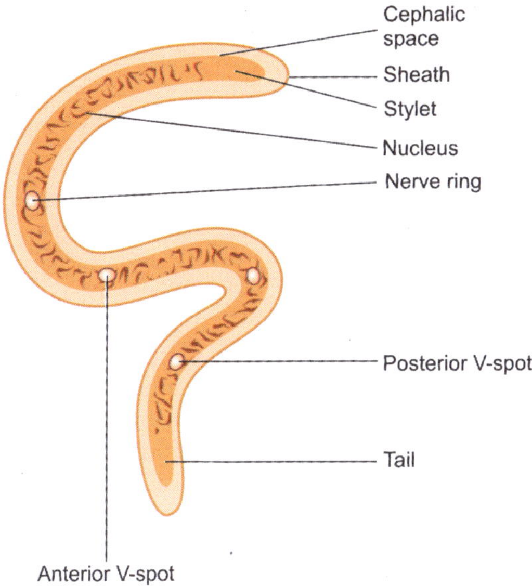

Fig. 19.2: Microfilaria of *Wuchereria bancrofti*

in peripheral circulation, being seen in large numbers in peripheral blood only at night between 10 PM and 4 AM. This correlates with the night biting habits of the vector mosquito and the sleeping habits of the hosts. If the sleeping habits are reversed over a period of time, the microfilariae will also change their periodicity from nocturnal to diurnal. The microfilariae spend their day time mainly in the capillaries of the lung and kidneys or in the heart and blood vessels.

Life Cycle

Wuchereria bancrofti passes its life cycle in two hosts namely man (the definitive host) and mosquito (the intermediate host), mosquitoes are specific in different geographical areas. Culex is the major vector in India and other parts of Asia.

Microfilariae do not multiply or undergo any further development in the human body. If they are not taken up by a female vector mosquito, they die. When a vector mosquito feeds on a carrier, the microfilariae are taken in with the blood meal and reach the stomach of the mosquito. Within 4 to 6 hours they cast off their sheath and within 4 to 12 hours migrate to the thoracic muscles, where they develop into first stage larvae, the second stage larvae and third stage larvae (in 16 to 20 days), which is actively motile and infective. It enters the proboscis sheath of the mosquito awaiting opportunity for infecting humans on whom the mosquito feeds.

There is no multiplication of the microfilariae in the mosquito and one microfilaria develops into one infective larva only.

When a mosquito with infective larvae in its proboscis feeds on a person, the larvae gets deposited usually in pairs on the skin near the puncture site. The infective larvae penetrates the skin and reach the lymphatic channels and settle down usually in the inguinal, scrotal and abdominal lymph nodes, where they develop into adult worms and become sexually mature. The male fertilizes the female, the gravid female give birth to embryo (microfilariae) and the life cycle is repeated.

The characteristic manifestations of filariasis are due to the obstruction of the lymph nodes. The essential features are lymphadenopathy, lymphopharyngitis, lymphedema, elephantiasis and hydrocele.

Elephantiasis is a feature unique to human filariasis caused by man's erect posture and consequent hydrodynamic factors affecting lymph flow. Elephantiasis is seen most commonly in the leg, but also may involve other parts of the body including the arm, breast, scrotum, penis and vulva.

Diagnosis

By staining the blood drawn between 10 PM and 4 AM.

Prevention and Control

1. Eradication of vector mosquito.
2. Detection and treatment of causes.

Ascariasis (Roundworm Infection)

ASCARIS LUMBRICOIDES

As an Etiological Agent

Roundworm infestation or ascariasis is caused by a nematode, *Ascaris lumbricoides*.

Habitat

The adult worm lives in the lumen of the small intestine mainly in jejunum.

Morphology

The mature worm is cylindrical with tapering ends resembling an ordinary earthworm. It is creamy white to brown in color. The male measures 12 to 30 cm × 2 to 4 mm (Fig. 20.1A). The female worm measures 20 to 35 cm in length and 3 to 6 mm in width (Fig. 20.1B). Round worm is the largest intestine nematode infecting man. The mouth opens at the anterior end and possess three finely toothed lips, one dorsal and two ventral. The body contains an irritating fluid called ascaron or ascarase.

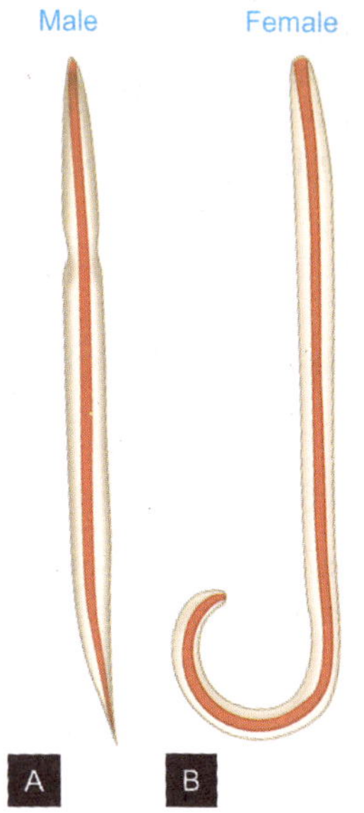

Characteristics of Egg

Fertilized Egg

Smaller in size, 45 to 75 μ × 30 to 50 μ, always bile stained. The shell has innermost very thin vitelline membrane, a thick glycogenous middle layer and coarsely laminate outermost layer, is unsegmented and made up of coarse lecithin granules. Floats in saturated salt solution (Fig. 20.2).

Unfertilized Egg

Always bile stained. Larger in size, 88 to 94 μ × 45 μ. The shell is relatively thin. The innermost layer vitelline is absent. Embryo contains disorganized mass containing refractile granules (Fig. 20.3). It does not develop into larvae. Does not float in saturated salt solution.

Figs 20.1A and B: Morphology of mature worm.
A. Male worm; **B.** Female worm

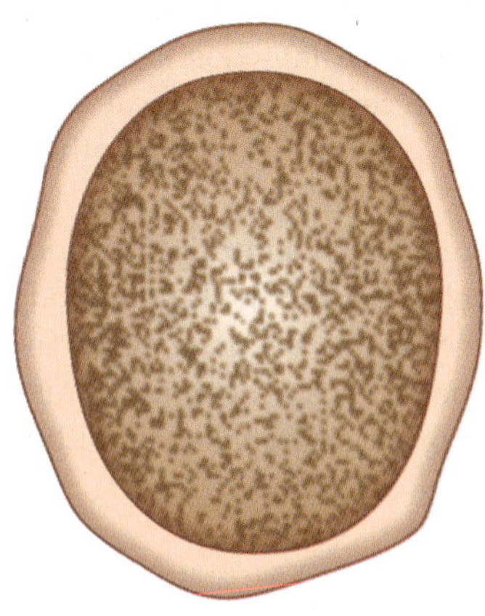

Fig. 20.2: Fertilized egg showing unsegmented ovum surrounded by three layers of coats (bile stained)

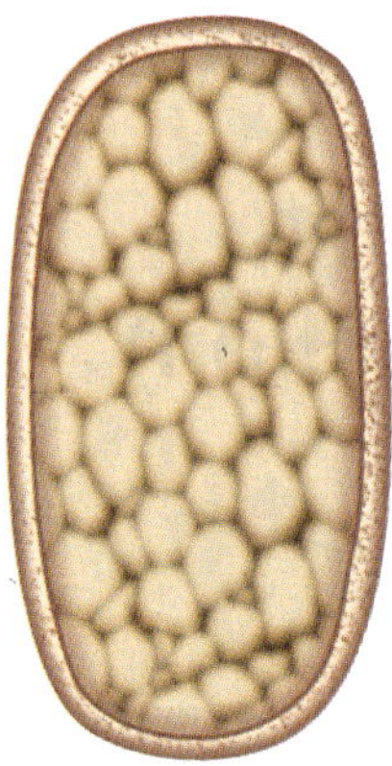

Fig. 20.3: Unfertilized egg elongates with atrophied ovum (bile stained)

Life Cycle

The female adult worm liberates fertilized eggs, which are passed with stools. The freshly passed fertilized eggs contain unsegmented ovum. At this stage, they are not infective to man.

Infection occurs from ingestion of embryonated eggs. The infective larvae hatch out in the small intestine and penetrate the intestinal wall to enter portal circulation. From the liver they are carried out to the heart and via the pulmonary artery to the lungs. In the lungs, these break out of the capillaries into the alveoli and undergo another moulting to become the fourth-stage larvae. These larvae move up to the bronchi and either swallowed with saliva or crawl up the epiglottitis to enter the digestive tract. In the intestine, these again undergoes moult to become sexually mature worms (Fig. 20.4). The life span of an adult worm is about 1 year after which it is spontaneously expelled.

Laboratory Diagnosis

Both fertilized and unfertilized eggs can be present in the feces of a patient suffering from ascariasis.

Examination of blood shows eosinophilia in the initial stages. Adult worms can be detected when they are passed out spontaneously in stools, anum, mouth or nose.

Detection of eggs can be done by direct examination of stool or after concentration. Typical fertilized or unfertilized eggs can be seen in the stool.

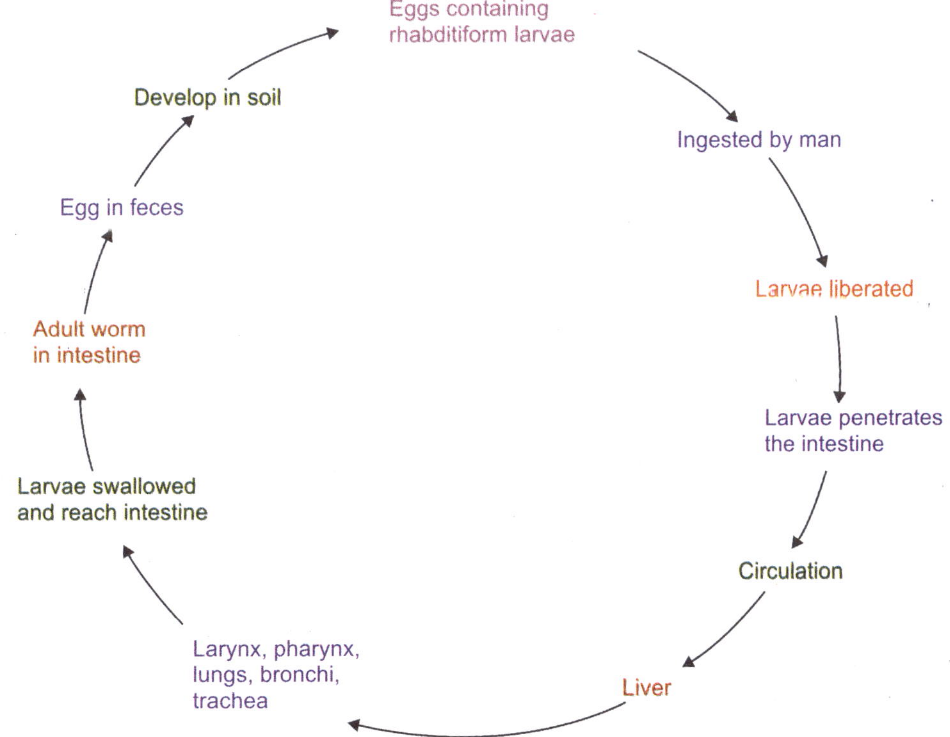

Fig. 20.4: Life cycle of roundworm

Ancylostomasis (Hookworm Infection)

ANCYLOSTOMA DUODENALE (HOOKWORM)

Geographical Distribution

Hookworm is widely found in tropical and subtropical countries.

Habitat

The adult worm resides in small intestine of man particularly in jejunum.

Morphology

Ancylostoma duodenale (A. duodenale) is small pinkish, fusiform in shape. The anterior end is curved. Female worm is 13 mm × 0.6 mm with pointed posterior end. Male worm is smaller, 11 mm × 0.4 mm having copulatory bursa with tripartite dorsal rays and a pair of long copulatory spicules. The oral cavity has single pair of dorsal teeth and two pairs of ventral teeth, which help the worm to get attached to the mucosa.

Eggs

Oval measuring 25 µ x 40 µ. It has thin outer shell enclosing a segmented ovum with four segments. There is a clear space between egg shell and segmented ovum. It floats in saturated salt solution. It is non-bile stained.

Life Cycle

The adult worm lives in small intestine of man attached to the mucosa. After fertilization, female lays eggs, which are passed out with stool. The larvae develop from eggs outside the body of host. Freshly passed egg contains segment-ed embryo and in 24 hours free living rhabditiform larvae is liberated. After 7 to 8 days, rhabditiform larvae moult twice (once in 3rd day and second in 5th day) and transforms into filariform larvae, which is infective. On coming in contact with the skin of foot, it penetrates into the hair follicle or bores through intact skin to reach right side of the heart (through lymphatics and venous blood). Thereafter, the larvae reaches the lung and after piercing capillary wall reach alveolar space. Third moulting occurs at this stage. From alveolar space larvae reaches bronchioles, trachea, larynx and swallowed back to stomach. On reaching duodenum and jejunum another moulting occurs. Here, in 5 to 7 weeks larvae grow to mature adult worms, which are also sexually mature (Fig. 21.1).

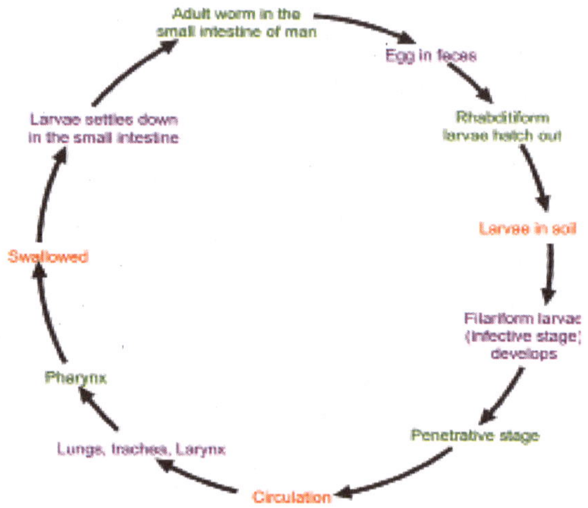

Fig. 21.1: Life cycle of hookworm

Pathogenicity and Clinical Picture

Ancylostomiasis or hookworm disease is characterized by anemia. At the site of filariform larvae penetration dermatitis may occur. The larvae then migrate to subcutaneous vessels and cause creeping eruption. When larvae reach lung, multiple hemorrhage and transient bronchopneumonia occur. Adult worms cause irritation and petechial hemorrhage in intestinal mucosa.

Laboratory Diagnosis

1. Stool examination for adult worm (naked eye).
2. Microscopic examination of stool for ova.
3. Study of duodenal contents for adult worms and ova.

Indirect Examination

1. Blood examination for anemia and eosinophilia.
2. Stool examination for occult blood for Charcot-Leyden crystals (CL crystals).

Stool Examination

Examination of stool forms an important part in the diagnosis of internal parasite infections and also those caused by parasites, which localize in the biliary tract and discharge their eggs into the intestine.

In protozoal infections, either the trophozoites or cystic forms may be detected; the former during the chronic phase. Examples are amebiasis, giardiasis and balantidiasis.

In helminthic infections either the adult worms or their eggs are found in the stool. For example are:

1. In ancylostomasis (hookworm infection), eggs are found. Adult worms are found affected by vermifuge.
2. In ascariasis (roundworm infection), adult worms and eggs are found.
3. In trichuriasis (whipworm infection), eggs are found.
4. In taeniasis (*Taenia saginatum* and *T. solium* tapeworm infections), segments (proglotides) of adult worms and eggs are found.

PRECAUTIONS

Precautions while collecting stool for examination are:

1. The stool must be fresh.
2. Receptacles must be clean and dry.
3. No antiseptics and disinfectants should be used to wash the receptacles.
4. Urine should not mix up with stool.
5. Oil, oil emulsions, barium and bismuth salts should not be given to the patient before stool examination.

TYPES OF STOOL EXAMINATION

The stool sample is usually subjected for:

1. Macroscopic examination usually done to note the following.

a. Amount.
b. Color.
c. Odor.
d. Form and consistency.
e. Mucus.
f. Blood.
g. Parasites.

The adult worms that can be seen with naked eye in stool include roundworm, thread worm, tapeworm and occasionally hookworm, whipworm and liver flukes.

2. Chemical examination is used to find out the presence of blood, bile pigments, fat contents and reaction.
3. Bacterial examination to isolate and identify pathogenic bacteria.
4. Microscopic examination is done in two ways:

a. Direct method using unstained (saline) and stained (iodine) wet cover slip methods.
b. Concentration method.

DIRECT EXAMINATION

Unstained Preparation

Requirements

Glass slide 3″ × 1″, coverslip 1″ × 1″, normal saline, stool sample, wooden tooth pick or broom stick.

Procedure

Place a drop of freshly prepared normal saline solution on a perfectly clean and grease-free glass slide. Transfer a minute amount of stool from the suspected portion, (i.e. mucus and blood stained part) with the aid of a broom stick and make a thin emulsion with the same stick. Remove coarse particles if any. Place a cover slip over it and spread out the emulsion into a thin film taking care to prevent inclusion of any air bubbles. The resulting preparation must be thin, uniform and transparent enough so that printed matter can be read through it, the excess of fluid should be removed by blotting either with a blotting paper or moistened cloth.

This preparation is specially used to demonstrate actively motile trophozoites of *Entameoba histolytica*.

Stained Preparation

Make a similar thin wet cover slip preparation using Lugol iodine (iodine 1 g, KI 2 g and 100 mL distilled water) instead of normal saline. Addition of iodine kills the organisms hence motility is lost. But it stains the nucleus of protozoa and glycogen mass, which enables the detailed study of nuclear characteristics. Both the preparations are examined under low power. Starting from one end, the entire slide is examined. If any suspicious object resembling ovum or cyst is seen, it is brought to the center of the microscopic field and then examined under high power for detailed diagrams.

Exercises

1. Examine the given sample of stool by preparing wet cover slip preparations using normal saline and Lugol iodine.
2. Concentrate the stool using the concentration method of Willis and examine.
3. Draw the diagrams of various ova and cysts observed and label the different parts.

Demonstration

The various trophozoites, cysts and ova of intestinal parasites of man.

HELMINTH OVA IN HUMAN STOOL

Eggs of Ascaris Lumbricoides (Roundworm)

Fertilized: Eggs measure 60 to 74 μm by 40 to 50 μm, always bile stained. Surrounded by thick coat of brown mammillations, contains large unsegmented ovum. Floats in saturated salt solution (Fig. 22.1).

Unfertilized: Eggs measure 90 to 45 μm in length, narrow and elliptical, bile stained. Thinner covering shell containing small atrophied ovum. Fails to float in salt solution (Fig. 22.2).

Question   : What are the usual constituents of stool seen under the microscope?

Answer 1   : Elastic fiber, muscle fiber, starch, Charcot-Leyden (CL) crystals.

Question 2 : List out the helminth ova that are found in stool.

Answer 2   : *Ascaris lumbricoides* (roundworm) *Ancylostoma duodenale* (hookworm [Fig. 22.3]) *Trichuris trichiura* (whipworm [Fig. 22.4]) *Taenia* (tapeworm, *Taenia solium* in pork sample and *Taenia saginatum* in beef sample [Fig. 22.5]) Cyst of *E. coli* (Fig. 22.6), *E. histolytica* (Fig. 22.7), *Giardia lamblia* (Fig. 22.8).

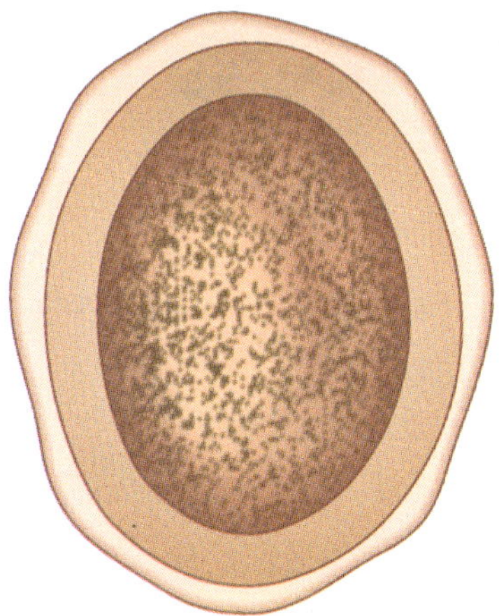

Fig. 22.1: Fertilized egg of *Ascaris lumbricoides*

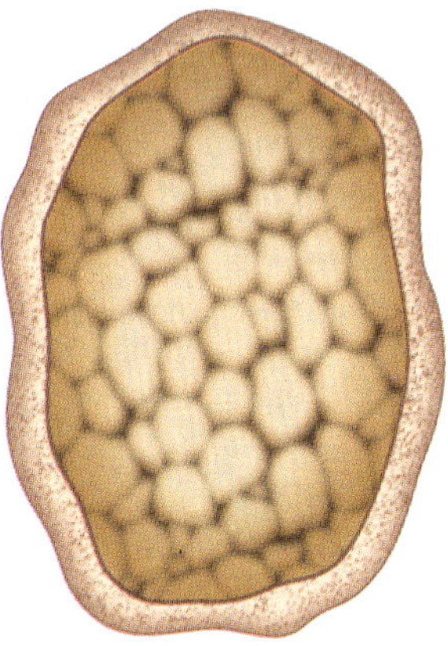

Fig. 22.2: Unfertilized egg of *Ascaris lumbricoides*

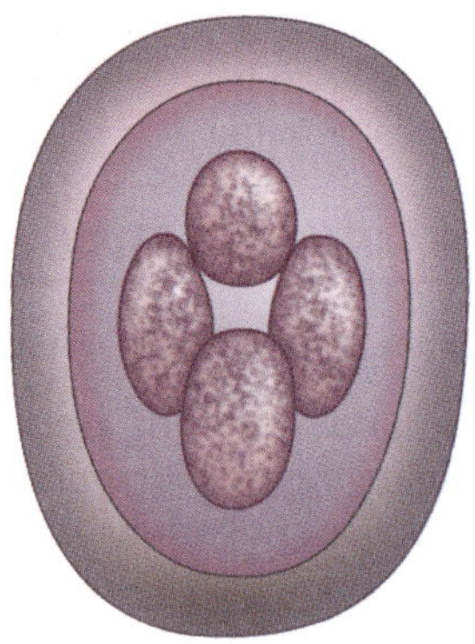

Fig. 22.3: Ovum of *Ancylostoma duodenale* (hookworm)

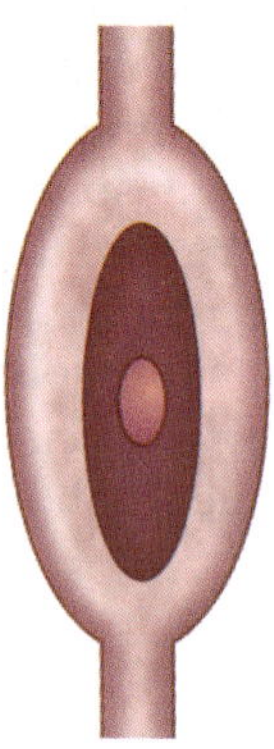

Fig. 22.4: Ovum of *Trichuris trichiura* (whipworm)

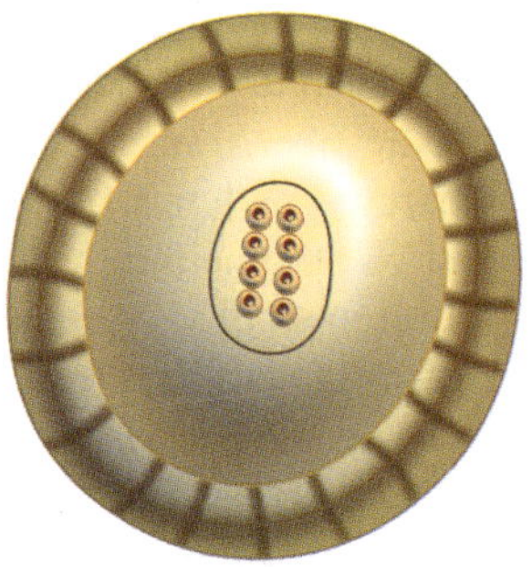

Fig. 22.5: *Taenia* (tapeworm ovum eight nuclei, bile stained)

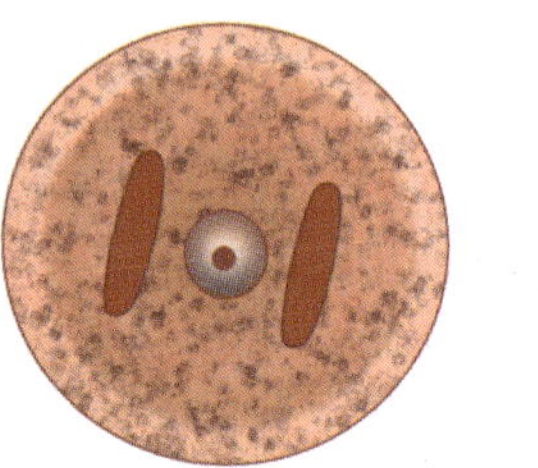

Fig. 22.6: Cysts of *Entamoeba coli*

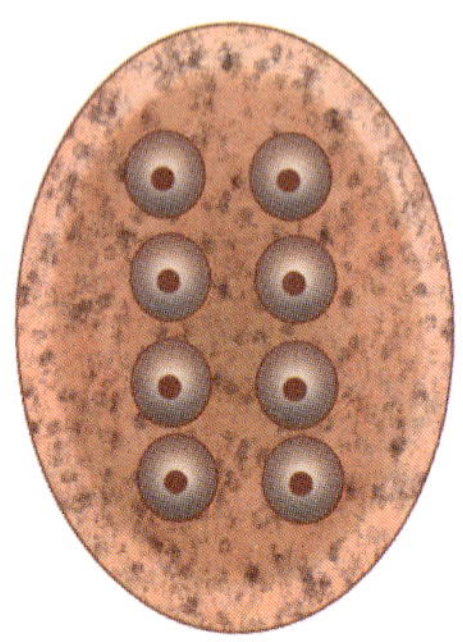

Fig. 22.7: Ovum of *Entamoeba histolytica*

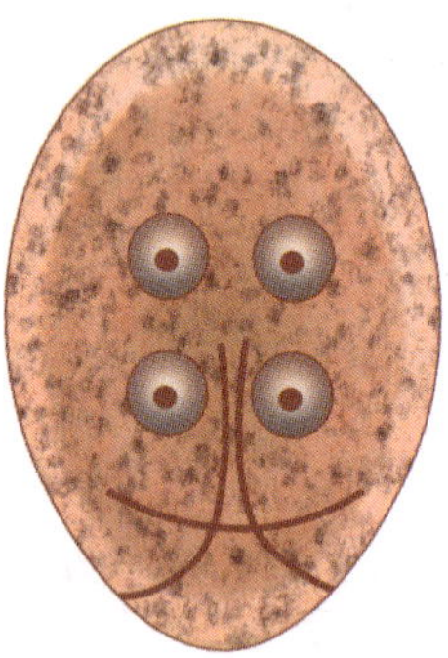

Fig. 22.8: Ovum of *Giardia lamblia*

Clinical Microbiology

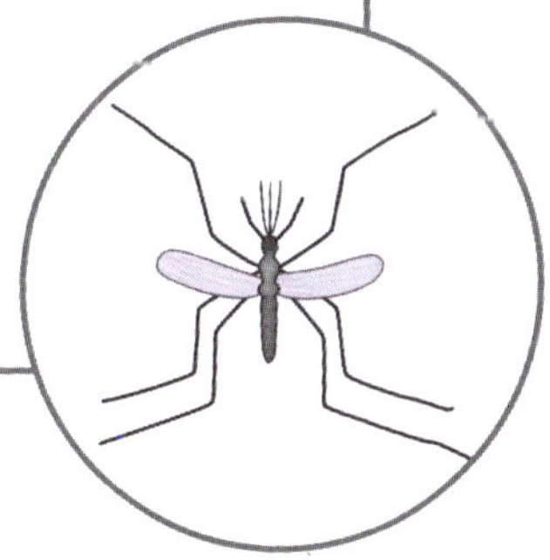

Normal Microbial Flora of Human Body

Human beings are not sterile. Normal microbrial flora refers to the population of microorganisms that inhabit the skin and mucous membrane of healthy normal individuals. It varies from person to person depending on age, general health, temperature and specific local conditions such as acidity of the stomach. The normal flora is acquired during and shortly after birth and changes continuously throughout life. It is basically environmentally determined. Man has about ten to fourteen types of bacteria associated with him, most of them in the large intestine.

TYPES OF NORMAL FLORA

The normal body flora are of two types namely:

1. Resident flora.
2. Transient flora.

The resident flora consist of relatively fixed types of microorganisms regularly found in given area at a given age.

Transient flora consists of non-pathogenic microorganisms that inhabit a particular part of the body for a limited period. Many pathogenic organisms generally do not cause disease, but are opportunistic. They cause disease when the normal flora is destroyed or body defence is weakened as in diabetes mellitus and immunodeficiency states. Some organisms are harmless in their natural residential area, but can cause disease in another area. For example, *Escherichia coli* which is a commensal organism, harmless in the colon are pathogenic in the urinary tract. The sites in the body, which are normally sterile are bone marrow, blood, cerebrospinal fluid (CSF), serous fluids, tissues, urine, respiratory tract, middle and inner ear. Sites with normal flora are the skin, upper respiratory tract, gastrointestinal tract, female genital tract and conjunctiva.

LOCATION OF NORMAL FLORA

Normal flora are found in those parts of the body that are exposed to or communicate with the external environment. Internal organs and tissues are normally sterile.

Skin

Staphylococcus epidermidis is one of the most (90%) common species of aerobes occurring in densities of 10^3 to 10^4 per square centimeter. *Staphylococcus aureus* may be present in the moist regions of the body, e.g. axillae, perineum, between toes and scalp.

Anaerobic diphtheroids are found below the skin surface in hair follicles, sweat and sebaceous glands, e.g. *Propionibacterium acnes*. *Candida* may occur on scalps and around nails. They are harmless on exposed skin, but can cause infection in moist skin folds (intertrigo).

Nose and Mouth

Nose and mouth are heavily colonized by streptococci, staphylococci, diphtheroids and gram negative cocci. Some of the species found as a part of the flora in healthy persons are potentially pathogenic, e.g. *Staphylococcus aureus, Streptococcus pneumoniae, Streptococcus pyogenes, Neisseria meningitidis, Lactobacillus, Candida*, etc. The teeth gingival surfaces carry large number of anaerobic bacteria. Plaque is a thin film of bacteria attached with polysaccharide matrix, which the bacteria secrete. When teeth are not cleaned regularly there is increased activities of certain bacteria like *Streptococcus mutans*, which leads to dental carries. Acid fermented by these organisms from carbohydrates can invade dental enamel.

Pharynx and Trachea

The pharynx and trachea carry their own normal flora, e.g. alpha and beta streptococci and staphylococci, *Neisseria* and diphtheroids.

Gastrointestinal Tract

The stomach contents give shelter to transient organisms, the acidic pH providing unfavorable environment. Gastric mucosa may be colorized by acid tolerant lactobacilli and streptococci. The upper intestine is colorized by streptococci, lactobacilli, enterobacteria and bacteroides. In large intestine, the majority (95%–99%) are anaerobes, bacteroides being common and major component of stool matter. A number of harmless protozoa occur in the intestine, e.g. *Entamoeba coli*.

Urogenital Tract

Urethra in male and female is highly colonized with *Staphylococcus epidermidis*, *Enterococcus faecalis* and diphtheroids. In females, before puberty the predominant organism are staphylococci, streptococci, diphtheroids and *Escherichia coli*. Subsequently *Lactobacilli* predominates its fermentation of glycogen, being responsible for maintenance of an acid pH, which prevents over growth by other vaginal organisms. *Candida* may overgrow causing a condition called thrush.

ADVANTAGES AND DISADVANTAGES OF NORMAL FLORA

Advantages

1. They prevent colonization of potential pathogens, e.g. skin bacteria provides fatty acids, gut bacteria release bacterocin and colicin, vaginal lactobacilli maintain acid pH, etc.
2. Gut bacteria release vitamin B and K.
3. Antigenic stimulation provided by the intestinal flora is important in providing normal development of the immune system.
4. Antibodies produced in response to normal flora cross react with pathogens, thus raising the immune status of the host. The endotoxins liberated by normal flora trigger alternative complement pathway.

Disadvantages

1. The disadvantages of the normal flora lie primarily in the potential hazard for the spread into the previously sterile parts of the body, e.g. when intestine is perforated, skin is broken, extraction of teeth. *E. coli* from the perineal skin ascend the urethra to cause urinary tract infection.
2. Over growth by pathogenic members of normal flora may occur in conditions like after administration of antibiotics, increase in stomach or vaginal pH or when immune system becomes ineffective.
3. Isolation of normal flora may cause confusion in the diagnosis.

Medical Entomology

Many pathogens are able to infect both man and animals. Animals may therefore act as sources of human infection. In some instances, infections in animal may be asymptomatic. Such animals serve to maintain the parasite in nature and act as the reservoir of human infections. They are therefore called reservoir hosts. Infectious diseases transmitted from animals to man are called zoonoses.

Zoonotic diseases may be bacterial, (e.g. plague from rats), viral (e.g. rabies from dogs), protozoal (e.g. leishmaniasis disease from dogs), fungal (e.g. zoophilic dermatophytes from cats and dogs) and spirochetal (e.g. leptospirosis from rats and other animals).

SOURCES OF INFECTION

Animals

Domestic Animals

1. Cow (e.g. beef tapeworm).
2. Pig (e.g. pork tapeworm).
3. Dog (e.g. hydatid disease, leishmaniasis).
4. Cat (e.g. toxoplasmosis, opisthorchiasis).

Wild Animals

1. Wild game animals (e.g. trypanosomiasis).
2. Wild felines (e.g. *Paragonimus westermani*).
3. Fish (e.g. fish tapeworm).
4. Molluses (e.g. liver flukes).
5. Copepods (e.g. guinea worm).

Insects

Blood sucking insects may transmit pathogens to man. The disease so caused are called arthropod-borne diseases. Insects such as mosquitoes ticks, mites, flies, fleas and lice that transmit infections are called vectors. Transmission may be mechanical, e.g. transmission of typhoid bacilli and amebic dysentery by the domestic fly. Such vectors are called mechanical vectors. In other cases, pathogen multiplies in the body of the vector when undergoing part of the developmental cycle in it. Such vectors are termed biological vectors, (e.g. *Aedes aegypti* mosquito in yellow fever, *Anopheles* female mosquito in malaria). Biological vectors transmit infection only after the pathogen has multiplied in them sufficiently or undergone a developmental cycle. The interval of time required for the biological vector to become infective, beginning from the time of entry of the pathogen into it, is termed extrinsic incubation period (EIP).

Beside acting as vectors, some insects may also act as reservoir hosts (e.g. ticks in relapsing fever and spotted fever). Infection is maintained in such insects by transovarial or transstadial passage.

Some ticks produce paralysis in some persons, presumably due to toxins in their secretions. Venom introduced into the skin by the bite of the scorpion or spider or bee at times produce both local reactions and profound systemic shock.

Blood-sucking flies, by depositing droplets on the skin, may provoke serious allergic reactions.

Bed Bugs (Cimicidae)

1. Have a length of 13 mm.
2. Broad flat reddish brown insects.
3. In males, the abdomen is pointed at the tip.
4. In females, abdomen is evenly rounded.
5. The major part of the body is covered with bristles.
6. Eggs are pearly white and oval with lid.

7. Complete life cycle is 15 to 50 weeks.
8. Life span varies from many months to about 1 year.
9. Bed bugs may be naturally infected with hepatitis B virus, which can transmit this virus mechanically or via feces.
10. Bed bugs can cause dermatitis or asthma.
11. Control includes:
    a. Pouring of boiling water to kill egg and nymph.
    b. Use of kerosene, benzene, turpentine or petroleum.

House Fly (Musca Domestica)

1. Male measures 5 to 6 mm and female 6 to 7 mm.
2. Dusky gray in color.
3. The head is broad, frons straw and dark brown, antenna brown.
4. Possess squarish ovoid thorax having four dark stripes.
5. Wings are transparent having straw colored base.
6. Foot or terminal segment at the end of each leg is provided with a pair of horny claws, pair of ventral cushion, each with many glandular hair.
7. Eggs are pearly white and 1 mm long.
8. Completes life cycle in about 2 weeks.
9. Responsible for transmitting microorganisms mechanically, e.g. *Salmonella, Mycobacterium tuberculosis, Yersinia pestis, Bacillus anthracis, Brucella abortus* and *Chlamydia.*
10. There is a close association with house flies and myiasis.
11. Control includes:
    a. Fly paper and fly traps.
    b. Garbage to be kept in closed fly proof containers, which is incinerated at frequent intervals.
    c. Insecticidal spray, e.g. chlorinated hydrocarbons (1% water emulsion) to be sprayed twice a week over breeding area of house flies.

Mosquitoes

1. Six-legged, delicate forms with 3,071 species all over the world.
2. Elongated piercing sucking mouth parts adapted for sucking blood, especially in female mosquito.
3. Long antennae, feathery in male and hairy in female.
4. Scales on wings look spotted in *Anopheles* mosquitoes and uniformly black in *Culex.*
5. Life span of male mosquito is about 7 days and for female mosquito it is 1 month. Life cycle of different mosquitoes is shown in Figure 24.1.
6. Responsible for transmission of diseases, i.e. malaria (*Anopheles*), yellow fever (*Aedes*), eastern equine encephalomyelitis (*Aedes*), western equine encephalomyelitis (*Aedes*), Venezuelan equine encephalitis (*Aedes, Anopheles*), chikungunya fever (*Aedes*), dengue fever (*Aedes*), Japanese encephalitis (*Culex*), filariasis (*Aedes, Culex* and *Anopheles*).
7. Prevention and control
    a. Reduction of breeding places of mosquitoes like drainage, clearing or filling of ditches and elimination of water containers.
    b. Use of insecticides.
    c. Use of mosquito repellents, e.g. residual sprays or lotion, gases or vapours.
    d. Diversion of mosquitoes from man to animals (cattle). This is called zooprophylaxis, a method hardly practiced deliberately, but often naturally effective.
    e. Introduction of larvicidal fishes like *Gambusia* and gold fish to breeding places of mosquitoes.
    f. Genetic control is successful by introducing sterile male mosquito (by radiation or exposure to UV light) into natural population.
    g. Many birds eat adult mosquitoes, e.g. swifts, nighthawks, etc.
    h. Wall lizards, frogs and spiders destroy mosquitoes.
    i. Many aquatic plants, e.g. *Chara* is poisonous to mosquitoes. *Utricularia* kills mosquito larvae.
    j. Certain bacteria help destroy larvae.

Lice Pubic or Crab Louse

1. Have dorsoventrally flattened body.
2. Size is 2 to 4 mm, elongated and grayish-white with piercing and sucking mouth parts.

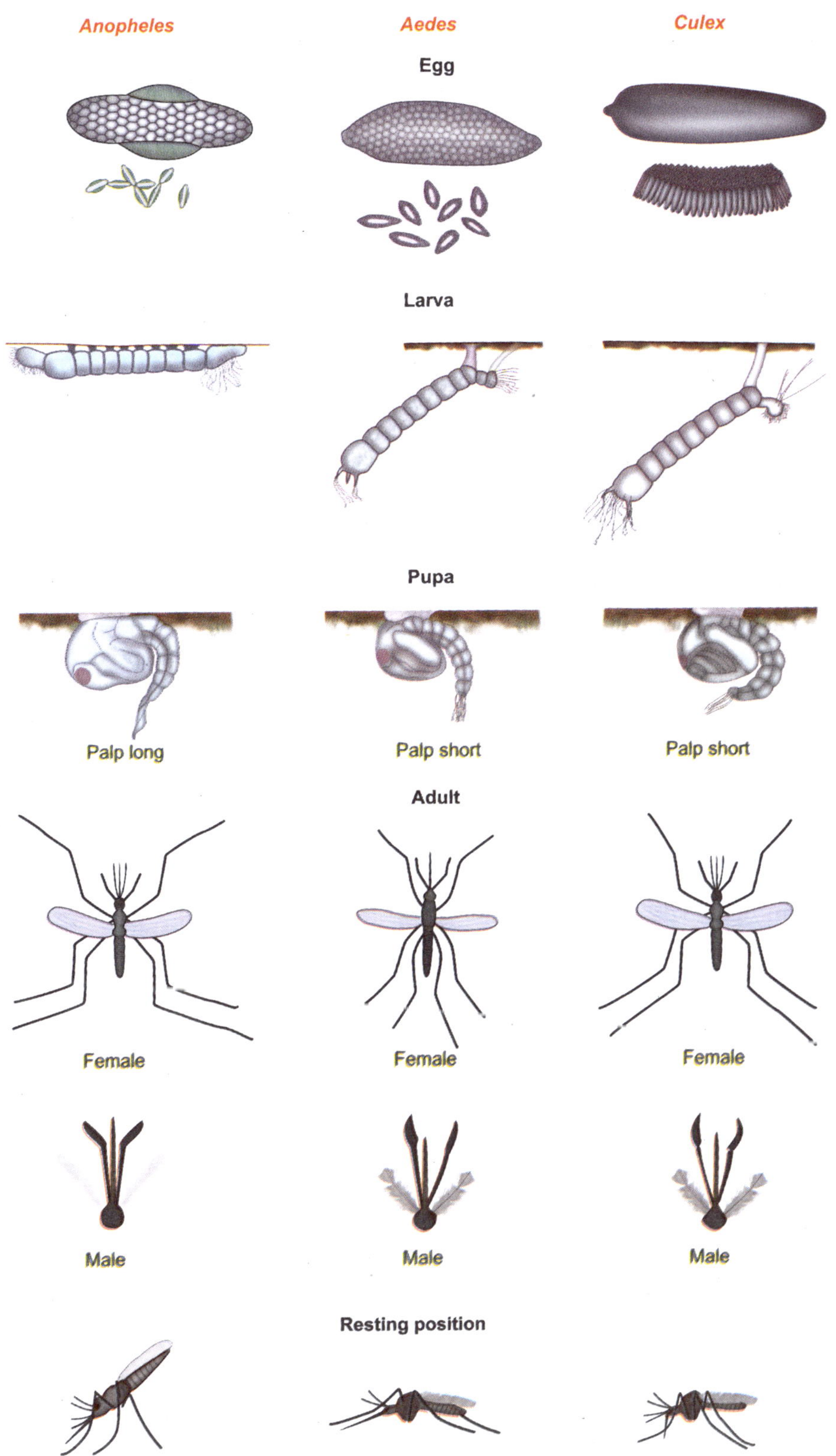

Fig. 24.1: Life cycle of mosquitoes

3. Lack wings, but have clawed legs.
4. Eggs are 0.8 mm long.
5. Principal habitat is human body and hair.
6. Life span of adults up to 1 month.
7. Many transmit typhus fever and cause irritating dermatitis. Transmit *Rickettsia* species.
8. Control includes:
   a. Use of benzyl benzoate, dichlorodiphenyl trichloroethane (DDT), benzocaine.
   b. Mixture of olive oil and kerosene oil.
   c. Kerosene having 0.12 percent pyrethrins.

Fleas

1. Adults are small oblong, compressed, hard skinned, bristly, wingless and dark brown in color.
2. They have concealed antennae and long jumping legs.
3. The head is broadly joined to thorax.
4. The abdomen consists of ten segments, the last three are modified for sexual purposes.
5. All parts of body are furnished with backward projecting bristles and spines, which prevent it from slipping backwards.
6. Male fleas are easily identified by rakish upward tilt of abdomen. In case of female, it is rounded.
7. The eggs are deposited in dark and dry places in the haunts or in its hosts, which takes about 70 to 75 days to mature.
8. Fleas transmit plague (*Yersinia pestis*), endemic typhus fever, etc.
9. Flea bite causes flea dermatitis.
10. For control: Dichlorodiphenyltrichloroethane (DDT), rotenone (1%), malathion (4%) or pyrethrin (1%) may be used. In case of infested floor, rugs, carpet, pillows, etc. spray of kerosene solution or emulsions of 3 percent malathion or 1 percent diazinon are useful. Rodent control can check fleas.

Sandfly (Phlebotomus)

1. Small, about 2 mm long.
2. Humpback, fawny in color with prominent black eyes.
3. Body, wings and legs are hairy.
4. Veins in the wings do not cross with each other.
5. Oval lanceolate wings are carried erect.
6. Only the females feed on blood.
7. Feeding usually occur at night and flies hide in dark, damp places during day time.
8. Have long slender antennae, long maxillary palpi and a proboscis longer than head.
9. The egg (long, ovoid) laying starts after 30 to 36 hours after blood meals. Life cycle is completed in 60 to 65 days.
10. Responsible for transmitting cutaneous leishmaniasis, visceral lieshmaniasis, viral 3 days fever, tularemia and loasis.
11. Control:
    a. Elimination of breeding grounds, cracks, crevices from walls and floors.
    b. Use of insecticides like DDT.
    c. Oiling pools of water can kill adult females who dive to lay eggs.

Cockroaches

1. Body is narrow elongated, symmetrical, smooth and flattened dorsoventrally.
2. Adult measures 2.5 to 5 cm in length and 2 cm in width.
3. The color is reddish brown.
4. The body is segmented into head, thorax and abdomen.
5. The body bears two pairs of wings (outer pair leathery and inner pair membranous).
6. Development from egg through nymph to adult requires 32 to 90 days depending on species and temperature.
7. Domestic cockroaches are intermediate host of *Hymenolepis diminuta*, etc. They may transmit enteric viruses and many bacteria. About 40 species of pathogenic bacteria have been isolated from contaminated cockroaches. *Aspergillus fumigatus* and *Asperigillus niger* have also been isolated from cockroaches. Cysts of *Giardia* and *Entamoeba histolytica* have also been found. An interesting report proposes the transport of *Toxoplasma gondii* from the feces of domestic cat by cockroaches. They can serve as a source of contactant, inhalant and ingestant allergens, hence they can cause, itching, dermatitis, localized necrosis, asthma and hay fever.
8. Control measures are:
   a. Kerosene oil spray on cockroaches hiding place. Care must be taken to protect food.

b. Use of suitable insecticides, e.g. fenitrothion, propoxur or dioxacarb at 1 percent.

Ticks

There are two types of ticks:
1. Soft-bodied ticks (argasidae) and hard-bodied ticks (ixodidae).
2. In the soft-bodied ticks, there is no hard dorsal plate, the mouth parts are situated ventral to the anterior extremity and the spiracles are usually located directly behind the third pair of coaxial segments, e.g. otobius, antricola.

In ixodidae, body is ovoid dorsoventrally flattened and unsegmented capitulum projects from the anterior end of the body. Dorsal surface of the body is covered by shield-like scutum bearing eyes. Walking legs are four pairs with adhesive pads and claws. Female is larger than male. They produce ixodine, which acts as an anesthetic agent and host does not feel pain.

Ticks are responsible for causing many human diseases. They also act as vectors of many human. Pathogens including *Rickettsia*, viruses and protozoa are thus responsible for tick-borne rickettsial infection (rocky mountain spotted fever, queensland tick typhus, etc.) viral (encephalitis, hemorrhagic fever, severe myalgia with fever, etc.) protozoal (babesiosis) and other diseases like Lyme disease, erythema chromicum migrans, etc.

Mites

1. Usually a millimeter greater in length or breadth than ticks.
2. They have hypostome unarmed with tooth-like anchoring processes.
3. Parasitic form, feeds on blood, lymph, digested tissues or sebaceous secretions on/near the surface of the skin.
4. Some tunnels subcutaneously causing an intense prurites.
5. Certain mites may serve as both reservoir and vector of *Rickettsia tsutsugamushi*.
6. House dust mites either produce or concentrate potent allergens commonly found within the home.
7. Control of ticks and mites: Insecticides are used like DDT, chlordane, dieldrin lindane, malathion and toxaphene. Animals like dogs are protected with insecticidal sprays or dust. Exposed workers should wear protective clothing impregnated with an insect repellant like indalone, diethyltoluamide and benzyl benzoate.

Fly Maggots

1. The adult fly is dirty yellowish brown with the tip of abdomen rusty black.
2. The life cycle is completed in about 10 weeks. Eggs are transformed into larvae in 2 weeks. Larva takes several weeks to become pupa and finally to adult.
3. There are many species of fly maggots, but the only larva that sucks blood by puncturing skin of man is Congo floor maggot, causes myiasis (infestation of living organs and tissues involving oral, nasal, aural, vaginal, urethral, skin and intestine).
4. Control includes:
   a. Proper disposal of carcasses to prevent laying their eggs.
   b. If possible maggots are removed using forceps after spray of 5 percent chloroform in light vegetable oil and lesion dressed with antiseptics.
   c. Adult flies of both sexes are attracted and they are intoxicated by 2 percent dichlorous.
   d. A genetic control measure using mass-trapping method by swomlure-2 for chemically defined trial and reared sterile male.

Rodents

Rodents may be classified into two groups:
1. Domestic.
2. Wild.

Domestic Rodents

Rodents of chief public health concern are those who live in close proximity to man.
1. The black rat (*Rattus rattus*).
2. The Norway rat (*R. norvegicus*).
3. The house mouse (*Mus musculus*).

Rattus rattus is a domestic animal whose area of movement is restricted. It readily infests ships. It is a good climber and infestation generally occurs in house roofs, even though in some places it does burrow. *R. norvegicus* is a semidomestic animal, which frequents sewers, drains and houses. Their characteristics are illustrated in Table 24.1.

Wild Rodents

The common wild rodents in India are *Tatera indica*, bandicoots (*Bandicota bengalensis*). In India, *Tatera indica* is found to be the natural reservoir of plague.

Rodents and Diseases

A number of diseases are associated with rodents, which are as follows:

Bacterial: Plague, tularemia, salmonellosis.

Viral: Lassa fever, hemorrhagic fever and encephalitis.

Rickettsial: Scrub fever, murine typhus, rickettsial pox.

Parasitic: *Hymenolepis diminuta* (*H. diminuta*) leishmaniasis, amebiasis, trichinosis, Chagas disease.

Others: Rat bite fever, leptospirosis, histoplasmosis, ringworm disease.

Mode of transmission: May be directly through rat bite, e.g. rat bite fever, some through contamination of food or water (e.g. salmonellosis, leptospirosis) and some through rat fleas, e.g. plague and typhus.

Sanitation Measures

Environmental sanitation should be effective. Rats require food, water and shelter. If these are derived, the rat population will come down. The environmental sanitation measures comprise by:

1. Proper storage, collection and disposal of garbage.
2. Proper storage of food stuffs.

3. Construction of rat-proof buildings, godowns and ware houses.
4. Elimination of rat burrows by blocking them with concrete.

Trapping

Trapping of rats is a simple operation, but it causes temporary reduction in the number of rodents. The number of traps should be more than 5 percent of the human population. According to Mumbai municipal authorities about four lakhs rats were trapped and killed this year.

Rodenticides

Rodenticides are divided into three groups:

1. Those requiring ordinary care:
   a. Red squill.
   b. Norbromide.
   c. Zinc phosphate.
2. Those requiring maximal precautions:
   a. Sodium fluoroacetate.
   b. Fluoroacetamide.
   c. Strychnine.
3. Too dangerous for use:
   a. Arsenic trioxide.
   b. Phosphorus.
   c. Thallium sulfate.

Fumigation

Very effective for destroying rats and fleas. Fumigants used are calcium cyanide, carbon disulfide, sulfur dioxide and methyl bromide. Trained personnel are required for fumigation. It is very effective for ships.

Chemosterilants

Chemosterilant is a chemical that can cause temporary or permanent sterility in either sex or both sexes of rats.

Table 24.1: Characteristics of house rat and sewer rat

SI No	Features	*Rattus rattus* (house rat)	*Rattus norvegicus* (sewer rat)
1.	Body	Slim and slender	Heavy, large
2.	Muscle	Long and sharp	Broad and blunt
3.	Tail	Longer than the combined length of the head and body	Shorter than the combined length of the head and body
4.	Ears	Large	Small
5.	Eyes	Big and prominent	Small

Specimen Collection

COLLECTION OF SPECIMEN

Collection of material for bacteriological examination is the responsibility of the nurse. The specimen should be collected in such a manner that it does not become contaminated with other organisms.

Preferably specimen should be obtained before antibiotic or other antimicrobial agents are administered. If culture has been taken after initiation of antimicrobial therapy, laboratory should be informed so that specific counteractive measures such as adding penicillinase or merely diluting the sample may be carried out.

Material should be collected from a region where the suspected organism is most likely to be found and with as little external contamination as possible.

Another important point to remember is the stage of the disease. Enteric pathogens are present in much larger number during the acute diarrheal stage of intestinal infections and they are most likely to be isolated at that time.

Specimen should be quantitatively sufficient to permit complete examination and should be kept in sterile containers. Arrangements should be made for prompt delivery of specimens to the laboratory. The laboratory should be provided with sufficient clinical information to guide the microbiologist in the selection of suitable media and appropriate techniques.

Important points to remember are:

1. Strict aseptic precautions.
2. Use always sterile containers labelled with patient's hospital number.
3. Avoid soaking outside of containers.
4. Proper transport. If delay is expected, refrigerate the specimens.

After microscopy, the microbiologist proceeds immediately to culture the specimen for pathologic bacteria in appropriate media. The cultures are grown at 37°C in an incubator.

Adhesives are refixed carefully. If anaerobic infection is suspected in the patient, additional media are to be used. After proper collection, the culture bottles are incubated at 37°C and are never to be refrigerated.

Urine

Midstream or clean-catch specimen is to be obtained. The specimen must be collected in a sterile, wide mouthed screw capped bottle, after thorough cleaning the genitalia with soap and water. Improperly collected urine specimens will lead to incorrect lab report. The specimen must reach the laboratory within 15 minutes of collection. If not, it should be refrigerated immediately.

If infection with tuberculosis is suspected, the entire early morning sample of urine should be sent in large special sterile bottle.

Feces

A small quantity of formed stool is placed in a sterile specimen container. About one third of the container should be filled with the stool. The container should never be completely filled with stool. Special care should be taken to see that the outside of the container is not contaminated. If mucus or flakes of tissue is present in the feces, these should be included in the collected specimen. In certain cases like suspected bacillary dysentery or *Escherichia coli* diarrhea, rectal swab is preferred. Sterile swabs, moistened in sterile saline are introduced well beyond the internal sphincter, twirled well, gently withdrawn and placed in a sterile test tube and sent to the laboratory immediately.

Pus Other Than Purulent Body Fluid

About 1 mL of pus is placed in a sterile test tube. If this is not possible as much as pus as possible is collected on two sterile swabs and replaced in a sterile test tube. The end of the swab sticks are never to be broken off. The tips of the swab sticks should project beyond the mouth of the tube to facilitate handling. The mouth of the test tube with projected tips of the swab sticks must be secured with the sterile cotton or guaze fastened with adhesive tapes soon after collection.

Ear, Nose, Eye and Throat Swabs

Two small stick swabs in a sterile test tube are used for collecting pus.

The throat swabs are taken as follows:

The patient tongue is depressed and two swabs are passed well over the tonsils, surrounding areas and over the area where there is inflammation. The swabs with specimen are to be placed in the sterile test tube. Care should be taken not to touch inside the cheek or tongue.

Sputum

As far as possible, an early morning coughed-up specimen is preferred. Instruct the patient to wash the mouth with plain water, a few minutes before taking the specimen. A few milliliter of the coughed-up specimen is placed in a sterile wide mouthed, screw-capped bottle and despatched as early as possible.

Blood

Blood for Serological Tests

For investigation 10 mL of blood should be taken in a dry syringe and placed in a sterile test tube or bottle. The bottle should not contain any anticoagulant. The blood should be allowed to clot. The blood should be placed in the container directly from the syringe after removing the needle to avoid hemolysis due to frothing (forcing blood through the needle can cause hemolysis).

Blood for Cultures

Cultures are made to determine the presence or absence of bacteria and therefore should be taken by venipuncture under careful aseptic conditions. The blood is added to the culture media in glass tubes and cultivated. It is observed after a period of time usually 2 to 3 days. Some of the organisms that can be determined by means of blood cultures are typhoid bacilli, pneumococci, streptococci and staphylococci.

Blood for Widal Test

Widal test is a specific test for antibodies produced by typhoid and paratyphoid bacilli within the blood and tissues. Blood is collected by a sterile syringe and needle. The serum is allowed to separate from the clot. When various dilutions of the serum are made with normal saline and a standard antigen prepared with killed organism is mixed with the serum, agglutination will take place in a positive test.

Blood for Wassermann Reaction

Wassermann reaction is a test to detect the presence of an antibody in patients of syphilis. For this, 5 mL of blood is taken from the veins, test is done on blood serum and also venereal disease research laboratory (VDRL) tests performed.

Hospital Waste Management

Hospital waste is defined as all waste generated from medical facilities including laboratory, office and kitchen waste. Only a small fraction of the total waste generated by hospital is infective. Unlike radioactive or chemical waste, infective waste cannot be identified easily. Hospital waste management is of great importance for the safety of laboratory personnel and the community in general.

MANAGEMENT OF HOSPITAL WASTE

Concern about transmission of hepatitis B virus (HBV) and virus causing acquired immunodeficiency syndrome (AIDS), i.e. human immunodeficiency virus (HIV) led to the World Health Organizations's (WHO) introduction of the universal precautions to minimize the infection in medical laboratory personnel and health care workers.

Universal Precautions

1. Assume that all patients/specimens are potentially infective for HIV/HBV and other blood-borne pathogens.
2. All blood specimens and body fluids stored should be placed in a leak-proof impervious bag for transportation to the laboratory.
3. Use gloves while handling blood, body fluid specimens and other objects disposed to them. If there is likelihood of spattering, use face masks, gloves and goggles.
4. Wear laboratory coat or gown while working in the laboratory. Wrap-around gowns should be preferred. These should not be taken outside the laboratory.
5. Never try to pipette by mouth. Mechanical pipetting devices should be used.
6. Decontaminate the laboratory work surfaces with an appropriate disinfectant after spillage of blood or other body fluids and when the procedures are completed.
7. Limit use of needles and syringes to situations for which there are no alternatives.
8. Biological safety hoods should be used for lab work.
9. All the potentially contaminated material of the laboratory should be decontaminated before disposal or reprocessing.
10. Always wash hands after completing work and remove all protective clothing before leaving the laboratory.

Screening of Waste

1. Yellow plastic bags and containers with human anatomical and pathological waste are directly dispatched for deep burial or incineration.
2. Red plastic bags and containers having infectious waste are quickly sent for sterilization by autoclaving. Afterwards, they are disposed off by land filling.
3. Blue plastic bags, containers with plastic and rubber disposable material are first of all cut into small pieces to prevent reuse, followed by treatment with sodium hypochlorite. Then they are autoclaved and disposed of by land filling or burial. If feasible treated material may be transported to reputed plastic companies for reuse. They should not be incinerated or burnt. They contain polyvinyl chloride, which will emit dioxin gas into the air, which is highly carcinogenic.

4. Blue or white transparent puncture proof containers need a little different treatment before disposal. Sharps must be destroyed, disinfected with 1 percent sodium hypochlorite solution and then disposed of in sharp pits that are covered and protected from reuse.

However, the non-infectious waste can be collected in any appropriate container and despatched to municipal garbage bins. Black plastic bags are used for this purpose.

Infectious Waste

Includes microbiological waste (cultures, etc.) blood, body fluids contaminated laboratory waste, used sharps, pathological waste (samples, tissues, etc.) bedding and other wastes like bandages used, cotton swabs and animal carcasses used in laboratory experiments. Chemical wastes is also hazardous. Biomedical waste management is detailed in Table 26.1. Color coding and type of container used for disposal of biomedical wastes is given in Table 26.2.

Table 26.1: Biomedical waste management

Waste category number	Waste category type	Treatment and disposal options	Subject/year of study
Category number 1	Animal waste: Animal tissues, organs, body parts, carcasses, bleeding parts, fluid, blood, experimental animals used in research, waste generated by veterinary hospitals and colleges, discharge from hospitals and animal houses.	Incineration*/deep burial[†].	II year Unit III Community health nursing—1 hour
Category number 2	Microbiology and biotechnology waste: Waste from laboratory cultures, stocks of specimens of microorganisms, live or attenuated vaccines, human and animal cell cultures used in research, infectious agents from research and industrial laboratories, wastes from production of biological toxins, dishes and devices used for transfer of cultures.	Local autoclaving/ microwaving/ incineration*.	I year Unit IV Microbiology—1 hour
Category number 3	Waste sharps: Needles, syringes, scalpels, blades, glass, etc. that may cause puncture and cuts. This includes both used and unused sharps.	Disinfection (chemical treatment[‡]/autoclaving), microwaving and mutilation/shredding[§].	I year Unit III Nursing foundation—1 hour
Category number 4	Discarded medicines and cytotoxic drugs: Waste comprising of outdated, contaminated and discarded medicines.	Incineration*/destruction and drugs disposal in secured landfills.	
Category number 5	Soiled waste: Items contaminated with blood and body fluids including cotton, dressings, soiled plaster casts, liners, bleedings and other material contaminated with blood.	Incineration* autoclaving/ microwaving.	
Category number 6	Liquid waste: Waste generated from laboratory and from washing, cleaning, housekeeping and disinfecting activities.	Disinfection, chemical treatment and discharge into drains.	
Category number 7	Chemical waste: Chemicals used in production of disinfectants such as insecticides, etc.	Chemical treatment and discharge into drains for liquids and secured landfill for solids.	I year Unit III Biochemistry and biophysics—1 hour

*   There will be no chemical pretreatment before incineration. Chlorinated plastics shall not be incinerated.

†   Deep burial shall be an option available only in towns with population less than five lakhs and in rural areas.

‡   Chemical treatment using at least 1 percent sodium hypochlorite solution or any other equivalent chemical reagent. It must be ensured that chemical treatment ensures disinfection.

§   Mutilation/shredding must be used so as to prevent unauthorized reuse.

Table 26.2: Color coding and type of container for disposal of biomedical wastes

Color coding	Type of container	Waste category	Treatment options
Yellow	Plastic bag	Category 1, category 2 and category 5	Incineration/deep burial.
Red	Disinfected container/plastic bag	Category 2 and category 5	Autoclaving/microwaving and chemical treatment.
Blue/white translucent	Plastic bag/puncture proof container	Category 3	Autoclaving/microwaving/ chemical treatment and destruction/shredding.
Black	Plastic bag	Category 4 and category 7 (solid)	Disposal in secured landfill.

Appendices

A—Terms to Know

Abiogenesis: Origin of life from non-living organisms.

Abrasion: Superficial injury where skin mucous membrane is rubbed and torn.

Abscess: A localized collection of pus in cavity by tissue disintegration.

Aerobe: An organism that requires oxygen for growth and can grow under an air atmosphere.

Agar: A dried polysaccharide extract of red algae used as solidifying agent.

Agglutination: Clumping of cells.

Agglutinin: An antibody capable of causing clumping.

Algae: Any member of a heterogenous group of eukaryotic, photosynthetic and unicellular or multicellular organisms.

Allergy: A type of antigen-antibody reaction marked by a physiological, but exaggerated response to a substance in sensitive persons.

Anabolism: The synthesis of cell constituents from simpler molecules, usually require energy.

Anaerobe: An organism that does not use O_2 to obtain energy, can not grow under atmospheric air.

Anaphylatoxin: A complement derived peptide, C5a, that causes the release of histamine from mast cells.

Anaphylaxis: Hypersensitivity in an animal following the parenteral injection of an antigen.

Anaplasia: Structural abnormality in a cell or cells.

Antibiosis: An antagonistic association between two organisms in which one is affected.

Antibiotic: A substance of microbial origin that has antimicrobial activity.

Antibody: Antibodies are class of substances (proteins) produced by an animal in response to antigen.

Antigen: A substance that when introduced into animal body stimulates the production of specific substances that react or unite with the substance introduced.

Antiseptic: Acting against decay by either preventing or arresting growth of microorganisms.

Antiserum: Blood serum that contains antibodies.

Antitoxin: An antibody capable of neutralizing a specific toxin.

Asepsis: A condition in which harmful microorganisms are absent.

Attenuation: A weakening or reduction in virulence.

Bacteremia: A condition in which bacteria are present in bloodstream.

Bactericide: An agent that destroys bacteria.

Bacteriostatic: Inhibiting growth of bacteria without killing them.

Barophile: An organism that grows under conditions of hydrostatic pressure.

Basic dye: A dye consisting of basic organic group of atoms (cation), which is the actively staining part combined with an acid, usually inorganic; the dye has affinity for nucleic acids.

BCG vaccine: Bacille Calmette-Guérin vaccine, an attenuated strain of *Mycobacterium bovis* used against tuberculosis.

Beta hemolysis: A colorless clear, sharply defined zone of hemolysis surrounding certain bacterial colonies growing on blood agar.

Biogenesis: The production of living organisms only from other living organisms.

Brownian motion: A peculiar dancing motion exhibited by finely divided particles and bacteria in suspension due to bombardment by molecules of fluid.

Capsid: A protein coat of virus.

Capsomer: A morphological subunit of capsid.

Capsule: An envelope or slime layer surrounding cell wall.

Catabolism: The breakdown of complex organic molecules releasing energy.

Chemoautotroph: An organism that obtains energy by oxidizing inorganic compounds. Carbon dioxide is the sole source of carbon.

Chemostat: A device of maintaining organisms in continuous culture. It regulates the growth rate of the organism by regulating concentration of essential nutrient.

Chemotaxis: The movement of an organism in response to chemical stimulus.

Chemotherapeutic agent: A chemical used to treat cancer.

Coagulase: An enzyme produced by staphylococci that coagulates blood plasma.

Commensalism: A relationship between members of different species living in proximity in which one organism benefits from other, but the second is not affected.

Complement: A normal thermolabile protein constituent of blood serum that participates in antigen-antibody reaction.

Compromised host: A person already weakened by debilitating disease.

Dimorphic: Occurring in two forms.

Disinfectant: An agent that frees from infection by killing the vegetative cells of microorganisms.

Endemic: Disease that has low incidence, but is constantly present in that region.

Endotoxin: A heat stable toxin, which consists of lipopolysaccharide, it is located in the outer membrane of gram-negative bacteria.

Epidemic: Disease that displays a sudden increase in incidence in a particular region.

Episome: A plasmid of bacteria, which integrate or can multiply independently of the chromosome.

Etiology: The study of the cause of diseases.

Exergonic: Energy yielding, as in a chemical reaction.

Exotoxin: A toxic protein excreted by microorganism into surrounding medium.

Fermentation: An anaerobic oxidation of compounds by enzyme action of microorganisms.

Gelatin: A protein obtained from skin, hair or bones, used in culture media.

Gene: A segment of DNA located on chromosome.

Genome: A complete set of genetic material.

Halophile: A microorganism whose growth is accelerated by or dependent on high salt concentration.

Hapten: A substance that reacts like antigen, but cannot induce antibodies by itself.

Hemolysis: The lysis of blood cells.

Heterotroph: A microorganism that is unable to use carbondioxide as sole source of carbon, but require it in an organic form.

Immunity: A natural or acquired resistance to a specific disease.

Immunization: Any process that develops resistance to a specific disease in a host.

Immunoglobulin: Any of the serum protein, such as gamma globulin that possess antibody activity.

Inclusion bodies: Assembly of virions.

Infection: A pathological condition due to growth of microorganism in host.

Inoculum: The substance containing microorganisms or other material that is introduced by in-oculation.

Intercellular: Between cells.

Interferon: An antiviral substance produced by animal tissue.

Intracellular: Within cell.

Latent: A disease carrier who shows no symptoms.

Lithotroph: An organism, which uses reduced inorganic compounds, as electron donor.

Lophotrichous: Having polar tuft of flagella.

Lymph: The fluid within lymphatic vessesls.

Lymph node: Ovoid structures of lymphatic system and distributed throughout the body.

Lyophilization: The preservation of specimens by freezing and dehydration in high vacuum.

Meninges: Membrane that covers brain and spinal cord.

Metabolism: Chemical changes by which the nutritional and functional activities of an organism are maintained.

Microtubules: Thin rods that occur within all types of eukaryotic microbial cells.

Monotrichous: Having single polar flagellum.

Mycology: Study of fungi.

Mycosis: A disease caused by fungi.

Negri bodies: Minute pathological structures found in certain brain cells of animals infected with rabies virus.

Osmosis: The passage due to osmotic pressure through semipermeable membrane.

Parasite: An organism that derives its nourishment from living plant or animal host.

Parasitism: The relationship of parasite to its host.

Pathogen: An organism capable of producing disease.

Phagocyte: A cell capable of ingesting microorganisms.

Phycology: Study of algae.

Prokaryote: A cell whose nucleus is not enclosed in membrane.

Psychrophile: A cold-loving microorganism.

Pus: The fluid product of inflammation.

Pyemia: A form of septicemia caused by pyogenic organisms in bloodstream.

Pyrogen: A chemical, which affects hypothalamus.

Resolving power: The ability of microscope to distinguish fine details in a microscopic specimen.

Sanitizer: An agent that reduces contamination to levels judged safe by public health authorities.

Saprophyte: An organism living on dead organic matter.

Sepsis: Poisoning by the products of putrefaction.

Septicemia: A systemic disease caused by invasion and multiplication of pathogenic microorganisms in the blood.

Serology: The branch of science that deals with the study of serum.

Smear: A thin layer of material on slide.

Strain: All the descendants of pure culture.

Synergism: The ability of two or more organisms to bring about changes that neither can accomplished alone.

Thallophyte: A plant having no true stem, roots or leaves.

Therapeutic: Pertains to the treating or curing of disease.

Toxemia: Presence of toxins in the blood.

Toxin: A poisonous substance.

Toxoid: A toxin treated to destroy its toxic properties.

Undulating: Exhibiting a wave-like motion.

Vaccine: A preparation of killed or attenuated microorganisms or their components or their products that is used to induce active immunity.

Venereal: Sexually transmitted.

Viremia: Presence of virus in the blood.

Virion: The complete mature virus particle.

Yeast: A kind of fungus that is unicellular.

Zoonosis: An animal disease transmissible to human beings.

Zymogen: An inactive antecedent form of an active enzyme that becomes functional by the action of an appropriate kinase or other action.

B—Model Semester Question Papers

Long Essays (Any Two)

1. Mention the physical methods of sterilization and give an account of moist heat sterilization.
2. Define sterilization and disinfection and discuss the various methods of disinfection.
3. Mention the sources of disinfection and give an account of nosocomial infections.

Short Essays (Any Seven)

4. Nutritional requirements of bacteria.
5. Gram stain.
6. Urinary tract infection.
7. Sputum examination for pulmonary tuberculosis.
8. Laboratory diagnosis of diphtheria.
9. Gases used in sterilization.
10. *Staphylococcus aureus*.
11. Bacterial motility test.
12. *Pneumococcus*.
13. Morphological classification of bacteria.

Short Answers

14. Disinfection of the skin.
15. Bacterial growth curve.
16. Iatrogenic infection.
17. Teratogenic infection.
18. Carriers.
19. L-J medium.
20. Uses of phenol.
21. VR fluid.
22. Anaerobic.
23. Fumigation.

Additional Questions

1. Flagella.
2. Bacterial spores.
3. Name two commensals of the throat.

4. Name two disinfectants of the aldehyde group.
5. Diseases passed through blood transfusion.

II SEMESTER EXAMINATION

Long Essays (Any Two)

1. Define and classify immunity. Describe innate immunity.
2. Describe the various types of hypersensitivity reactions. Describe anaphylaxis.
3. What is enteric fever? Describe the laboratory diagnosis of typhoid fever.

Short Essays (Any Seven)

4. List the hepatitis viruses. Write briefly on hepatitis B.
5. VDRL test.
6. *Candida albicans.*
7. Transmission of HIV and prevention of AIDS.
8. National Immunization Schedule of India.
9. Leptospirosis.
10. Hepatitis.
11. Classification of viruses.
12. Rubella.
13. Pulse Polio Immunization of India.

Short Answers

14. ELISA test.
15. Diagram of HIV.
16. Mycetoma.
17. BCG vaccine.
18. Mantoux test.
19. Cultivation of viruses.
20. Cytopathic effect.
21. Name two sexually transmitted viral diseases.
22. Rabies and its prevention.
23. Name two spirochetal diseases.

III SEMESTER EXAMINATION

Long Essays (Any Two)

1. What is amebiasis? Discuss the pathogenicity and lab diagnosis of amebiasis.
2. Describe the malarial parasite and its life cycle.
3. Describe the life cycle of *Wuchereria bancrofti*, filariasis and its prevention.

Short Answers (Any Seven)

4. Life cycle of roundworm
5. Amastigotes of LD bodies.
6. Specimen collection.
7. Stool examination.

8. Compare amebic dysentery with bacillary dysentery.
9. Sheathed microfilaria.
10. *Plasmodium vivax.*
11. Characteristics and classification of parasites.
12. Normal flora.

Short Answers

13. Water-borne diseases.
14. Mosquito-borne diseases.
15. Amplifier host.
16. Definitive hosts.
17. CL crystals.
18. *Ascaris* ovum.
19. Name five biological vectors.
20. Name three bile stained ova.
21. Name two blood flagellates of India.
22. *Giardia intestinalis.*

C—University Question Papers

RAJIV GANDHI UNIVERSITY OF HEALTH SCIENCES, KARNATAKA

First Year BSc Nursing (Basic) Degree Examination, April 2005

MICROBIOLOGY

(Revised Scheme)

Long Essays (Any Two)

1. Classify mycobacteria. How will you diagnose a suspected case of pulmonary tuberculosis. Add a note on RNTCP.
2. Classify immunity. Discuss innate immunity in detail.
3. Name the malarial parasites. Describe the life cycle of any one of them.

Short Essays (Any Seven)

4. Sterilization using dry heat.
5. Bacteriophage.
6. Bacterial capsule.
7. Bacterial growth curve.
8. *Entamoeba histolytica.*
9. *Toxoplasma gondii.*
10. Widal test.
11. Polio vaccines.
12. Prophylaxis in rabies.
13. Varicella-zoster virus.

Short Answers

14. Name two hemoflagellates.
15. Components of MMR vaccine and dosage schedule.
16. Mention two sexually transmitted diseases.
17. Name two arboviral diseases seen in India.
18. Name the four different types of hypersensitivity.
19. Robert Koch.
20. Gram stain.
21. Pili.
22. Exotoxin.
23. LD body.

First Year BSc Nursing (Basic) Degree Examination, September 2005

MICROBIOLOGY

(Revised Scheme)

Long Essays (Any Two)

1. Classify vibrios. Discuss the laboratory diagnosis of cholera. How is this disease prevented?
2. Define sterilization. Discuss in detail the methods of sterilization using moist heat.
3. Describe the morphology, life cycle and laboratory diagnosis of *Entamoeba histolytica*.

Short Essays (Any Seven)

4. Acid-fast bacilli.
5. Bacterial spore.
6. Flagella.
7. Agglutination reaction.
8. Differences between bacteria and viruses.
9. Serum sickness.
10. Methods of culture of bacteria.
11. Laboratory diagnosis of streptococcal pharyngitis.
12. *Leishmania donovani.*
13. *Candida albicans.*

Short Answers

14. Name two tapeworms.
15. Draw a diagram of a hookworm egg.
16. Definitive host with an example.
17. Dermatophytes.
18. DPT vaccine.
19. *Leptospira.*
20. Weil-felix test.
21. Mantoux test.
22. Hepatitis B virus.
23. Satellitism.

First Year BSc Nursing (Basic) Degree Examination, April 2006

MICROBIOLOGY

(Revised Scheme)

Long Essays (Any Two)

1. Classify streptococci. Describe the pathogenicity and laboratory diagnosis of infections caused by streptococci.
2. Describe the morphology and life cycle of *Entamoeba histolytica*.
3. Classify viruses. Write in detail viral diagnosis in the laboratory.

Short Esssays (Any Seven)

4. Laboratory diagnosis of *Corynebacterium diphtheriae*.
5. Bacterial capsule.

6. Tyndallization.
7. Bacterial toxins.
8. Laboratory diagnosis of pulmonary tuberculosis.
9. Labeled diagram of immunoglobulin G (IgG).
10. Type IV hypersensitivity.
11. Candidiasis.
12. Gram staining.
13. Antirabies vaccines.

Short Answers

14. Robert Koch.
15. Catalase test.
16. Name two intestinal parasites.
17. Pasteurization.
18. Name four selective media.
19. Sterilization controls.
20. BCG vaccine.
21. Name two methods of antibiotic sensitivity test.
22. Draw immunoglobulin A (IgA).
23. Inclusion bodies.

First Year BSc Nursing (Basic) Degree Examination, October 2006

MICROBIOLOGY

(Revised Scheme)

Long Essays (Any Two)

1. Define immunity, classify immunity with examples and write in detail on active immunity.
2. Define infection, classify infections and discuss in detail on hospital infection.
3. Describe the morphology, cultural characteristics and laboratory diagnosis of *Corynebacterium diphtheriae*.

Short Essays (Any Seven)

4. Bacterial growth curve.
5. Hepatitis A virus.
6. Bacterial spore.
7. Labelled diagram of *Giardia intestinalis*.
8. Autoclave.
9. Fumigation.
10. *Candida albicans*.
11. Laboratory diagnosis of pulmonary tuberculosis.
12. Draw immunoglobulin M (IgM).
13. Gram stain.

Short Answers

14. What is septicemia?
15. Negative staining.
16. Catalase test.

17. Classify hypersensitivity.
18. Labelled diagram of hookworm ova.
19. Enumerate spirochetes.
20. Morphological classification of bacteria.
21. MMR vaccine.

First Year BSc Nursing (Basic) Degree Examination, May 2007

MICROBIOLOGY

(Revised Scheme)

Long Essays (Any Two)

1. Classify culture media and write in detail on selective media with examples.
2. Define antigen-antibody reaction, enumerate with examples and add a note on Widal test.
3. Classify mycobacteria, laboratory diagnosis of pulmonary tuberculosis and add a note on RN-TCP.

Short Essays (Any Seven)

4. Bacterial filters.
5. Bacterial spore.
6. Laboratory diagnosis of amebiasis.
7. Hepatitis A virus.
8. VDRL Test.
9. Morphological classification of bacteria.
10. Chemical sterilization.
11. Bacillary dysentery.
12. Stool examination for parasites.
13. Viral cultivation in laboratory.

Short Answers

14. Name DNA viruses.
15. Fumigation.
16. Define sterilization and anitseptic.
17. Labelled diagram of *Giardia intestinalis.*
18. Infections caused by *Candida albicans.*
19. Uses of candle jar.
20. Name two diseases casued by spirochetes.
21. DPT vaccine.
22. Name bile stained ova.
23. Collection of urine for culture.

First Year BSc Nursing (Basic) Degree Examination, October 2007

MICROBIOLOGY

(Revised Scheme)

Long Essays (Any Two)

1. Define and classify sterilization. Write in detail on hot air oven.
2. Enumerate sexually transmitted diseases and laboratory diagnosis of gonococcal infections.
3. Enumerate hepatitis viruses. Write in detail on hepatitis B virus.

Short Essays (Any Seven)

4. Widal test.
5. Bacterial growth curve.
6. Sterilization by radiation.
7. Draw cyst and trophozoite of *Entamoeba histolytica*.
8. Laboratory diagnosis of *Corynebacterium diphtheriae*.
9. Syphilis.
10. Hospital infection.
11. Ziehl-Neelsen stain.
12. Anaphylaxis.
13. Robertson cooked meat medium (RCM).

Short Answers

14. Name four tapeworms.
15. Name four transport media.
16. Draw a spore.
17. Name two zoonotic diseases.
18. Define selective media.
19. Define antibody and name them.
20. Name dermatophytes.
21. Draw bacteriophage.
22. Exotoxin.
23. Write contributions of Robert Koch.

First Year BSc Nursing (Basic) Degree Examination, Aug/Sept 2009

MICROBIOLOGY

(Revised Scheme — 3)

Long Essays (Any Two)

1. Describe the morphology of a bacterial cell with a neat labeled diagram.
2. What is immunity? Classify immunity. Describe the mechanisms of innate immunity.
3. Classify staphylococci. Describe the pathogenicity and laboratory diagnosis of *Staphylococcus aureas*.

Short Essays (Any Seven)

4. Universal precautions with highly infectious patient.
5. Bacterial growth curve.
6. Widal test.
7. MMR vaccine.
8. Bacterial capsule.
9. Hepatitis B virus.
10. Prokaryotes and eukaryotes.
11. Immunoglobulin E (IgE).
12. Koch's postulates.

Short Answers

13. Name two RNA viruses.
14. Name a screening and confirmatory test for HIV infection.
15. Name two gaseous disinfectants.
16. Anaerobic culture media.
17. CSSD.
18. DPT vaccine.
19. Name two diseases caused by spirochetes.
20. Infections caused by herpes simplex virus.
21. Name two bacterial sexually transmitted diseases.
22. Define sterilization and disinfection.

First Year BSc Nursing (Basic) Degree Examination, August 2010

MICROBIOLOGY

(Revised Scheme—3)

Long Essays (Any Two)

1. Classify streptococci. Describe pathogenicity and laboratory diagnosis of *Streptococcus pyogenes.*
2. Classify culture media and write in detail on selective media with examples.
3. Classify *Mycobacterium.* Describe the pathogenesis and laboratory diagnosis of pulmonary tuberculosis.

Short Essays (Any Seven)

4. Amebic dysentery.
5. Hot air oven.
6. Agglutination reactions.
7. Roundworm.
8. Bacterial flagella.
9. Prophylaxis of needle prick injuries.
10. Nosocomial infection.
11. Immunoglobulin E (IgE).
12. Gram stain—principle, theories and procedure.

Short Answers

13. Name two DNA viruses.
14. Name a screening and a confirmatory test for HIV.
15. Name two chemical disinfectants.
16. Louis Pasteur.
17. Name the color coding of bags used for segregation of hospital waste.
18. DPT vaccine.
19. *Candida albicans.*
20. Name four hepatitis viruses.
21. Name two infections transmitted by mosquitoes.
22. Name two viruses causing CNS infections.

First Year BSc Nursing (Basic) Degree Examination, August/September 2011

MICROBIOLOGY

(Revised Scheme — 3)

Long Essays (Any Two)

1. Define the anatomy of the bacterial cell with a neat labeled diagram.
2. Classify antigen-antibody reactions. Describe agglutination reaction in detail.
3. Describe the pathogenesis and laboratory diagnosis of *Vibrio cholerae.*

Short Essays (Any Seven)

4. Anaerobic culture methods.
5. Principle and applications of autoclaving.
6. Anaphylaxis.
7. Differences between active and passive immunity.
8. *Staphylococcus aureus.*
9. Laboratory diagnosis of pulmonary tuberculosis.
10. Cultivation of viruses.
11. Prophylaxis of type B hepatitis.
12. Dermatophytes.

Short Answers

13. Define sterilization and disinfection.
14. Mention two contributions of Robert Koch.
15. Name two important properties, which make a substance antigenic.
16. Draw a neat labeled diagram of immunoglobulin M.
17. Mention two zoonotic diseases.
18. Name the vectors involved in the transmission of epidemic and endemic typhus fevers.
19. Mention two RNA and two DNA viruses.
20. Mention four opportunistic infections associated with HIV infection.
21. Mention two important complications of falciparum malaria.
22. DPT vaccine.

First Year BSc Nursing (Basic) Degree Examination, February/March 2012

MICROBIOLOGY

(Revised Scheme)

Long Essays (Any Two)

1. Name the etiologic agent of cholera. Write in detail on the pathogenesis and laboratory diagnosis of cholera.
2. Define and classify hypersensitivity. Write in detail on type I hypersensitivity.
3. Name the malarial parasites. Describe the life cycle and laboratory diagnosis of any one of them.

Short Essays (Any Seven)

4. Gas gangrene.
5. Food poisoning.
6. Pneumococci.
7. Blood culture.
8. Relapsing fever.
9. Use of embryonated egg in virology.
10. Hepatitis B virus.
11. *Balantidium coli.*
12. *Trichinella spiralis.*
13. *Candida albicans.*

Short Answers

14. Name two bacteria causing diarrhea.
15. Antibiotic sensitivity test.
16. Phagocytosis.
17. Structure of IgG.
18. Name two bacterial zoonotic diseases.
19. Flagella.
20. Log phase of bacterial growth.
21. Tyndallization.
22. DPT vaccine.
23. Name two bacteria causing nosocomial infections.

First Year BSc Nursing (Basic) Degree Examination, September 2012

MICROBIOLOGY

(Revised Scheme — 3)

Long Essays (Any Two)

1. Draw a neat labeled diagram of bacterial cell. Write about bacterial flagella?
2. Enumerate the causes of diarrhea and write the laboratory diagnosis of cholera.
3. Discuss the source and mode of transmission of hospital infection and add a note on preventive measures.

Short Essays (Any Seven)

4. Agglutination reaction.
5. Widal test.
6. Bacterial growth curve.
7. Antirabies vaccine.
8. Prophylaxis of tetanus.
9. Laboratory diagnosis of HIV.
10. Oral thrush.
11. Life cycle of *Plasmodium falciparum.*
12. Anaphylaxis

Short Answers

13. Name two gaseous disinfectants.
14. Acid-fast staining.
15. Define selective media. Give an example.
16. Mention four differences between active and passive immunity.
17. Name four congenitally transmitted infections.
18. DPT vaccine.
19. Draw a neat labeled diagram of IgM molecule.
20. VDRL test.
21. Name four intestinal nematodes.
22. Mention four contributions of Robert Koch to microbiology.

First Year BSc Nursing (PC) Degree Examination, August 2010

MICROBIOLOGY

(Revised Scheme—3 and Revised Scheme—4)

Long Essays (Any Two)

1. Define sterilization. List the methods of sterilization. Discuss the autoclave.
2. Define and classify hypersensitivity. Describe in detail anaphylaxis.
3. Name the organisms causing meningitis. Describe the laboratory diagnosis of bacterial meningitis caused by *Mycobacterium tuberculosis*.

Short Essays (Any Seven)

4. Bacterial growth curve.
5. Widal test.
6. Bacterial capsule.
7. Laboratory diagnosis of intestinal amebiasis.
8. MMR vaccine.
9. Passive immunity.
10. Acid-fast staining.
11. *Candida*.
12. Food poisoning.

Short Answers

13. Name two bacteria having flagella.
14. Four contributions of Robert Koch.
15. Name two sexually transmitted diseases.
16. Draw immunoglobulin G.
17. Pasteurization.
18. Draw hookworm and roundworm ova.
19. Name two fungal infection.
20. Blood culture.
21. Name two RNA viruses.
22. VDRL test.

First Year BSc Nursing (PC) Degree Examination, February/March 2011

MICROBIOLOGY

(Revised Scheme — 3 and Revised Scheme — 4)

Long Essays (Any Two)

1. Define viruses. Classify viruses. Explain life cycle of viruses.
2. Classify mycobacteria. Explain pathogenicity and laboratory diagnosis of pulmonary tuberculosis. Add a note on RNTCP.
3. Define hypersensitivity. Classify hypersensitivity and write about type I hypersensitivity.

Short Essays (Any Seven)

4. Different shapes of bacteria with examples.
5. Bacterial capsule composition and functions.
6. Explain bacterial growth curve.
7. Radiations in sterilization.
8. Widal test.
9. Food poisoning.
10. Koch's postulates.
11. Mumps.
12. Intestinal amebiasis.

Short Answers

13. Name any two bacterial respiratory diseases.
14. Name the dermatophytes.
15. Steps of gram staining.
16. BCG vaccine.
17. Name any four RNA viruses.
18. Mention any two zoonotic diseases.
19. Mention any two DNA viruses.
20. Mention any two food poisoning causing bacteria.
21. Mention any four modes of transmission of HIV.
22. Mention any two types of infectious wastes in hospital.

First Year BSc Nursing (PC) Degree Examination, August/September 2011

MICROBIOLOGY

(Revised Scheme — 3 and Revised Scheme — 4)

Long Essays (Any Two)

1. Define and classify sterilization, discuss in detail the autoclave.
2. Classify enterobacteriaceae. Discuss the morphology and laboratory diagnosis of typhoid fever.
3. Define and classify hypersensitivity. Discuss in detail type IV hypersensitivity reaction.

Short Essays (Any Seven)

4. Gram stain.
5. LJ media.

6. Hospital infection.
7. Bacterial spore.
8. Laboratory diagnosis of diphtheria.
9. MMR.
10. Laboratory diagnosis of HIV.
11. *Candida albicans.*
12. Cultivation of viruses.

Short Answers

13. Prophylaxis of rabies.
14. Name four bacteria causing food poisoning.
15. State four contributions of Robert Koch.
16. Name four organisms causing UTI.
17. Name four toxins of streptococci.
18. Name two gaseous disinfectants.
19. Name two blood parasites.
20. Name two bile stained ova.
21. IGA.
22. Indole test.

First Year BSc Nursing (PC) Degree Examination, February/March 2012

MICROBIOLOGY

(Revised Scheme—3 and Revised Scheme—4)

Long Essays (Any Two)

1. Describe the pathogenesis, clinical features and laboratory diagnosis of poliomyelitis.
2. Define immunity, classify immunity and write in detail on innate immunity.
3. List the various physical methods of sterilization. Discuss the principle and uses of sterilization by autoclave.

Short Essays (Any Seven)

4. Type I hypersensitivity.
5. Widal test.
6. Gram staining.
7. Bacterial spore, diagram and description.
8. *Candida albicans.*
9. ELISA and its uses.
10. Different treatment methods of biomedical wastes.
11. Bacillary dysentery.
12. Syphilis.

Short Answers

13. Name two methods of pasteurization.
14. Name any two viral sexually transmitted diseases.
15. Draw a neat diagram of *Trichomonas vaginalis.*
16. Draw a neat labeled diagram of bacterial flagella.

17. MMR vaccine.
18. RNTCP.
19. Name any two biological vectors.
20. Name any two zoonotic diseases.
21. Mention any two selective media and two differential media.
22. Tyndallization.

First Year BSc Nursing (PC) Degree Examination, September 2012

MICROBIOLOGY

(Revised Scheme—3 and Revised Scheme—4)

Long Essays (Any Two)

1. Define sterilization, describe the different methods of dry heat sterilization.
2. Classify mycobacteria. Discuss is detail the morphology, pathogenesis and laboratory diagnosis of pulmonary tuberculosis.
3. Name the malarial parasites, explain the life cycle and laboratory diagnosis of *Plasmodium falciparum*.

Short Essays (Any Seven)

4. Albert stain.
5. Blood culture.
6. Laboratory diagnosis of UTI.
7. Bacterial flagella.
8. Oral thrush.
9. Active immunity.
10. Kala-azar.
11. Compound microscope.
12. VCRL test.

Short Answers

13. Name four bacteria causing meningitis.
14. Prophylaxis of hepatitis B.
15. Fumigation.
16. Name four bacteria causing diarrhea.
17. Name four agents causing STD.
18. IGG
19. DPT
20. Name two transport media.
21. Name two intermediate hosts in parasitic infections.
22. Name two agglutination tests.

D—Multiple Choice Questions (MCQs)

1. The term microbiology was introduced by
   a. Louis Pasteur
   b. Robert Koch
   c. Alexander Fleming
   d. Antonie van Leeuwenhoek.
2. Who is considered as the father of aseptic and antiseptic surgery?
   a. Louis Pasteur
   b. Robert Koch
   c. Joseph Lister
   d. Alexander Fleming.
3. Attenuated live vaccine was first developed by
   a. Louis Pasteur
   b. Lazier
   c. Paul Ehrlich
   d. Loeffler.
4. Transmission of malarial parasites by anopheles mosquitoes was discovered by
   a. Lowenstein
   b. Louis Pasteur
   c. Sir Ronald Ross
   d. Joseph Lister.
5. The word vaccination was coined by
   a. Edward Jenner
   b. Ronald Ross
   c. Louis Pasteur
   d. Ferdinand Cohn.
6. Which of the following are not prokaryotes?
   a. Bacteria
   b. Fungi
   c. *Rickettsia*
   d. *Chlamydia.*
7. The diameter of the smallest structure that can be resolved and seen clearly by naked eye is
   a. 20 µm
   b. 60 µm
   c. 100 µm
   d. 200 µm.

8. Fimbriae are found in
    a. Motile organisms
    b. Non-motile organisms
    c. Both of the above.
9. The bacterial flagellum originate from
    a. Nucleus
    b. Protoplasm
    c. Cytoplasmic membranes
    d. Capsule.
10. The organs of adhesion in bacteria are
    a. Slime layer
    b. Fimbriae
    c. Flagella
    d. Capsule.
11. Organisms that grow better in presence of traces of oxygen and prefer increased concentration of CO_2 are called
    a. Facultative anaerobes
    b. Facultative aerobes
    c. Microaerophilic
    d. Obligate aerobe.
12. Minimum time required for sterilization by moist heat at 121°C is
    a. 2 hours
    b. 1 hour
    c. 45 minutes
    d. 3 minutes.
13. Temperature commonly used for sterilization in hot air oven is
    a. 120°C for 3 hours
    b. 140°C for 2 hours
    c. 160°C for 2 hours
    d. 180°C for 30 minutes.
14. All the following are motile except.
    a. *Shigella*
    b. *E. coli*
    c. *Vibrio cholerae*
    d. *Enterobacter.*
15. The following pathogen does not satisfy Koch's postulates
    a. *Bacillus anthracis*
    b. *Mycobacterium*
    c. *Clostridium tetani*
    d. Lepra bacilli.
16. One of the following is an example of negative staining
    a. Gram staining
    b. India ink preparation
    c. La Fontaine staining.
17. The optimum temperature for the growth of *Bacillus stearothermophilus* is
    a. 35°C

b. 37°C
c. 42°C
d. 55°C.

18. Fiberoptic instruments like endoscope should be sterilized by
    a. Formaldehyde
    b. Glutaraldehyde
    c. Gamma radiations
    d. Ethylene oxide gas.

19. Disposable medical articles are generally sterilized by
    a. Autoclaving
    b. Chemical treatment
    c. Gamma radiation
    d. Dry heat.

20. Mesophilic organisms are those that grow best at temperatures of
    a. - 20°C to -7°C
    b. - 7°C to + 20°C
    c. 25°C to 40°C
    d. 55°C to 80°C.

21. The response to treatment of syphilis is best measured by
    a. VDRL test
    b. TPHA test
    c. FTA-Abs test
    d. None of above.

22. The animal most commonly used for pathological studies of *Treponema pallidum* is
    a. Guinea pig
    b. Rabbits
    c. Mouse
    d. Monkey.

23. Which is a zoonotic disease?
    a. Coryza
    b. Anthrax
    c. Typhoid
    d. Tetanus.

24. Which of the following is not transmitted by an arthropod?
    a. Q fever
    b. Scrub fever
    c. Typhus fever
    d. Trench fever.

25. Least important mode of cross-infection by *Staphylococcus aureus* is
    a. Direct contact
    b. Indirect contact
    c. Droplet spray
    d. Insect vectors.

26. Most reliable test for diagnosis of typhoid fever is
    a. Feces sample
    b. Widal test

c. Blood culture

d. Urine culture.

27. The commonest bacterial cause of primary urinary tract infection is

a. *Staphylococcus aureus*

b. *Pseudomonas aeruginosa*

c. *Escherichia coli*

d. *Proteus* species.

28. The bacterial agent causing infection endocarditis is

a. *Streptococcus viridans*

b. Enterococci

c. *Haemophilus* species

d. *Streptococcus.*

29. The main cause of septicemia in hospital acquired infection is

a. *Escherichia coli*

b. *Staphylococcus aureus*

c. *Streptococcus*

d. *Bacteroides* species.

30. Penicillin can be used against the following infections except

a. Streptococcal

b. Staphylococcal

c. Pneumococcal

d. Meningococcal.

31. All the following are live attenuated vaccines except

a. OPV

b. Mumps vaccine

c. Measles vaccine

d. Pertussis vaccine.

32. Nosocomial infection due to *Mycobacterium tuberculosis* occurs due to

a. Droplets

b. Blood

c. Direct contact

d. Via equipment.

33. Hepatitis B can spread in a hospital through

a. Droplets

b. Skin scales

c. Food

d. Blood.

34. *Staphylococcus aureus* is differentiated from *Staphylococcus epidermidis* by

a. Color of colonies

b. Shape of bacteria

c. Coagulase test

d. Catalase test.

35. Food poisoning has occurred due to ingestion of contaminated fried rice, most likely organism is

a. *Yersinia*

b. *Staphylococcus*

    c. *Bacillus cereus*

    d. *Vibrio parahaemolyticus.*

36. *Clostridium tetani* is
    a. Gram-positive bacillus
    b. Gram-negative bacillus
    c. Gram-positive coccus
    d. Gram-negative coccus.

37. Which is the transport medium for cholera bacilli?
    a. Tellurite medium
    b. Chacko-Nair medium
    c. Venkatraman Ramakrishnan medium
    d. McLeod medium.

38. Dark ground microscopy is useful to identify the following microbe
    a. Spirochetes
    b. Fungi
    c. Mycoplasma
    d. Rickettsia.

39. Which of the following is caused by rats urine?
    a. Plague
    b. Brucellosis
    c. Leptospirosis
    d. Legionellosis.

40. The immunoglobulin that can cross the placenta is
    a. IgG
    b. IgM
    c. IgD
    d. IgA
    e. IgE.

41. Which of the following contains lysozyme?
    a. Cerebrospinal fluid
    b. Human tears
    c. Urine
    d. Sweat.

42. Herd immunity is not available in
    a. Tetanus
    b. Measles
    c. Diphtheria
    d. Pertussis.

43. The course of hepatitis B vaccine is completed in
    a. 2 weeks
    b. 2 months
    c. 4 months
    d. 6 months.

44. Which of the following spreads through skin?
    a. Measles
    b. Tuberculosis

   c. Pneumonia
   d. Blood.
45. VDRL is a
   a. Slide agglutination test
   b. Tube flocculation test
   c. Gel precipitation test
   d. Indirect hemagglutination test.
46. Which of the following vaccines should not be given to an immunodeficient patient?
   a. Rubella vaccine
   b. Influenza vaccine
   c. Pneumonia vaccine
   d. Trivalent oral polio vaccine.
47. Which of the following is an example of type IV hypersensitivity?
   a. Arthus reaction
   b. Serum sickness
   c. Schwartzman reaction
   d. Granulomatous reaction.
48. One of the following is not type III hypersensitivity
   a. TB
   b. Rheumatoid arthritis
   c. SLE
   d. Arthus reaction.
49. Delayed hypersensitivity reaction involves
   a. Neutrophils
   b. Monocytes
   c. Eosinophils
   d. Lymphocytes.
50. Carriers are not found in
   a. Cholera
   b. Typhoid
   c. Measles
   d. Poliomyelitis.
51. Nosocomial organisms are all except
   a. *Streptococcus*
   b. *Pseudomonas*
   c. *Salmonella*
   d. *Proteus*
   e. *Klebsiella.*
52. Antisera is prepared from
   a. Guinea pig
   b. Rabbit
   c. Horse
   d. Rat.
53. Hepatitis B is considered persistent if HBsAg is present for more than
   a. 2 months
   b. 3 months

   c. 6 months
   d. 12 months.
54. Which of the following viruses can cross the placenta?
   a. Varicella
   b. Human herpes virus
   c. Epstein-Barr virus
   d. None of the above.
55. Blood is a source of infection for
   a. Hepatitis A
   b. Hepatitis C
   c. Hepatitis E
   d. All the above.
56. How many doses of tissue culture vaccines are recommended for post exposure immunization against rabies?
   a. 1
   b. 2
   c. 4
   d. 6.
57. Classical congenital rubella syndrome consists of abnormalities of the following organs except
   a. Brain
   b. Eyes
   c. Ear
   d. Heart.
58. Protection with attenuated rubella vaccine last for
   a. 1 year
   b. 5 years
   c. 10 years
   d. 15 years.
59. The number of which cells decrease dramatically in AIDS
   a. B cells
   b. T4 cells
   c. T8 cells
   d. None of the above.
60. Circulation HIV is found in
   a. T4 cells
   b. Monocytes
   c. Macrophages
   d. All the above.
61. Interferon is a product of
   a. Viral cell
   b. Host cell
   c. Synthetic copolymer
   d. Bacterial cell.
62. Rubella vaccination is contraindicated in all except
   a. Patient on immunosuppressive drugs
   b. Girls with leukemia

   c. Girls between 11 to 14 years of age

   d. Pregnancy.

63. The most common mode of AIDS transmission in India is by

   a. Vertical transmission

   b. IV drug addicts

   c. Heterosexual promiscuity

   d. Homosexual promiscuity.

64. Virion is defined as

   a. An extracellular infectious virus particle

   b. Smallest virus

   c. A smallest particle similar to viruses

   d. None of the above.

65. Refrigerated blood stored up to 48 hours before transfusion can destroy

   a. HIV

   b. Hepatitis B

   c. *Treponema pallidum*

   d. *P. vivax.*

66. Which is the best source of complement for use in complement fixation test

   a. Guinea pig

   b. Sheep

   c. Rabbit

   d. Mice.

67. All are general properties of viruses except

   a. May contain both RNA and DNA

   b. Form extracellular infectious particles

   c. Heat-labile

   d. Not affected by antibodies.

68. Amastigote forms of *Leishmania* parasite are seen in

   a. Vertebrate host

   b. Sandfly

   c. Culture media

   d. All above.

69. Which of the following parasites can be transmitted vertically?

   a. *Entamoeba histolytica*

   b. *Toxoplasma gondii*

   c. *Giardia lamblia*

   d. *Echinococcus granulosus.*

70. In which of the following condition the microfilaria are present in the peripheral blood

   a. Elephantiasis

   b. Occult filariasis

   c. Classical filariasis

   d. In early allergic manifestations.

71. In systematic classification, *Entamoeba histolytica* belongs to which of the following classes

   a. Mastigophora

   b. Sporozoa

   c. Rhizopoda

   d. Ciliata.

72. How many amebulae develops from cyst of *Entamoeba histolytica*?

   a. 2

   b. 4

   c. 6

   d. 8.

73. Which is the best method of staining the chromatoid bars in the cyst of *Entamoeba histolytica*?

   a. JSB

   b. Iodine

   c. Iron hematoxylin

   d. Methylene blue.

74. At which of the following sites, the encystations of cysts of *Entamoeba histolytica* occur

   a. Sigmoid colon

   b. Large intestine

   c. Lower part of ileum

   d. Duodenum.

75. Which of the following causes hepatic amebiasis

   a. Cyst of *Entamoeba histolytica*

   b. Trophozoite of *Entamoeba histolytica*

   c. Toxin liberated by diphtheria

   d. Antoimmune mechanism.

76. *Leishmania donovani* is primarily an infection of

   a. Reticuloendothelial system

   b. White blood cells

   c. Red blood cells

   d. Musculoskeletal system.

77. Which of the following causes malignant malaria

   a. *P. falciparum*

   b. *P. vivax*

   c. *P. malariae*

   d. *P. ovale.*

78. Multiple invasion of erythrocytes is commonest with

   a. *P. falciparum*

   b. *P. vivax*

   c. *P. malariae*

   d. *P. ovale.*

79. The following statements are true of malaria except

   a. Albumin-globulin ratio is reversed

   b. Plasma potassium level rises

   c. ESR is raised

   d. Blood pH rises.

80. In *Plasmodium* infection of man

   a. Erythrocytes are increased in size

   b. All stages of erythrocytic schizogony are seen in peripheral blood.

   c. Multiple infection of erythrocytes are seen

   d. Each erythrocytic cycle lasts 72 hours.

81. All of the following are yeast like fungi except

   a. *Candida*

   b. *Geotrichum*

   c. *Cryptococcus*

   d. *Trichophyton.*

82. Culture medium for fungi

   a. Tellurite medium

   b. NNN medium

   c. Chocolate agar medium.

83. *Candida albicans* is associated with the following diseases except

   a. Oral thrush

   b. Mycetoma

   c. Endocarditis

   d. Meningitis.

84. The most common cause of food poisoning is

   a. *Clostridium*

   b. *Salmonella*

   c. *Staphylococcus*

   d. *Campylobacter.*

85. Which of the following can cause food poisoning?

   a. *Staphylococcus aureus*

   b. *Clostrium perfringens*

   c. *Bacillus cereus*

   d. *Vibrio parahaemolyticus*

   e. All the above.

86. In transmission of malaria, mosquito bite transfers

   a. Trophozoite

   b. Merozoite

   c. Hypnozoite

   d. Granulocyte.

87. An anxious mother brought her 4-year-old daughter to the pediatrician. The girl was passing loose bulky stools for the past 20 days. This was often associated with pain in abdomen. The stool examination gave the following organisms. Identify the organisms

   a. *E. coli*

   b. *E. histolytica*

   c. *Giardia lamblia*

   d. *Cryptosporidium.*

88. A patient with semisolid stool with an offensive odor mucus and little blood. The organism likely responsible is

   a. *E. histolytica*

   b. *Giardia lamblia*

   c. *Strongyloides stercoralis*

   d. *Cryptococcus neoformans.*

89. The cystic stage is seen in man in all except
    a. *E. histolytica*
    b. *Giardia*
    c. *Toxoplasma*
    d. *Trichomonas.*
90. Which of the following is most severly affected in kala-azar?
    a. Spleen
    b. Liver
    c. Adrenal gland
    d. Bone marrow.
91. The following tests help in the laboratory diagnosis of kala-azar except
    a. Blood examination
    b. Bone marrow examination
    c. Aldehyde test
    d. Immobilization test.
92. A 42-year-old farmer present with multiple discharging sinus in leg. The diagnosis is
    a. Actinomycetes
    b. Syphilis
    c. Tuberculosis
    d. LGV.
93. *Aspergillus* infection in tissue is characterized by
    a. Budding cell
    b. Septate hyphae
    c. Pseudohyphae
    d. Metachromatic granules.
94. What is the most probable portal of entry of *Aspergillus*?
    a. Puncture wound
    b. Lungs
    c. Blood
    d. Gastrointestinal tract.
95. Which egg does not float in a saturated solution of saline
    a. *Ancylostoma* eggs
    b. *Trichuris* eggs
    c. Unfertilized eggs of *Ascaris.*
96. A young boy complains of upper abdominal distension and reports also that he passed worm per rectum, nose and mouth. Examination of stool showed eggs. The most likely worm is
    a. Hookworm
    b. Roundworm
    c. Tapeworm
    d. Guinea worm.
97. In disinfection procedures all is true except
    a. Dettol is good at reducing the level of bacteria at floor
    b. Dettol destroys spores
    c. 80 percent formaldehyde in ethanol kills the spores of bacteria and many viruses, though it may take many hours.
    d. Glutaraldehyde 2 percent kills tubercle bacillus.

98. Bacteria is not shed in
    a. Carrier state
    b. Incubation period
    c. Latent infection
    d. Subclinical infection.
99. The best urine sample for culture of pyogenic organism is
    a. First voided sample in the morning
    b. Midstream urine
    c. Catheterization sample
    d. 24 hour collection.

Answers to Multiple Choice Questions (MCQS)

1. a	26. c	51. c	76. c
2. c	27. c	52. c	77. d
3. a	28. a	53. c	78. a
4. c	29. a	54. a	79. d
5. c	30. b	55. b	80. c
6. b	31. d	56. d	81. d
7. c	32. a	57. a	82. d
8. b	33. d	58. d	83. b
9. b	34. c	59. b	84. b
10. b	35. c	60. d	85. e
11. c	36. a	61. b	86. a
12. d	37. c	62. c	87. c
13. c	38. a	63. c	88. b
14. a	39. c	64. a	89. d
15. d	40. a	65. c	90. a
16. b	41. b	66. a	91. d
17. d	42. a	67. a	92. a
18. b	43. d	68. a	93. b
19. c	44. d	69. b	94. b
20. c	45. a	70. c	95. c
21. a	46. a	71. c	96. b
22. b	47. d	72. d	97. b
23. b	48. a	73. c	98. c
24. a	49. d	74. c	99. b
25. c	50. c	75. b	

Index

Page numbers followed by *f* refer to figure and *t* refer to table

A

Acid-fast staining 15
Acquired
    immunity 77, 77*f*
    immunodeficiency syndrome 39, 41, 45, 89, 107,
        121
Acridine
    dyes 33
    orange 32
Acriflavin 32
Actinomycetes 10, 70
Acute
    brucellosis 66
    purulent meningitis 63
    respiratory disease 113
Adenovirus 110, 113, 113*f*
Aeruginosa sepsis 41
Agglutination 91, 102
    in VDRL test 101*f*
Albert
    stain 16, 17
    staining of *C. diphtheriae* 16*f*
Alcaligenes faecalis 12
Alcohol 32
Aldehydes 32
Algid malaria 143
Alkaline peptone water 22, 23
Alveolar macrophages 82
Amebic dysentery and bacillary dysentery 136*t*
Amikacin 45
Aminoglycosides 45
Amniotic sac 109
Anaerobic media 24
Anatomy of bacterial cell 10*f*
Ancylostoma duodenale 148
Ancylostomasis 148
Anthrax 4
Antibiogram 26
Antibiotic 44
    sensitivity 49
        method 63
        test 25, 59

B

Antibody mediated immunity 84
Antifungal
    drugs 45
    polyene antibiotics 45
Antigen 78
    antibody reactions 90, 90*f*, 99
    structure 115
Antigenic structure 47, 50, 60
Antimicrobial therapy 44
Antirabic vaccines 117
Antiseptic 27
Antitumor antibiotics 46
Antiviral chemotherapy 45
Antonie van Leeuwenhoek 4
Appearance of spherules of *Coccidioides immitis* 128*f*
Application of
    agglutination reactions 102
    microbiology in health science 3
Arboviruses 118
Arrangement of flagella 12*f*
Artificially acquired passive immunity 77
Asbestos disc filters 28
Ascariasis 146
Ascaris lumbricoides 146
Asepsis 27
Aspergilloma 128
Aspergillosis 128
Aspergillus asthma 128
Athlete's foot 129
Autoclave 28, 29
Autoimmune
    diseases 88
    hemolytic anemia 86, 89

Bacillus 9, 55
    anthracis 36, 55, 55*f*, 99
    cereus 56
    stearothermophilus 13, 30
Bacitracin 45
Bacterial
    growth curve 19
    spore 12, 13*f*

staining 14

wall 10*f*

Bactericidal agents 27

Bacteriophage typing 48

Basal body 12

BCG vaccine 97

Biochemical tests 49

Biomedical waste management 166*t*

Black sickness 138

Blackwater fever 143

Blastomyces dermatitidis 127, 128*f*

Blastomycosis 127

Blood 164

agar 22, 47

culture 61

Boiling 29

Bone marrow 83

Bordetella pertussis 65

Bordet-Gengou medium 65

Borrelia 68

burgdorferi 69

recurrentis 69

vincentii 69

Bronchitis 64

Browne tubes 30

Brucella 65

abortus 36

Bubonic plague 64

Buffered glycerol saline 24

Burkitt lymphoma 110

Bursa of fabricius 83

C

Campylobacter 36

Candida albicans 129, 130*f*

Candidiasis 129

Capsular K antigen 65

Carbon dioxide 19

Cary-Blair medium for feces 24

Cell

and organs of immune system 80

mediated immunity 84

of immune system 80

wall 10, 50

Cellular immunity 84, 85*f*

Central lymphoid organs 83

Cephalosporins 45

Cerebral malaria 143

Cerebrospinal fluid 51, 114, 155

Chemical

methods 32

structure of sulfa drugs 44*f*

Chemotherapy 112

Chicken cholera 4

Chickenpox 124

glandular fever 110

Chikungunya fever 123

Chinese letters 9

Chlamydia 10, 70

pneumoniae 71

psittaci 71

trachomatis 70

Chloramphenicol 45

Chlorine 33

Chloroform 32

Chlorohexidine 33

Chloroxylenol 33

Chocolate agar 22

Cholera 4

Chromatoidal bars 134

Chromosome 9

Chronic

brucellosis 66

carriers 38

Classification of

human fungal infections 126*f*

hypersensitivity 87*t*

immunity 76, 76*f*

infections 35

microorganisms/microbes 5

parasites 133*f*

streptococci 49*f*

Clinical manifestation of herpes 112

Clostridium 56

botulinum 24, 57

perfringens 24, 56

tetani 24, 57, 57*f*

Cluster arrangement of staphylococci 49*f*

Coccidioides immitis 128

Coccidioidomycosis 128

Coccobacilli 9

Cold sores 110

Collodion membrane filters 28

Combined immunization 54

Common

cold 123

respiratory tract infections 41

types of hospital infections 41*t*

Comparison of exotoxins and endotoxins 40*t*

Competitive ELISA 94, 94*f*

Complement

fixation test 92, 104

system 75, 84

Complex symmetry in viruses 109*f*

Condenser

adjustment screw 6

centering screws 6

Continuous cell lines 109

Control of

diseases of silkworms 4

microorganisms 27

Conventional vaccines 97

Coomb test 104, 105*f*

Corynebacterium 53
    diphtheriae 9, 16, 17, 54*f*
Crab louse 158
Cryptococcosis 127
Cryptococcus neoformans 127, 127*f*
Cultivation of viruses 108
Cutaneous infection 48, 112, 126
Cycloserine 45
Cysts of *Entamoeba coli* 152*f*
Cytomegaloviruses 112
Cytopathic effect 110
Cytoplasm 9, 11
Cytoplasmic membrane 11, 45

D

Dark ground microscopy 7
Dark-field
    illumination 12
    microscopy 6, 7
Deep
    infections 48
    mycoses 127
Denature proteins 32
Dendritic cells 82
Dengue fever 36, 123
Deoxycholate citrate agar 23
Deoxyribonucleases 50
Deoxyribonucleic acid 9, 10*f*
Deoxyribonucleoprotein 9
Detection of functions 12
Development of resistance 46
Diagnosis of
    diphtheria in laboratory 16
    enteric fever 103
Diarrhea 59, 113
Different microscopic methods 8*f*
Digestive tract 37
Diphtheria 97
Diploid cell lines 109
Direct
    contact 37, 38, 41
    immunofluorescence 92, 93*f*
    transmission 38
Discovery of streptococci 4
Disease transmission 37
Disseminated aspergillosis 128
DNA
    vaccines 97
    viruses 110*t*, 111
Dog tapeworm 36
Draughtsman appearance of pneumococci 51*f*
Dressing technique 42
Droplet infection 38
Drug resistance 46
Dry heat 27, 28
Drying 27, 28
DTP vaccine 97

E

Earthenware candles 28
Ectoplasm 134
Eggs of *Ascaris lumbricoides* 151
Electron microscopy 6, 8, 12
Elek test 55*f*
Embryonated egg 109*f*
Encephalitis 36
Endemic syphilis 68
Endoplasm 134
Endoplasmic reticulum 9
Enriched media 23
Entamoeba histolytica 134
Enterobacteriaceae 58
Enterobacterial
    diarrhea 41
    sepsis 41
Enterohemorrhagic *E. coli* 59
Enteroinvasive *E. coli* 59
Enteropathogenic *E. coli* 59
Enterotoxigenic *E. coli* 59
Enzyme-linked immunosorbent assay 93, 105, 106*f*
Epidemic jaundice 119
Epiglottitis 64
Epstein-Barr virus 113
Erythroblastosis fetalis 105
Erythrocytic schizogony 140
Escherichia coli 23, 35, 41, 58, 75
Ethylene oxide 32-34
Exoerythrocytic schizogony 140, 141
Exotoxins 41
Eye infections 63

F

Factors influencing growth of bacteria 18
Facultative aerobes 18
Father of
    antiseptic surgery 4
    bacteriology 4
    microbiology 4
    microscopy 4
Fatty acids 33
Feces culture 61
Fertilized egg 146
    of *Ascaris lumbricoides* 151*f*
Fiberglass filters 28
Filament 12
Filariasis 36, 144
Fimbriae 12
Fine adjustment screw 6
Flagella 11
Florence nightingale 5
Fluorescent
    microscopy 6, 7
    treponemal antibody absorption test 68
Food poisoning 36, 48
Footwear of persons with athlete foot 33

Formaldehyde 32, 33
   gas 32, 33
Fragment
   antigen binding 79*f*
   crystallization 79*f*
Fumigation of wards and operation theater 33
Functions of cell wall 10
Fungal infection 33, 41
Fungi 5

G

Gametogony 140
Gastroenteritis 61
Gastrointestinal
   diseases 110
   infections 41
   tract 76, 156
Genital
   herpes 110
   infection 50
Genitourinary tract 37
Gentamicin 45
Germ tube formation 130
German measles 124
Glutaraldehyde 32, 33
Glycogen mass 134
Golgi apparatus 9
Grading of smears of bacilli 66*t*
Gram
   negative bacteria 15*f*
   positive bacteria 15*f*
   staining 13, 14
Granulocytes 82, 83*f*
Graves' disease 86, 88
Growth
   cycle of chlamydia 71*f*
   of staphylococci on various media 47*t*
   on MacConkey media 58

H

H1N1 flu 123
Haemophilus influenzae 11, 22, 41, 64, 65*f*
Hands spread disease 42
Hanging drop method 8, 8*f*
Hashimoto disease 88
Heavy
   and light chains 79
   metals 32
Helical symmetry in viruses 108
Helminth ova in human stool 151
Helminthology 3
Hemagglutination 12
Hemolytic uremic syndrome 59
Hepadnaviruses 110
Hepatitis

A 36, 119
   and C 118
B 39, 41, 118, 119
   virus 31, 110
C 120
   and D 118
D 120
E virus 120
   virus 118, 120*f*
Herd immunity 78
Herpes
   simplex virus 111
   virus 110, 111
   zoster 112
Herpetic stomatitis 110
Hexachlorophene 33
Hide Porter's disease 55
Histoplasma capsulatum 36
Histoplasmosis 127
HLA complex 86
Hookworm infection 148
Hospital
   acquired infections 41
   waste management 165
Hot
   air oven 28, 28f
   water boiler 28
House fly 158
Human
   cycle 140
   immunodeficiency virus 31, 121
Humoral immunity 84, 85
Hydatid disease 36
Hydrochloric acid 16
Hydrogen
   ion concentration 18
   peroxide 32, 33
Hydrophobia 117
Hyperimmune serum 117
Hypersensitivity 87
   phenomenon of mycobacterium tuberculosis 4

I

Iatrogenic and laboratory infections 37, 39
Icosahedral symmetry in viruses 108*f*
Identification of bacteria/staining 14
Immune deficiency diseases 88
Immunization 95
Immunoelectrophoresis 91, 91*f*
Immunofluorescence 92
Immunoglobulin
   A 80
   D 80
   E 80
   G 80
   M 80

Important functions of capsule 11t
In vitro test 54
Inactivation of complement in serum 101
Incineration 28
Incubation 104
Indian leishmaniasis 138
Indirect
    ELISA 93, 93f
    immunofluorescence 92, 93, 93f
    transmission 38, 39
Infantile diarrhea 63
Infection control committee 43
Infective hepatitis A virus 36
Influenza virus 115f
Infrared radiation 31
Ingested red blood cells 134
Ingestion 37, 38
Inhibition of
    protein synthesis 45
    synthesis of cell wall peptidoglycan 45
Innate immunity 76
Inoculation 24, 37, 38
Inorganic acids hydrogen chloride 32
Insects 38, 157
Interdigitating dendritic cells 83
Intermediate host 134
Interpretation of complement fixation text 92f
Interstitial cells 83
Intestine amebiasis 137
Intracutaneous test 54
Intraplasmic inclusions 11
Inulin fermentation 51
Ionizing radiation 31
Iris diaphragm lever 6
Isolation of bacilli 61

J

Japanese encephalitis 122

K

Kala-azar 138
Kanamycin 45
Killed
    oral vaccine 63
    parental vaccine 63
    polio vaccine 114
Kirby-Bauer method 25
Klebsiella pneumoniae 11, 41, 59
Koch's
    phenomenon 4
    postulates 4
Kupffer cell 82

L

Lamina propria 84
Laminar airflow 31

Langerhans cells 82
Latex agglutination test 92f
Legionnaires disease 41
Leishmania 138, 138f
Length of bacilli 9
Leptospira 36, 69, 69f
Leptospirosis 36
Lice pubic 158
Life cycle of
    Entamoeba histolytica 136f
    hookworm 149f
    malarial parasites 141f
    mosquitoes 159f
    roundworm 147f
Live
    polio vaccine 114
    vaccine 63
Location of normal flora 155
Lowenstein-Jensen medium 22, 23, 67
Lower respiratory tract infection 41
Lyme disease 69
Lymph node 83, 84f
Lymphoid cells 80
Lysis of cells 84

M

MacConkey
    agar 22
    liquid medium 21
Macrophage cell 82f
Madura foot 127
Major histocompatibility complex 85f, 86
Malaria 36, 39
Malarial parasites 140, 142f
Management of hospital waste 165
Manifestation of immune reaction 90t
Mannitol salt agar 47
Mast cells 82
Measles 124
    virus 41, 116, 116f
Mechanism of
    gram staining 15
    precipitation 99
Member of enterobacteriaceae 41
Meningitis 48, 64
Mercuric chloride 33
Mercurochrome 33
Methods of transfer of infection 37
Microbial theory of fermentation 4
Microfilaria of *Wuchereria bancrofti* 145f
Microglial cells 82
Mitochondria 9
MMR vaccination 98
Modes of transmission 41t
Modified Ziehl-Neelsen staining 13
Moist heat 28, 29
Moisture 18

Mononuclear phagocytes 82
Monotrichous 12
Morphological classification of bacteria 9
Morphology of
	bacteria 9
	mature worm 146*f*
	spores 12
Mosquito
	borne diseases 36
	cycle 141
Mucormycosis 128
Mucosal-associated lymphoid tissue 83
Mucous membrane 75, 76
Mumps virus 116
Muramic acid 9
Musca domestica 158
Mutation 46
Myasthenia gravis 86, 89
Mycobacterium tuberculosis 4, 16, 20, 23, 66
Mycology 3, 126
Mycoplasma 5, 10, 71, 72*f*

N

National immunization schedule 95
Natural immunity 74
Naturally acquired
	active immunity 77
	passive immunity 77
Negative staining 14
Neisseria 52
	gonococcus 16
	gonorrhoeae 52
	meningitidis 52, 155
	meningococcus 16
	pneumoniae 22
Neomycin 45
Nervous system 112
Netilmicin 45
Neural vaccines 117
Nicotinamide adenine dinucleotide 50
Nitric acid 16
Nocardia asteroides 36
Non-ionizing radiation 31
Non-lactose fermenters 22
Non-specific reagin antibody tests 68
Non-suppurative complication 50
Nosocomial
	infections 35, 41
	pneumonia 41
Nuclear apparatus 9, 11
Nucleic acid 108
Nucleolus 9
Nutrient
	agar 22, 47
		slope 47
	broth 21, 23
Nutrition 18

O

Obligate
	aerobes 13
	anaerobes 13, 19
	parasite 133
Opportunistic mycoses 128
Organic acids 32
Organs of
	adhesion 12
	immune system 83
Orthomyxoviruses 115
Osmotic pressure 19
Osteoclasts 82
Ovum of
	Ancylostoma duodenale 152*f*
	Entamoeba histolytica 152*f*
	Giardia lamblia 152*f*
	Trichuris trichiura 152*f*
Oxidizing agents 32, 33

P

Papillomavirus 110, 114
Papovaviruses 110, 114
Para-aminobenzoic acid 44
Paracoccidioides brasiliensis 128*f*
Paracoccidioidomycosis 128
Parainfluenza viruses 116
Paramyxoviruses 115
Parasite 35, 133
Paratyphoid fever 61
Parts of autoclave 30*f*
Parvoviruses 114
Passive
	agglutination test 91
	immunity 77
	immunization 54
Pasteurization 28, 29
Pathogenesis of enteric fever 103*f*
Penicillin 45
Penicilliosis 129
Penicillium 129*f*
	griseofulvum 46
	notatum 45
Peptone water 21
Peripheral lymphoid organs 83
Pernicious malaria 143
Pertussis 98
Peyer's patch 84
Pharyngitis 113
Pharyngoconjunctival fever 113
Phenol derivatives 32
Phenylpropanolamine 60
Picornaviruses 114
Plasmodium
	falciparum 140
	malariae 140
	ovale 140

vivax 140
Pneumococci 51
Pneumococcus and *Streptococcus viridans* 51*t*
Pneumonia 41, 59, 64, 113
Pneumonic plague 64
Polio 97
    vaccine 125
Poliomyelitis 36, 124
Poliovirus 114
Polyomavirus 114
Potassium permanganate 32, 33
Potassium tellurite medium for *Corynebacterium diphtheriae* 23
Povidone iodine 33
Poxvirus 110, 111
Pre-erythrocytic schizogony 140
Preparation of antigen emulsion 101
Primary
    cell
        culture 109
        lines 109
    stain 14
Proteolytic clostridia 24
Protozoa 5, 134
Protozoology 3
Pseudomonas aeruginosa 26, 41, 63
Pseudopodia 134
Pulmonary aspergillosis 128
Pulse polio immunization 125
Purified antigen vaccines 97
Pyogenic infection 59
Pyrogenic exotoxin 50

Q

Q fever 72
Qualitative VDRL test 101
Quantitative
    serum test 101
    VDRL test 102*f*
Quaternary ammonium compounds 32, 33
Quellung test 51

R

Rabies 4, 117
Radial immunodiffusion 91, 91*f*
Recombinant vaccines 97
Red heat 27, 28
Reiter protein complement fixation test 68
Relapsing fever 69
Removal of immune complex 84
Resistance 13
Respiratory
    infections 41, 50
    syncytial virus 116
    tract 37, 76
    viruses 41

Retrovirus 121, 121*f*
Rhabdovirus 116, 116*f*
Rheumatoid arthritis 86, 88
Rhinosporidiosis 127
Rhinoviruses 115
Ribonucleic acid 9
Rickettsia 5, 72, 72*f*
Rickettsial diseases 72
RNA viruses 110t, 114
Robertson cooked meat medium 21, 24
Rotavirus diarrhea 125
Roundworm infection 146
Rubella virus 118

S

Sabin vaccine 114
Sabouraud dextrose agar medium 22
Sacrolytic clostridia 24
Salmonella 29, 36, 61, 101
    typhi 8, 12, 23, 41, 46, 61, 102
Salts of heavy metals 33
Sandfly 160
Sandwich ELISA 93, 94*f*
Saprophytes 35
Science of
    infectious viruses 3
    pathogenic bacteria 3
Screening
    of waste 165
    tests 69
Scrub typhus 72
Septicemia 48, 61, 63
Septicemic plague 64
Serological tests 69, 164
Serum hepatitis 110, 119
Sexual intercourse 121
Sheathed microfilariae 144
Sheep red blood cells 92*f*
Sintered glass filters 28
Size of bacteria 6
Skin
    exfoliative diseases 48
    resistance 75
Slide
    agglutination 91
    coagulase test 48
    test 101
Small pox 110
Sodium
    chloride 21
    hypochlorite 33
Solid media 21, 22
Specific *Treponema pallidum* tests 68
Spirilla 10
Spirillum 12
    minus 10
Spirochetes 10, 67

Sporothrix 127*f*
Sporotrichosis 127
Spotted fever 72
Stages of *Entamoeba histolytica* 135*f*
Stained preparation 14, 151
Staining techniques 14
Staphylococci smear and diagnosis 48*t*
Staphylococcus
　　aureus 26, 41, 44, 48, 155
　　epidermidis 41
Sterilization 27, 42
Stokes method 25, 25*f*
Streptococcal sepsis 41
Streptococcus
　　pneumoniae 41, 155
　　pyogenes 50, 155
　　viridans 35
Streptokinase 50
Streptomyces noursei 46
Streptomycin 45
Structure of
　　capsule 11*f*
　　immunoglobulin 79, 79*f*
Stuart transport medium 24
Study of
　　fungi 3
　　helminths 3
　　insects 3
　　parasites 3
　　pathogenic protozoa 3
Subcutaneous mycoses 127
Sulfuric acid 32
Superficial mycoses 126
Suppurative lesion 48, 64
Swine flu 123
Symptoms of athlete's foot 129
Syphilis 39
Systemic
　　bacteriology 47
　　mycoses 127

T

Techniques of microscopy 6
Teratogenic infections 39
Tetanus 98
Tetracyclines 45
Tetrathionate broth 23
Thiosulfate-citrate-bile salts-sucrose 22
Three genera of dermatophytes 127*f*
Thymus 83
Thyrotoxicosis 86
Tincture of iodine 33
Tissue culture vaccines 117
Tobramycin 45
Toxic shock syndrome 48

Toxoplasma gondii 36
Toxoplasmosis 36
Transmission of
　　AIDS 121
　　resistance 46
Trench fever 72
Treponema pallidum 67, 67*f*, 76, 101
　　hemagglutination assay 68
　　immobilization 68
Trophozoite 134
Tube
　　agglutination 91, 102
　　coagulase test 48
Tuberculosis 4, 41
Tumor of jaw 110
Tyndallization 28, 29
Type
　　A hepatitis 120
　　B hepatitis 120
　　C hepatitis 121
Types of
　　antibodies 79
　　chemicals 32
　　container 167
　　normal flora 155
　　stool examination 150
Typhoid
　　and paratyphoid fevers 36
　　fever 61

U

Unclean hands and fingers 38, 40
Unfertilized egg 146
　　of *Ascaris lumbricoides* 151*f*
Urinary
　　infection 59
　　tract infections 35, 37, 41, 48, 59, 63, 74
Urine 163
Urogenital tract 156
Uses of spores 13

V

Vaccination 97
　　schedule 117
Vaccines 96
Vaccinia virus 109, 111*f*
Vancomycin 45
Varicella 124
　　zoster virus 112
Variola virus 110
Vector borne infection 38, 39
Vehicle borne infection 38, 39
Venereal disease research laboratory test 67, 68, 101
Verocytotoxin producing *E. coli* 59

Vibrio cholerae 8, 10, 12, 21, 24, 36, 62, 62*f*
Vincents angina 69
Viral hepatitis 36, 118
Virulence tests 54
Virus 5, 107, 108*f*

W

Wassermann reaction 104, 164
Water-borne diseases 36
Weak organic acids 33
Widal test 103, 164
Woolsorter's disease 55
Wound and
    burn infections 63
    skin sepsis 41

Wuchereria bancrofti 144, 144*f*, 145
Wurtz and human skin cancer 110

Y

Yellow fever 36
Yersinia 63, 64*f*
    pestis 36, 63
Yolk sac 109

Z

Zidovudine 45
Ziehl-Neelsen staining 15, 16
Zone phenomenon 99, 100*f*
Zoonotic disease 157
    in India 36*t*